LYNN Ritter

Springer Series: Focus on Men

Jordan I. Kosberg, PhD, Series Editor
James H. Hennessy, PhD, Founding Editor

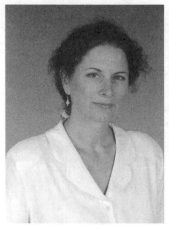

Betty J. Kramer, PhD, is an Associate Professor in the School of Social Work at the University of Wisconsin-Madison. She received her MSSW from the Raymond A. Kent School of Social Work at the University of Louisville, and her PhD in Social Welfare from the University of Washington (Seattle). Her research efforts to date have enhanced understanding of three aspects of caregiving that have emerged as unique areas of inquiry: positive aspects of caregiving, transitions in caregiving, and men as caregivers. She is currently engaged in research on innovations and enhancements to end-of-life care. Her clinical experiences have been in multiple settings including hospitals, nursing homes, family practice clinics, and community-based social service agencies. She team teaches a course on Family Caregiving, and teaches other graduate social work courses on the topics of grief and loss, and gerontological social work practice.

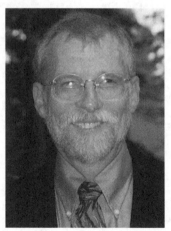

Edward Thompson, PhD, is a Professor of Sociology and Director of the Gerontology Studies Program at Holy Cross College. He received his BA in sociology from California State University, Sacramento, and his PhD in sociology in 1980 from Case Western Reserve University (Cleveland). He has long been interested in issues of gender and family life, publishes on men and masculinity, and teaches courses on the family, sociology of men, aging and society, sociology of mental health, and medical sociology. Dr. Thompson studies the social worlds of older men and has published on men's caregiving, religious experiences of older men, and later life masculinity. He edited the first collection of original articles examining older men (*Older Men's Lives,* 1994). He serves as the organizer of the men's issues interest group for the Gerontological Society of America, and enjoys working closely with students.

Betty J. Kramer, *PhD*
Edward H. Thompson, Jr., *PhD*
Editors

Men as Caregivers

Theory, Research, and Service Implications

 Springer Publishing Company

Springer Publishing Company, Inc.
536 Broadway
New York, NY 10012-3955

Acquisitions Editor: Sheri W. Sussman
Production Editor: Jeanne Libby
Cover design by Susan Hauley

02 03 04 05 06 / 5 4 3 2 1

Library of Congress Cataloging-in-Publication Data

Men caregivers : theory, research, and service applications /
Betty J. Kramer, Edward H. Thompson, editors.
        p. cm. — (Springer series, focus on men ; v. 13)
    Includes bibliographical references and index.
    ISBN 0-8261-1472-5
    1. Male caregivers. 2. Social work with men. I. Kramer,
Betty J. II. Thompson, Edward H. III. Series

    HV1441.4 .M44 2002
    362'.0425—dc21

                                                    2001042874

Printed in the United States of America by Sheridan Books, Inc.

This book is dedicated to Dale Bruhn, Kurt Bergen, Hank Hoover, and Ralph Osmun, who, as caregivers, have served as profound role models for other men caregivers and family members; and to the other husbands, sons, partners, friends, brothers, and fathers who have become providers of care.

Contents

Part IV Services and Interventions

Contributors

Karen A. Adler, ScB, is a third-year graduate student in the San Diego State University, University of California, San Diego, joint Doctoral Program in Clinical Psychology, San Diego, California.

Susan M. Allen, PhD, is an Associate Professor of Medical Science in the Department of Community Health, at the Center for Gerontology and Health Care Research at Brown University, Providence, Rhode Island.

Jamila Bookwala, PhD, is an Assistant Professor in the Psychology Department at Lafayette College, Easton, Pennsylvania.

Elizabeth H. Carpenter, MSW, is a doctoral candidate at the Mandel School of Applied Social Sciences at Case Western Reserve University, Cleveland, Ohio.

Joan Chohan, MSN, RN, is an Assistant Professor at Trinity College of Nursing, Moline, Illinois.

Desirée Ciambrone, PhD, is a Post Doctoral Research Fellow at the Center for Gerontology and Health Care Research at Brown University, Providence, Rhode Island.

Aimee Coonerty-Femiano, BA, is a graduate student in Psychology at Boston College, Boston, Massachusetts.

Elizabeth Lehr Essex, MSS, PhD, is an Assistant Professor at the Jane Addams College of Social Work, University of Illinois at Chicago, Chicago, Illinois.

Sam Femiano, ThD, EdD, is a Psychologist in private practice in Northampton, Maine.

Igor Grant, MD, is a Professor and Vice Chair of Psychiatry at the University of California, San Diego School of Medicine and the San Diego Veteran's Administration Healthcare System, La Jolla, California.

Jan S. Greenberg, MSSW, PhD, is a Professor of Social Work at the University of Wisconsin-Madison, Madison, Wisconsin.

Phyllis Braudy Harris, MSW, PhD, is a Professor of Sociology and Director of the Aging Studies Program at John Carroll University, Cleveland, Ohio. She is also co-editor of "Dementia: The International Journal of Social Research and Practice."

Lenard W. Kaye, MSW, DSW, is a Professor of Social Work at the University of Maine, Orono, Maine.

Marty Wyngaarden Krauss, PhD, is the John Stein Professor of Disability Research and the Associate Dean for Faculty at the Heller School for Social Policy and Management at Brandeis University, Waltham, Massachusetts.

Sarah H. Matthews, PhD, is a Professor of Sociology at Cleveland State University, Cleveland, Ohio.

Baila H. Miller, MSSW, PhD, is a Professor of Social Work at Case Western Reserve University, Cleveland, Ohio.

Judith L. Newman, PhD, is an Associate Professor of Human Development and Family Studies at the Pennsylvania State University-Abington College, Abington, Pennsylvania.

Thomas L. Patterson, PhD, is a Professor in residence of Psychiatry at the University of California, San Diego School of Medicine, and the San Diego Veteran's Administration Healthcare System, La Jolla, California.

Richard Schulz, PhD, is a Professor of Psychiatry, and Director of the University Center for Social and Urban Research, University of Pittsburgh, Pittsburgh, Pennsylvania.

Marsha Mailick Seltzer, PhD, is a Professor of Social Work at the University of Wisconsin, Madison, and Acting Director of the Waisman Center, Madison, Wisconsin.

Carolyn Sidwell Sipes, DNSc, is a member of the adjunct faculty at the Rush University, Adult Health Nursing School in Chicago, Illinois, and at the University of Colorado, School of Nursing, Denver, Colorado.

Eleanor Palo Stoller, PhD, is the Selah Chamberlain Professor of Sociology and Associate Director of the Center for Aging and Health at Case Western Reserve University, Cleveland, Ohio.

Jacqueline M. Stolley, PhD, RN, CS, is a Professor at Trinity College of Nursing, Moline, Illinois.

Richard G. Wight, MPH, PhD, is an Assistant Research Sociologist in the Department of Community Health Sciences, School of Public Health, University of California, Los Angeles, California.

Acknowledgments

The idea for this volume has been ruminating for several years and has emerged as a result of the contributions and support of caregivers, colleagues, and family members. We gratefully acknowledge the contributions of many groups and individuals. First, personal and professional experiences with men caregivers inspired our attention to this topic, because they often defied the stereotypical representation of men as uninvolved bystanders in family care. In professional presentations to family caregivers in many communities, men repeatedly showed up to express their unique concerns, challenges, and sense of isolation. One gentleman angrily responded to a presentation on "Gender Differences in Caregiving," which reported patterns of higher perceived burden among adult daughters than among sons caring for parents with chronic or physical impairments. He expressed immense frustration and concern about his experiences as a sole provider of care to his parents, in the absence of support from his five siblings. This experience was an important reminder that mean differences do not account for individual suffering and unique differences. Bearing witness to the strokes, heart attacks, back distress, depression, and isolation experienced by numerous husband caregivers participating in spousal support groups, community social service agencies, and research studies of community dwelling elders over the years left impressions of tremendous devastation among this population of caregivers. It is these men who have heightened our sense of awareness and compassion for the many thousands of men who fulfill caregiving roles. We have felt privileged to learn from them and acknowledge their contributions as the impetus for this text.

Second, we were influenced by the budding academic interest in caregiving men by our esteemed colleagues in family caregiving research. In the mid- and late-1990s we were beginning to see several prominent scholars initiating efforts to understand the experience of caregiving men. As a way to profile these efforts and highlight the topic, a symposium entitled "The Male Caregiver" was presented at the 51st Annual Scientific Meeting of the Gerontological Society of America (GSA) on

November 23, 1998. This symposium, coordinated by Betty Kramer, was cosponsored by the "Men's Interest Group" (with Ed Thompson serving as Chair). The interest generated by this topic resulted in a second symposium on "Men as Caregivers" for the 53rd Annual Meeting of GSA, on November 18, 2000, at which several contributors to this volume presented their research. We are grateful to the following persons for their contributions to these two symposiums: Baila Miller, Elizabeth Essex, Marsha Mailick Seltzer, Marty Wyngaarden Krause, Phyllis Braudy Harris, Lenard W. Kaye, Thomas L. Patterson, Karen A. Adler, Igor Grant, Sarah H. Matthews, Desirée Ciambrone, Susan M. Allen, and Jordan I. Kosberg. A special thanks to Nadine F. Marks for introducing us and for providing her insightful observations to the topic.

Third, we would like to thank the distinguished scholars who have contributed their chapters to this volume. Without their expertise, commitment, hard work, and patience, this text would not be possible. Working within tight time constraints and amid many other pressures, the authors worked diligently to write and rewrite their drafts according to specified guidelines. Their professionalism has resulted in what we believe is a real contribution to the family caregiving literature.

Finally, our partners (Jim Kramer and Ruth Thompson) and children (Jenner Kramer, Clariel Kramer, Stephen Thompson, and Natalie Thompson) have graciously provided allowances for missed soccer and baseball games, evenings and weekends away from family, and other related distractions related to working on the book. Their support and encouragement to pursue our academic passions make this text possible.

Introduction

I

Men Caregivers: An Overview

1

Betty J. Kramer

INTRODUCTION AND PURPOSE: WHY FOCUS ON MEN CAREGIVERS?

This volume was planned for six primary reasons. First, the experience of caregiving men has been largely neglected, and their contributions have been often marginalized. Despite the proliferation of caregiving research over the past three decades, the vast majority of research has centered on the experience of the female caregiver. When included in caregiving studies, men have tended to serve as a contrast group to illustrate the additional challenges and disadvantages female caregivers face in contrast to their male peers. This focus on women is not unwarranted, nor surprising given that women generally predominate in caregiving roles. Yet comprehensive, responsive, and responsible social policies and programs for families may only develop when we openly acknowledge and understand the contributions and challenges of all caregivers.

Second, as noted by Kaye and Applegate (1994), "although our understanding of the challenges and rewards of family caregiving for men remains grossly underdeveloped, recent evidence suggests that there may be more males engaged in helping other relatives than previously assumed" (p. 219). As will be illustrated later in this chapter, men currently provide care in substantial numbers and provide important contributions to family and society. Men make up approximately 30% of all caregivers, and may individually and collectively have unique experiences and needs. Indeed, in some caregiving contexts males provide the bulk of care. For example, 41 to 53% of all primary caregivers to persons with AIDS in the United States are relatively young males (Turner & Catania, 1997; Turner, Catania, & Gagnon, 1994). Many of these men have extensive responsibilities that are not acknowledged. Frequently cited reports from gender comparative studies documenting lesser involvement in parent care among sons, as compared to daughters, appears to have fostered the belief that men are not fulfilling caregiving roles and their contributions are insignificant. Yet there are sons who are fully devoted to their parents' care needs and other caregiving males who are substantially involved in demanding caregiving functions. For example, 70% of husband caregivers help their wives with personal care and hygiene tasks (Stone, Cafferata, & Sangl, 1987). We believe it is important to avoid the tendency to stereotype the male caregiving experience, seek to understand gender similarities in the caring experience, and reexamine our assumptions about gender and care. As Fisher (1994) so eloquently states, "we will have to develop a new appreciation of the caring capacities of men . . . There are circumstances where men accept the obligation to care, undertake intimate personal care, and derive identity and reward from their caring work. In doing so, they seem driven by similar motives and to experience similar struggles as do women" (p. 677).

Third, as will be discussed more fully below, several demographic trends, and trends in family and kinship, the social environment, and health conditions and policy, are reconstructing the nature of family roles and responsibilities and are likely to put increasing pressure on men as caregivers in the future. For example, the current national prevalence of male caregiving and projected demographic trends (cf., Himes, 1992; Marks, 1996) suggest that increased longevity for men and women will significantly increase the numbers and proportion of male caregivers across the life course in the immediate future. It is important that multidisciplinary educators, researchers, practitioners, and students better understand the ramifications of these trends in order to respond proactively.

Fourth, a body of literature is beginning to develop that suggests that caregiving is not the benign experience for men that is often presumed from gender comparative findings. Drawing upon a national probability sample of U.S. adults who were primary respondents to the National Survey of Families and Households, my colleague and I recently reported that older men who transitioned into the spousal caregiving role reported a greater decrease in emotional support, marital happiness, and psychological well-being than husbands with well spouses (Kramer & Lambert, 1999). Upon entering the caregiving role, husbands experienced a decline in their happiness and elevated levels of depression. This parallels other studies affirming higher levels of depression among male caregivers when compared to their non-caregiving peers (Folkman, Chesney, & Christopher-Richards, 1994; Fuller-Jonap & Haley, 1995). In another longitudinal study, I recently discovered that although husbands who placed their wives in nursing homes reported fewer physical strains and more time for social and recreational activities, 50% of these older men had depression scores indicative of risk of clinical depression (Kramer, 2000). Schulz and

Williamson (1991) found that male caregivers became significantly more depressed over time. As noted in chapter 5, there is emerging and growing recognition that the caregiving experience engenders significant challenges and detrimental impacts among males. Similarly, as will be discussed in chapter 6, there may be reason to believe that caregiving has serious physical health consequences for men. Men have a greater level of physiological disturbance, and may be more physiologically reactive to psychosocial stressors when compared to women. Fuller-Jonap and Haley (1995) reported that caregiving males had more respiratory problems, more difficulty with sleep, and greater use of over-the-counter medications than non-caregiving males.

Fifth, there may be unique challenges faced by caregiving men that we need to better understand. Many older men are unaccustomed to dealing with welfare agencies and have been socialized to have a strong sense of self-reliance. Other cultural expectations may hinder the ease with which they seek support or may constrain their options for responding to caregiving. Men in our society are often expected to be in control, confident, more concerned with thinking than feeling, providers, rational, assertive, courageous, competitive, concerned with achieving goals and tasks, action oriented, and able to endure stress and bear pain (Staudacher, 1991). As a result, it is not uncommon for them to respond to stress differently than women typically do. For example, they may guard their feelings, remain silent, engage in solitary mourning or keep their grief "secret," feel anger and aggression, or become immersed in activity (Staudacher, 1991). None of these behaviors are inherently good or bad; nevertheless, when men are faced with profound losses and challenging emotions that are typically associated with caregiving, internal expectations or expectations of others may hinder their providing the typical cues women do to seek professional or informal assistance for these personal challenges. Another unique challenge for men is that they tend to have more acquaintances but fewer confidants, other than their spouse, than women do. Indeed, wives are often the sole source of emotional support to married men (Chappell, 1990). Traditionally, women are the ones who keep in touch with other relatives and friends by maintaining family rituals, phoning others, and writing letters. When wives become ill, husbands frequently experience tremendous isolation and loss of social connectedness. This may be one explanation offered for the fact that older men are seven to eight times more likely to die within six months of their spouses' death than married people matched for age (Fasey, 1990). In addition, there are a great many skills involved in the caregiving role and caregivers often are confronted with taking on new tasks and learning new skills. Some men have expressed tremendous anxiety in working to handle the multiple demands of care, while simultaneously tackling entirely new skills.

Finally, we wanted to furnish service providers with an understanding of the male caregiver in an effort to enhance gender-relevant interventions. We know that men are dramatically underrepresented in interventions designed to assist caregivers (cf., DeVries, Hamilton, Lovett, & Gallagher-Thompson, 1997; Toseland & Rossiter, 1989). There has been little concerted effort to design therapeutic approaches for working specifically with men in the caregiving role. Many of the interventions used to support family caregivers may be gender biased. Support groups and counseling modalities that focus on sharing and expression of feelings may be more appealing to women than men in caregiving roles. In fact, the terminology used to describe these interventions may deter participation of male caregivers. Ways of therapeutically working with the caregiving male and interventions designed in the context of gender sensitivity have not been explicated well in light of the emerging body of research focusing on this population.

In sum, we developed this volume to acknowledge the contributions of male caregivers and to enhance knowledge regarding their needs and experiences. Fisher (1994) suggested that "Rather than seeking maximum distance between the motives and experiences of women and men carers, one important way to promote non-sexist community care will be to explore the conditions where men's caring is undertaken and how it can be understood and developed" (p. 677). We envisioned a text that would provide a centralized resource of contemporary theory, research, and service-related issues relevant to men as caregivers, in order to improve understanding of this unique subpopulation of caregivers. The spotlight of this text on men as caregivers is in not intended to diminish the contributions, challenges, and needs of female caregivers. Clearly we must continue to understand and to advocate for responsive and compassionate policies that will lessen the burden of all caregivers and seek to enhance kinship and family relationships in the caregiving context. Our intention, rather, is to explicitly acknowledge and honor the unique contributions, challenges, and needs of the many sons, husbands, brothers, lovers, and friends who have become providers of care.

INFORMAL CAREGIVING AMONG MEN

Caregiving Defined

Prior to examining the nature and extent of caregiving among men, it is necessary to clarify what is meant by the term "caregiving." In the broader literature, there is a great deal of analytic confusion generated by the myriad definitions of informal caregiving. The "choice of definition greatly influences estimates of the number of family caregivers, the magnitude of burden on individuals, families, employers, and the society, and the costs of different policy options" (Stone, 1991, pp. 724–725). The definition of "caregiver" has includee the type of care provided, the amount, volume, intensity, and duration of care provided, the living arrangements and relationship of the caregiver to the care receiver, and self or other identification as a caregiver (Barer & Johnson, 1990; Malonebeach & Zarit, 1991).

Caregivers may adopt primary caregiving functions in which they handle all or the bulk of responsibility for meeting the care receiver's needs, or they may serve a secondary role by supplementing care provided by others. Because of the greater potential for strain among primary caregivers, most research has centered on the needs and experiences of these individuals. Yet evidence suggests that secondary caregivers have an important and valuable role to play in familial caregiving. For example, as Essex, Seltzer, and Krause note in chapter 11, although fathers of adult children with developmental disabilities are not typically identified as primary caregivers, they are nevertheless involved, socially engaged, and providers of critical emotional and financial support to their wives.

In this text, we consider caregiving to include informal (i.e., unpaid) care arrangements and efforts that move beyond customary and normative social support provided in social relationships. We view caregiving broadly, as a dynamic process that entails a social transition in one form or another. These transitions may be life changes or long-term "processes" that influence both external (e.g., changes in behavior, role arrangements, social and interpersonal relationships) and internal (e.g., shifts in perceptions) aspects of one's life (Cowan, 1991). As such, men become caregivers when they are called upon to consider the physical or psychological needs of others, and in so doing experience changes in their expected and accustomed roles, behaviors, social or interpersonal relationships, and perceptions about themselves or others. We know that some become caregivers suddenly (following stroke, accidents), but more often transitioning into a caregiver role is an insidious process for which it is difficult to identify beginnings (Pearlin & Aneshensel, 1994; Seltzer & Li, 1996). We do not consider the "fatherhood" role in and of itself to be indicative of "caregiving." However, there are two circumstances addressed in this text in which fatherhood enters the caregiving realm. The first involves fathers of adult children with developmental disabilities. The second involves fathers of adult children who develop schizophrenia. In chapter 11, Essex et al. note that the role of caregiving emerges in these contexts because the adult child's illness fosters dependency beyond the time that children traditionally become independent, or requires additional care than what is typically provided by parents.

Contemporary Prevalence of Caregiving Among Men

Several national surveys providing estimates of informal caregiving in the United States suggest that men "provide care in substantial numbers" (Marks, 1996, p. 34). Using the National Survey of Families and Households to generate populations estimates of in- and out-of-household caregiving for persons of all ages, Marks (1996) reported that 14% of all U.S. males aged 19 or older provided care to a family member or friend with a serious illness or disability in 1987–1988. Across the life course, rates of caregiving varied. During young adulthood (ages 19–34), approximately 11% of men were giving care to dependent relatives or friends. By early middle age, more than one in seven men were providing care. By later middle age more than 18% were in caregiving roles. In the age group 75 and older, there were more husbands in caregiving roles than wives. National estimates of elder caregiving indicate nearly one in three caregivers are men (Cantor, 1983; Chang & White-Means, 1991). Forty-five percent of these men are husbands, 30% are sons, and 25% are other nonrelatives or friends (Stone et al., 1987). As noted previously, there are some caregiving contexts in which men predominate in the caregiving role. For example, within central cities, over 50% of caregivers to persons with AIDS are men and over 83% are under 50 years of age (Turner et al., 1994). These caregivers are not only partners but also brothers and friends.

In other national surveys of employees, substantial numbers of men indicated that they provide care. In the Transamerica Life Companies survey, 33% of male employees indicated that they were currently "providing special assistance (physical, financial, or emotional) to a person at least 60 years old" (Scharlach, Sobel, & Roberts, 1991, p. 779). Eighteen percent of male Americans aged 65 and over who participated in the 1991 Commonwealth Fund survey reported providing more than 20 hours of care during the previous week to a relative, friend, or neighbor with a disability or illness (Doty, 1995).

As mentioned previously, the range of estimates provided in these studies are influenced by the definitions used to identify caregivers. Some of these figures may be underestimates of care provided by men. For example, studies that identify caregivers only by reports of providing assistance with Activities of Daily Living (e.g., bathing, dressing, eating) exclude caregivers who provide other forms of care. Studies that recruit self-defined caregivers may exclude those who provide significant assistance, but view such help as a normal part of their marital or familial role.

In sum, substantial numbers of men currently provide various forms of care to others. Some of these men draw upon a rich support network to facilitate their efforts. Some supplement the caregiving efforts of others. And some are sole caregivers shouldering the burden of care alone.

DEMOGRAPHIC AND HEALTH TRENDS: IMPLICATIONS FOR FUTURE MALE CAREGIVING

A variety of convergent demographic and health trends have important consequences for twenty-first century families and are likely to influence not only the prevalence of male caregiving in the future, but also the roles, functions, and stressors experienced by caregiving men.

Social Demographic Trends

In the coming years, we will experience striking changes in the population structure by age. The prospective and historical shifts in the number of births (including the baby boom of 1946–1964), and the level and age pattern of death rates in the United States will contribute to dramatic increases in the number and proportion of older adults after 2010 (Siegel, 1996). The 65 and over age group is expected to grow from 31 million in 1990 to 79 million by the year 2050 (Day, 1992). A 240% increase is expected in the growth of the oldest old (aged 85 and over) by 2040, dramatically enlarging future demands for informal care (Peterson, 1999).

The majority of elders in need of long-term care are women and 50% of all care provided to older adults is provided by spouses (Soldo & Myllyluoma, 1983). Since the majority of older men are married (due to their high remarriage rates following divorce and widowhood, should these events occur), it is likely that more husbands will enter the caregiving role in the future. Among older populations, men who are divorced or widowed are six times more likely to remarry than women (Treas & VanHilst, 1976). As a result, the majority of these men (i.e., 73%) live with their spouses (Federal Interagency Forum on Aging-Related Statistics, 2000). Using the National Survey of Families and Households to generate population estimates of caregiving, Marks (1996) reported that males in the oldest old group were proportionately predominant in the caregiving role, and attributed this finding to the fact that more older men are married than women. We know that husbands play a major and important role in caring for older women with chronic illness. They are the first persons called upon to meet their wives' needs for care, they are the oldest subgroup of caregivers, they report spending the greatest number of extra hours fulfilling caregiver responsibilities, and they are more likely than other men to be the primary caregivers without assistance from others (Chang & White-Means, 1991; Dwyer & Seccombe, 1991; Stone et al., 1987). The current national prevalence estimates of male caregiving described above, combined with these demographic trends and the health care trends noted below enhance the likelihood of increasing numbers and proportion of male caregivers (particularly husbands) in the future (Himes, 1992; Marks, 1996).

Changes in family and kinship structures because of declining family size, and delayed ages of child bearing, may influence the availability of family caregivers in the future and bring more men into this role. Several factors have contributed to substantial declines in family size. Medical advances and court rulings have made childbearing discretionary, and the availability of oral contraceptives, widespread use of surgical steriliza- tion, and legalization of abortion have contributed to the sharp decline in births between 1960 and 1995 (Hutchinson, 1999). According to Census Bureau data, there are currently more married couples without children than married couples with children (Ahlburg & De Vita, 1992). In addition to having few children, women in higher socioeconomic groups are wait- ing longer to have children. Couples without children will be more reliant on one another for care, and there may be fewer children available to assist parents in the future. Peterson (1999) predicts that "with each pass- ing decade, the number of adult child 'caregivers' available to help each dependent elder will decline steadily, increasing the time and money burden on mature adults and putting extra pressure on governments to pick up the slack" (p. 58). These trends are likely to necessitate greater involvement of sons in family caregiving.

Studies show a rapid increase in the labor force participation of women since 1950. The greatest influx has occurred among married women with small children who combine work and family responsibilities (Kain, 1990). As brothers and husbands continue to bear witness to the similar demands faced by working women, there may be gradual erosion in the expectation that female family members will automatically assume care- giving responsibilities, and do so without assistance. The increasing num- bers of women in the labor force, combined with the aforementioned trends, may challenge twenty-first century families to balance and share child and elder care responsibilities (Himes, 1992). As more women seek professional careers that demand intensive time commitments more men may take active roles in caregiving responsibilities.

Another social trend that may influence the future of male caregiving involves changing gender roles and norms relevant to social relationships. While total gender equality in responsibilities is far from reality in most families, evidence suggests that change is taking place (Pleck, 1993). For example, Willinger (1993) found that men of the 1990s found greater accep- tance of their involvement in family roles and of women's employment than did men of the 1980s. Recently published results generated from the National Long Term Care Survey reported "participation of sons as pri- mary caregivers increased by 50% between 1984 and 1994" (Spillman & Pezzin, 2000, p. 362). More men are demonstrating participation in nur- turing and caring roles traditionally ascribed to women and serving as role models for their young children. For example, the number of single fathers who have primary caregiving responsibility for their children grew from 390,000 in 1970 to 1,351,000 in 1990 (U.S. Bureau of the Census, 1990). Time-use studies show long-term trends with a slow shift toward greater equality in the allocation of domestic work and time spent in family roles among men and women (Gershuny et al., 1986; Miles, 1989; Robinson, Andreyenkov, & Patrushev, 1988). As women's level of educational attainment and labor force participation in more diverse occupations continues to expand, and families seek to accommodate these changes, we may witness further shifts in gender roles and expectations, including more participation of men in all types of caregiving (Kain, 1990).

Migration and the increasing geographic mobility of adult children and older parents, that has accompanied the trend from a communal to an individualistic culture (Pipher, 1999), may have implications for future caregiving demands. Data indicate that 20% of Americans change their residence each year (Vanzetti & Duck, 1996). There has been a 40% reduction in the average number of people in an American household from 1900 to 1980 (Vanzetti & Duck). In these scenarios where people are moving frequently and are less likely to live with their relatives, fewer supports may be available to help persons with caregiving needs, and available men may be more frequently recruited into caregiving roles.

Health Care Trends

As new technologies and improved health care continue to extend life expectancy, there are some population groups who will require more informal care from men as well as women caregivers in the future. We have already witnessed a notable increase in the life expectancy of persons with developmental disabilities (Seltzer & Seltzer, 1992). As adults, these individuals typically live with their fathers and mothers who provide ongoing and long-term care (Fujiura & Braddock, 1992).

There has been a shift in the epidemiology of disease from acute to chronic diseases. Several of these chronic physical and mental health conditions that are more common among women, may increase the demands placed on older husbands and adult children (including sons) in the future. Older women report higher levels of functional impairment and more chronic disabling conditions than older men (Federal Interagency Forum on Aging-Related Statistics, 2000; Thomas & Kelman, 1990). Women have higher prevalence than men of affective disorders, anxiety disorders, and nonaffective psychosis, and have both lifetime and 12-month comorbidity of three or more psychiatric disorders (Kessler et al., 1994). More women than men are diagnosed with dementia, and unless a cure is found for Alzheimer's disease, projections suggest that 14 million persons will have this illness by the year 2050 (Evans et al., 1989). Gaps in death rates among men and women have narrowed in recent years for several illnesses. For example, there has been a 400% increase in respiratory cancer death rates among women since 1960 (Furner, Maurer, & Rosenberg, 1992).

AIDS is another disease that will undoubtedly influence the caregiving efforts of males in the future. Nearly 85% of the adolescents and adults reported with AIDS have been men, and the majority of these are homosexual males (Ward & Drotman, 1998). Although HIV prevalence appears to have stabilized, the prevalence of HIV infection among the homosexual population of men remains unacceptably high and new infections continue to occur (Ward & Drotman). Currently there are 400,000 to 600,000 persons living with HIV, but not diagnosed with AIDS (Rosenberg, 1995). Male partners, friends, and brothers will continue to enter the caregiving role in the coming years. This population of caregivers often experience particularly severe stressors, stigma, chronic mourning, and a sense of both personal and collective trauma (Dean, Hall, & Martin, 1988).

Health care expenditures have increased at alarming rates. Health care reforms designed to contain and reduce these costs have and are likely to continue to exacerbate informal caregiving responsibilities. For example, the prospective reimbursement associated with Diagnostic-Related Groups (DRGs) which reduces and limits the length of hospital stays, often require informal helpers to care for very sick family members with complex care needs, and minimal training. The expansion of managed care as a mechanism to slow cost increases, and the "corporatization of health care" is likely to continue well into the twenty-first century (Ginzberg, 1996; Vladeck, 1996). Unfortunately, profit-driven health care pays little attention to the very serious and detrimental experiences incurred by patients and their family members who interface with this system (e.g., see Baer, Fagin, & Gordon, 1996). In addition, the numbers of persons without access to health care is growing at an alarming rate with approximately a hundred thousand people a month being added to the numbers of the uninsured in the United States (see Vladeck). Indeed, over 40 million Americans are without health care coverage at some point during a year (see Ginzberg). Persons who become ill and who don't have access to health care are likely to rely on their family members (male and female) for care and support.

In sum, these social and health care trends taken together are likely to place increasing pressures on men in their families and communities to take on more caregiving roles in the future. Many men will not be prepared for this. Caregivers tend to have little preparation for the tasks and demands of this role. It is incumbent upon social and health care providers to ensure the development and implementation of gender-sensitive and responsive policies and services to prepare and support caregiving men as well as their caregiving women peers.

ORGANIZATION AND STRUCTURE OF THE BOOK

The book is organized into four main parts. Part I—the "Introduction," consists of two chapters, which together provide the rationale and an overview of the issues relevant to men as caregivers. This first chapter articulates the purpose of this volume and the nature and extent of men as caregivers, and identifies the fundamental social demographic and health trends that are changing the nature of familial roles with implications for the future of male caregiving. Chapter 2 explores styles of caregiving and critiques the premise that men do not do hands-on care. These two chapters set the stage for the issues covered in this text and help to explain why it is essential that we gain a better understanding of the male caregiver experience if we hope to develop gender-relevant supportive services and interventions to respond to their needs.

Part II—"Conceptual, Theoretical, and Methodological Insights," includes two chapters that highlight theoretical and methodological issues relevant to the study of male caregivers. Chapter 3 reviews theoretical explanations of the gendered division of labor in family care. Specially, the author examines the strengths and weaknesses of theories relevant to three explanatory domains (i.e., individual, institutional, and interactional), and proposes a multilevel and integrated theoretical approach to explain the gendered work of elder care. Chapter 4 provides a critical review of the methods used in studies that focus exclusively on male caregivers. The authors evaluate the strengths, limitations, and challenges of this research and set an agenda for future research on male caregiving.

Part III—"Research," consists of nine chapters that both review the literature and present original research on men caregivers. Although this text is unable to provide an exhaustive review of all forms of male caregiving, we have tried to capture in these chapters the divergent male caregiving subpopulations that are frequently identified. Chapters 5 and 6 shed light on the potential impacts and effects of caregiving experienced by men in the caregiving role. Chapter 5 critically reviews 18 published studies to uncover and underscore the methodological limitations and key findings relevant to psychosocial challenges and rewards of male caregivers. The authors use a conceptual model, consisting of stressors, moderating resources, and outcomes to structure the review of findings. Given the absence of research that focuses on ethnic variation in male caregiving, the authors provide data from a study of husbands caring for wives with dementia to examine distress levels among African American and Caucasian males. Chapter 6 reviews research examining the effects of caregiving on men's physical and physiological well-being, and related studies examining physiological responses to acute stressors in men more generally. The authors provide evidence that caregiving men may be at greater risk for developing stress-related illnesses than women, and suggest that additional attention to the physical health of male caregivers is warranted.

Chapters 7 and 8 focus on men caring for persons with AIDS. Chapter 7 reports findings from a qualitative study that employed grounded theory methodology to richly describe the complexity of experiences and relationships among gay male caregivers. Chapter 8 reviews findings from a longitudinal quantitative study of 376 gay-identified men to uncover the mechanism by which the caregiving stress process unfolds distinctively among caregivers with AIDS-related health problems in comparison to HIV-negative caregivers. Chapter 9 offers a comparative analysis of husbands and sons as caregivers to family members with cognitive impairments. The author reports findings from a qualitative study of 30 husbands and 30 sons to review the common strengths, challenges, similarities, and differences reported by these two subpopulations of caregivers. Implications for service providers are also discussed. Chapter 10 reviews brothers' involvement in caring for older parents. The author offers an explanation for why brothers are differentially involved in parental care that takes into consideration sibling and gender composition, as well as size of the sibling network. The author reviews research focusing on brothers' involvement in parent care and summarizes research findings from interviews with 149 pairs of siblings who answered questions about how they and their siblings meet the needs of their parents. Rather than emphasizing the experience of the primary caregivers, this chapter encourages us to take sibling relationships and care approaches into account. Chapter 11 reviews the literature on fathers of children with disabilities and then synthesizes research findings relevant to paternal roles and well-being, generated from an extensive longitudinal study on older families of adults with mental retardation who live at home with their aging parents. This chapter highlights the contributions of fathers as socially engaged, active caregivers to adult children, who provide critical support (financial and emotional) to their wives. Recommendations for future research are highlighted. Chapter 12 reports findings from a large, statewide study that investigated the contributions of 95 couples (fathers and mothers) in caring for their adult children with mental illness, the types of challenges they faced, and the differential effects of these challenges on the well-being of fathers and mothers. The author notes that over 90% of the fathers were actively involved in the lives of their sons and daughters with mental illness and that fathers experienced levels of burdensome caregiving strains similar to mothers. Chapter 13 focuses on spousal caregiving to women with cancer with a focus on the nature of assistance provided, their perception of burden, barriers to optimal care provision, the nature of the marital relationship as it is tied to positive outcomes, and the challenges facing these husband caregivers. A research agenda for further understanding the husband caregiver is also put forth.

Part IV—"Services and Interventions," profiles gender-sensitive interventions, skills, supports, and services that draw upon research and clinical wisdom for working with the male caregiver. Chapter 14 focuses on the spiritual and religious needs of male caregivers. Attention is given to various assessment, diagnosis, intervention, and outcome measures and techniques that may assist service providers to identify, intervene, and evaluate the male caregiver's spiritual needs and experiences, and intervene appropriately when needed. Chapter 15 highlights common challenges facing male caregivers and articulates several suggested principles and interventions for responding to these challenges. This chapter serves as a resource for those in direct service roles, as it provides practical suggestions and direction for individual therapists and counselors, social service providers and facilitators of informal and formal support groups. Finally, Chapter 16 explores our understanding of male caregivers and their service consumption patterns, barriers to use of services, structural strategies for presenting and implementing supportive groups for men to make them more palatable to male caregivers, and highlights emergent trends and their implications for service utilization and support.

REFERENCES

Ahlburg, D. A., & De Vita, C. J. (1992). New realities of the American family. *Population Bulletin, 47* (August): 1–44.

Baer, E. D., Fagin, C. M., & Gordon, S. (1996). *Abandonment of the patient: The impact of profit-driven health care on the public.* New York: Springer.

Barer, B. M., & Johnson, C. L. (1990). A critique of the caregiving literature. *The Gerontologist, 30,* 26–29.

Cantor, M. (1983). Strain among caregivers: A study of experience in the United States. *The Gerontologist, 23,* 597–604.

Chang, C. F., & White-Means, S. I. (1991). The men who care: An analysis of male primary caregivers who care for frail elderly at home. *The Journal of Applied Gerontology, 10,* 343–358.

Chappell, N. L. (1990). Aging and social care. In R. H. Binstock & L. K. George (Eds.), *Handbook on aging and the social sciences* (3rd ed., pp. 438–454). New York: Academic Press.

Cowan, P. A. (1991). Individual and family life transitions: A proposal for a new definition. In P. A. Cowan & M. Hetherington (Eds.), *Family transitions* (pp. 3–30). Hillsdale, NJ: Lawrence Erlbaum Associates.

Day, J. C. (1992). Population projections of the United States, by age, sex, race, and Hispanic origin: 1992 to 2050. *Current Population Reports* (Series P25, No. 1092). Washington, DC: U.S. Government Printing Office.

Dean, L., Hall, W. E., & Martin, J. L. (1988). Chronic and intermittent AIDS-related bereavement in a panel of homosexual men in New York City. *Journal of Palliative Care, 4*(4), 54–57.

DeVries, H. M., Hamilton, D. W., Lovett, S., & Gallagher-Thompson, D. (1997). Patterns of coping preferences for male and female caregivers of frail older adults. *Psychology and Aging, 12*, 263–267.

Doty, P. (1995). Older caregivers and the future of informal caregiving. In S. A. Bass (Ed.), *Older and active: How Americans over 55 are contributing to society* (pp. 97–121). New Haven, CT: Yale University Press.

Dwyer, J. W., & Seccombe, K. (1991). Elder care as family labor: The influence of gender and family position. *Journal of Family Issues, 12*, 229–247.

Evans, D. A., Funkenstein, H. H., Albert, M. S., Sherr, P. A., Crook, N. R., Chown, M. J., Herbert, L. E., Hennakens, C. H., & Taylor, J. D. (1989). Prevalence of Alzheimer's disease in a community population of older persons: Higher than previously reported. *Journal of the American Medical Association, 262*, 2551–2556.

Fasey, C. N. (1990). Grief in old age: A review of the literature. *International Journal of Geriatric Psychiatry, 5*, 65–75.

Federal Interagency Forum on Aging-Related Statistics (2000). *Older Americans 2000: Key indicators of well-being.* Hyattsville, MD: National Center for Health Statistics.

Fisher, M. (1994). Man-made care: Community care and older male carers. *British Journal of Social Work, 24*, 659–680.

Folkman, S., Chesney, M. A., & Christopher-Richards, A. (1994). Stress and coping in caregiving partners of men with AIDS. *Psychiatric Clinics of North America, 17*, 35–53.

Fujiura, G. T., & Braddock, D. (1992). Fiscal and demographic trends in mental retardation services: The emergence of the family. In L. Rowitz (Ed.), *Mental retardation in the year 2000* (pp. 316–338). New York: Springer.

Fuller-Jonap, F., & Haley, W. E. (1995). Mental and physical health of male caregivers of a spouse with Alzheimer's disease. *Journal of Aging and Health, 7*, 99–118.

Furner, S. E., Maurer, J., & Rosenberg, H. (1992). Mortality. *Vital and health statistics: Health data on older Americans: United States, 1992* (pp. 77–112). (DDDS Publication No. PHS 93-1411). Washington, DC: U.S. Government Printing Office.

Ginzberg, E. (1996). *Tomorrow's hospital.* New Haven, CT: Yale University Press.

Gershuny, J., Miles, I., Jones, S., Mullings, C., Thomas, G., & Wyatt, S.

(1986). Time budgets: Preliminary analyses of a national survey. *Quarterly Journal of Social Affairs, 2,* 13–39.

Himes, C. L. (1992). Future caregivers: Projected family structures of older persons. *Journal of Gerontology: Social Sciences, 47,* S17–S26.

Hutchinson, E. D. (1999). *Dimensions of human behavior.* Thousand Oaks, CA: Pine Forge Press.

Kain, E. L. (1990). *The myth of family decline: Understanding families in a world of rapid social change.* Lexington, MA: Lexington Books.

Kaye, L. W., & Applegate, J. S. (1994). Older men and the family caregiving orientation. In E. H. Thompson, Jr. (Ed.), *Older men's lives* (pp. 218–236). Thousand Oaks, CA: Sage.

Kessler, R. C., McGonagle, K. A., Zhao, S., Nelson, C. B., Hughes, M., Eshleman, S., Wittchen, H., & Kendler, K. S. (1994). *Archives of General Psychiatry, 51,* 8–19.

Kramer, B. J. (2000). Husbands caring for wives with dementia: A longitudinal study of continuity and change. *Health and Social Work, 25,* 97–107.

Kramer, B. J., & Lambert, J. D. (1999). Caregiving as a life course transition among older husbands: A prospective study. *The Gerontologist, 39,* 658–667.

Malonebeach, E. E., & Zarit, S. H. (1991). Current research issues in caregiving to the elderly. *International Journal of Aging and Human Development, 32,* 103–114.

Marks, N. F. (1996). Caregiving across the lifespan: National prevalence and predictor. *Family Relations, 45,* 27–36.

Miles, I. (1989). Time use and information technology: Present and future developments of private households. In B. Strumpel (Eds.), *Industrial societies after the stagnation of the 1970s* (pp. 209–242). Berlin, Germany: Walter de Guyter.

Pearlin, L. I., & Aneshensel, C. S. (1994). Caregiving: The unexpected career. *Social Justice Research, 7,* 373–390.

Peterson, P. G. (1999). *Gray dawn: How the coming age wave will transform America and the world.* Westminster, NJ: Random House.

Pipher, M. (1999). *Another country: Navigating the emotional terrain of our elders.* New York: Riverhead Books.

Pleck, J. H. (1993). Are "family-supportive" employer policies relevant to men? In J. C. Hood (Ed.), *Men, work, and family* (pp. 217–237). Newbury Park, CA: Sage.

Robinson, J. P., Andreyenkov, V. G., & Patrushev, V. D. (1988). *The rhythm of everyday life: How Soviet and American citizens use time.* Boulder, CO: Westview.

Rosenberg, P. S. (1995). The scope of the AIDS epidemic in the United States. *Science, 270,* 1372–1375.

Scharlach, A. E., Sobel, E. L., & Roberts, R. E. L. (1991). Employment and caregiver strain: An integrative model. *The Gerontologist, 31*, 778–787.

Schulz, R., & Williamson, G. M. (1991). A 2-year longitudinal study of depression among Alzheimer's caregivers. *Psychology and Aging, 6*, 569–578.

Seltzer, M. M., & Li, L. W. (1996). The transitions of caregiving: Subjective and objective definitions. *The Gerontologist, 36*, 614–626.

Seltzer, M. M., & Seltzer, G. B. (1992). Aging in persons with developmental disabilities. In F. J. Turner (Ed.), *Mental health and the elderly: A social work perspective* (pp. 136–160). New York: The Free Press.

Siegel, J. S. (1996). *Aging into the 21st century*. Bethesda, MD: Administration on Aging.

Soldo, B., & Myllyluoma, J. (1983). Caregivers who live with dependent elderly. *The Gerontologist, 23*, 605–611.

Spillman, B. C., & Pezzin, L. E. (2000). Potential and active family caregivers: Changing networks and the "sandwich generation." *The Milbank Quarterly, 78*, 347–374.

Staudacher, C., (1991). *Men and grief: A guide for men surviving the death of a loved one: A resource guide for caregivers and mental health professionals*. Oakland, CA: New Harbinger.

Stone, R. (1991). Editorial: Defining family caregivers of the elderly: Implications for research and public policy. *The Gerontologist, 31*, 724–725.

Stone, R., Cafferata, G., & Sangl, J. (1987). Caregivers of the frail elderly: A national profile. *The Gerontologist, 27*, 616–626.

Thomas, C., & Kelman, H. R. (1990). Gender and the use of health services among elderly persons. In M. G. Ory & H. R. Warner (Eds.), *Gender, health, and longevity: Multidisciplinary perspectives* (pp. 137–156). New York: Springer.

Toseland, R. W., & Rossiter, C. M. (1989). Group interventions to support family caregivers: A review and analysis. *The Gerontologist, 29*, 438–448.

Treas, J., & VanHilst, A. (1976). Marriage and remarriage rates among older Americans. *The Gerontologist, 16*, 132–136.

Turner, H. A., & Catania, J. A. (1997). Informal caregiving to persons with AIDS in the United States: Caregiver burden among central cities residents eighteen to forty-nine years old. *American Journal of Community Psychology, 25*, 35–59.

Turner, H. A., Catania, J. A., & Gagnon, J. (1994). The prevalence of informal caregiving to persons with AIDS in the United States: Caregiver characteristics and their implications. *Social Science and Medicine, 38*, 1543–1552.

U.S. Bureau of the Census (1990). *Household and family characteristics: March 1990 and 1989* (Series P-20, No. 447). Washington, DC: U.S. Government Printing Office.

Vanzetti, N., & Duck, S. (1996). The future of interpersonal relationships. In N. Vanzetti & S. Duck (Eds.), *A lifetime of relationships* (pp. 487–508). Pacific Grove, CA: Brooks/Cole.

Vladeck, B. C. (1996). The corporatization of American health care and why it is happening. In E. Baer, C. M. Gagin, & S. Gordon (Eds.), *Abandonment of the patient: The impact of profit-driven health care on the public* (pp. 9–19). New York: Springer.

Ward, J. W., & Drotman, D. P. (1998). Epidemiology of HIV and AIDS. In G. P. Wormser (Ed.), *AIDS and other manifestations of HIV infection* (pp. 1–17). Baltimore: Lippincott-Raven.

Willinger, B. (1993). Resistance and change: College men's attitudes toward family and work in the 1980s. In J. C. Hood (Ed.), *Men, work, and family* (pp. 108–130). Newbury Park, CA: Sage.

What's Unique About Men's Caregiving?

2

Edward H. Thompson, Jr.

> *Once upon a time, a man, name Tang Ao, looking for the Gold Mountain, crossed an ocean, and came upon the Land of Women. The women immediately captured him . . . They plucked out each hair on his face, powdered him white, painted his eyebrows like a moth's wings, painted his cheeks and lips red. He served a meal at the queen's court. His hips swayed and his shoulders swiveled because of his shaped feet. "She's pretty, don't you agree?" the diners said.*
> Maxine Hong Kingston (1976)

> *Perhaps the sentiments contained in the following pages, are not yet sufficiently fashionable to procure them general favor; a long habit of not thinking a thing wrong, gives it a superficial appearance of being right, and raises at first a formidable outcry in defence (sic) of custom. But tumult soon subsides. Time makes more converts than reason.*
> Thomas Paine, *Common Sense*[1]

In *China Men*, Maxine Hong Kingston discloses how the social worlds of the men in her family evolved as the fathers and sons claimed America. The men with Chinese faces, Chinese eyes, noses, and cheekbones came to "do manhood" American style. Like Tang Ao, they were figuratively and literally transformed in the new land, becoming American in spite of the ongoing violence of racism and prejudicial exclusion. Caregiving men's transformation as men might not be so different. Husbands, gay partners, fathers, adults sons, brothers, sons-in-law, and other men engaged in the undertaking of caregiving come to "do caregiving," something many have never done before. They do it in men's style, but they become caregivers and transformed as men.

In a similar fashion to Thomas Paine's argument in *Common Sense*, I question how well we—the research community, policymakers, health and social service professionals—are prepared to think critically or objectively about men as caregivers. Not uncommonly, people actively engage in gender comparisons and thus stereotyping as they examine information about "male caregivers." The adjective "male" announces a predisposition to reframe caregiving to something different . . . generally something less . . . when the caregivers are men. This is a tyranny of sorts. As members of a culture, are we so conditioned by our beliefs and assumptions about gender that it becomes difficult to envision men as caregivers? As scholars and practitioners concerned with caregiving, are we guilty of ignoring men's styles of caregiving and thus minimizing the caregiving work men do? Think a moment about the number of ways we have tried to systematically outline gender differences in the caregiving experience—the burdens, the strains, the gains, the absence of psychological distress. By comparison, we have rarely stepped outside the typical gender difference approach and looked within to ask how gender constructions, societal reaction, and men's involvements and relationships shape their caregiving experience. What do men experience, and why? The imagination that underpins discovering what men and what *different* men do, feel, and contemplate as caregivers has been neglected. Perhaps a paradigm shift is needed.

Kramer (chap. 1) just explicated six reasons men caregivers need to be more thoroughly studied, as well as how trends in health care, family organization, and American demographics will soon affect their caregiving involvement. I begin this chapter by resetting the stage and reviewing three informal caregiving trends that beg attention and are worth revisiting. My primary objective in the chapter is to disclose what the research community and health and social service professionals already know about men's approach to caregiving. This chapter is designed to help (re)discover men's caregiving and styles of caregiving.

CAREGIVING TRENDS

The enterprise: Informal caregiving expectations are not shrinking.   Every year since 1993 a presidential proclamation designated the week of Thanksgiving as "National Family Caregivers Week." In one press release, President Clinton (1997) observed:

> Caregivers reflect family and community life at its best. Thanks to their efforts, Americans with disabilities and a growing number of elderly Americans are able to stay in familiar surroundings and to maintain their

dignity and independence. Caregivers not only enhance the quality of life for those they serve, but also greatly reduce the demands on the formal system of caregiving services in our Nation.

Approximately 80% of all home care is provided by family caregivers. For older adults, nearly 95% who needed help with daily activities and resided in the community during the 1990s relied in part or solely upon family members for their care (Administration on Aging, 1999; Tennstedt, 1999). This pattern is not unusual. From Colonial time to the present, informal (unpaid) caregivers have been a mainstay for meeting people's recuperative and long-term care needs (Abel, 1995; Cancian & Oliker, 2000; Litwak, 1985). Even though macroeconomic forces have shifted to the public a greater responsibility in matters related to older adults' health and welfare (e.g., Social Security, Medicare, Older Americans Act), the same social policies insure that caregiving by family and friends will continue to be the primary source of help-giving, especially to elders. The transformation in the Medicare system to a prospective fixed payment system, for example, redirected the responsibilities of recuperative care from paid hospital staff back to family members or other individuals in the community. Shorter hospital stays and greater use of outpatient and ambulatory care further compel family members, friends, and others to become caregivers (Robinson, 1996); family caregivers are an integral part of the U.S. health care delivery system (Haug, 1994). To insure the vitality of the unpaid caregiving, federal initiatives such as the Family and Medical Leave Act of 1993 compelled large employers to "assist" their employees who are involved as family caregivers with unpaid time off or paid sick days to care for a relative. Congress' enactment of the Older Americans Act Amendments of 2000 (Public Law 106-501) funds a new National Family Caregiver Support Program. Put simply, informal caregiving by intimates is, for varied reasons, what policymakers favor, whether the person in need is a frail elder, a mentally ill adult child cared for by aging parents, or a young adult or older adult with AIDS. The nation's macroeconomic structure is designed to first enlist, then assist and profit from family and friends' involvement in the caregiving enterprise.

The need: Caregiving requests are mounting. Despite the implication in media presentations of a healthier older adult population, the logical conjecture about the next generation of older adults' lesser dependency on informal caregiving needs to be reconsidered. Virtually one-half of the U.S. population now lives with a chronic health condition. Chronic conditions range from paralysis, Parkinson's disease, mental disorders, and HIV/AIDS to asthma, arthritis, diabetes, and hypertension. The conditions most common among older age groups are more disabling. Many with chronic conditions already require care from multiple physicians, take a variety of medications, and need the assistance of family caregivers; it is estimated that one-third of the people age 65–74 and 45% of people aged 75 and older are limited in their ability to work or to live independent because of their chronic condition (Robert Wood Johnson Foundation, 1996). The size of the Boomer generation and their increased longevity are two new pressure points on the caregiving enterprise; the proportion of adults whose lives will be restricted in some way by their health status is expected to double during the first two decades of the twenty-first century (see Robert Wood Johnson Foundation). Another recent study (Spillman & Pezzin, 2000) using the 1984 and 1994 National Long Term Care Surveys (NLTCS) found a decline in the prevalence of IADL-only disability between 1984 and 1994 was matched by no decline in the prevalence of ADL disability; this means there was a shift upward in the level of disability among those who received help. This translates, simply, to a "mounting need" that is analogous to the proverbial iceberg: What lies below the already visible threshold of informal caregiving is the expanding duration of caregiving and more people needing care. Caregiving networks are increasingly being put to the test. Men's involvement in caregiving is not likely to ebb, rather it is long term.

The caregiving landscape: Men's contribution. Most older adults do have several informal caregivers available. One estimate shows that for each person needing care in 1990, there were 11 *potential* caregivers—for example, spouses, adult children and their spouses, grandchildren, household mates. However, by 2020, that 11:1 ratio will be cut by more than half (Robert Wood Johnson Foundation, 1996). Spillman and Pezzin (2000) also observed a decrease in receipt of informal care, specifically care from spouses and children. The pool of potential informal caregivers is shrinking (cf., Hoffman, Rice, & Sung, 1996; Kramer, chap. 1; Wagner, 1997). It is thus predictable that women who need care will be turning to a husband, son, son-in-law, brother, or father for their care, more often than in the past. Men, too, will be looking to other men to provide care. Caregiving men could be drafted into their caregiving responsibilities or be volunteers. They could be sole caregivers or the principal care-manager or part of an informal team of caregivers. Whatever their manner of caregiving or motivation, men's presence among primary caregivers will become more significant.

It is already significant. In the late 1980s Stone, Cafferata, and Sangl (1987) estimated that one in five primary caregivers was either a husband or son, and Tennstedt, McKinlay, and Sullivan (1989) cautioned that the importance of men as secondary caregivers should not be dismissed. In the gay community, more than one-quarter of the men were caregiving, and most were assisting another working-age adult with an illness or disability (Fredriksen, 1999). Marks (1996) observed that among *midlife adults* involved in caregiving either in or out of their residence, the ratio of female to male caregivers was about four to three—a much higher prevalence of midlife men's involvement than most nonrepresentative sample studies indicate. Spillman and Pezzin (2000) also observed that contrary to past observations, the proportion of primary caregivers who were sons increased significantly between 1984 and 1994, and they offset the decrease in the proportion of caregivers who were wives. The National Alliance for Caregiving and AARP survey (1997) reported that more than a quarter of the caregivers were men, and among the Hispanic and Asian communities, the proportion of men to women caregivers increased to a third and nearly one-half, respectively. In a national sample of informal caregivers who *live with* their care recipient, about 47% of primary caregivers (those with the principal responsibility) and 55% of secondary caregivers were men (Kennedy & Walls, 1997). Those living-in caregivers were more often husbands, gay partners, and sole adult sons. Another nationally representative telephone survey conducted for the National Family Caregivers Association (2000) also observed that men's involvement in caregiving seems to have stepped up as the twentieth century closed. This new study found 27% of the 1,000 people surveyed actively provided care for a relative or friend in the past year, and 44% of the caregivers of an elderly, disabled, or chronically ill friend or relative were men. The study did not identify which men were husbands, sons, or friends, but it did show that half the caregivers (39% of whom were men) provided physical care. They rolled up their sleeves to help loved ones in need of personal assistance, including helping with dressing, bathing, toileting, eating, and mobility. Almost half the caregivers (41% of them men) were involved in performing some type of nursing activity such as managing medications, changing dressings, or monitoring vital signs. Whether or not they are self-defined caregivers or counted as caregivers, men quietly adapt to accommodate the person-in-need, provide care, and assist other caregivers. Men are vital to caregiving networks.

MEN AS CAREGIVERS

Old precepts. The nation, and the research community too, has come to normalize the caregiving work performed on behalf of families in essentialist terms. That is, women's greater involvement in caring is not just their disproportionate representation in unpaid family labor (Dwyer & Seccombe, 1991; Finley, 1989; Lee, 1992; Shanas, 1979), caring is envisioned as the essence of womanhood (Gilligan, 1982) and women's learned predisposition (Chodorow, 1978). When this gendered lens frames observation, the image of a largely sex-segregated division of labor is subtly replaced by a gendered definition of family work. Caregiving becomes more than women's delegated work in a patriarchal society (Walker, 1992); it is women's badge of courage and a woman's issue (Hooyman & Gonyea, 1999).

Without doubt, throughout the twentieth century the bulk of family caregiving was provided by women, largely because of the "breadwinner mandate" and "cult of true womanhood" that arose in the mid-nineteenth century. According to the separate spheres ideology, men's duty was to separate from family, engage in paid labor outside the home, and bring home the family wage. Women's work became making and mending interpersonal relations (or "connections") as well as the unpaid home-based responsibilities that include eldercare and childcare; poor and working-class families women were also expected to engage in paid piecework. Underpinning this division of labor was the nineteenth century precept that men and women are "naturally" suited to their respective spheres (Abel, 1990; Kimmel, 1997). Today, still, women are sometimes described as better suited for caregiving for elders because they are "more responsive to pain and suffering and more willing to take on arduous and often unrewarding personal duties" (Wilson, 1990, p. 417). The gender model that long ago helped script a breadwinner-caregiver family system and assigned caregiving to be "women's work," remains part of the culture and many social institutions. It has some researchers expecting women's caregiving to be "natural." Men engaged in caregiving thus are thought to be valiant (Murray, 1996) and deviant (Thompson, 2000) simply because they cross over the stereotypical masculine-feminine boundary into a female-dominated area.

Twenty-five years ago Doll, Thompson, and Lefton (1976), for example, extolled the virtues of the way mothers could fight through their doubts and unconditionally care for their deinstitutionalized adult children with psychiatric diagnoses (or mental illness). According to the authors, it was mothers, not fathers, who had "the knack" to be caregivers. Either the special bond between spouses or the contracted relationship that wives and husbands make through their marriage vows appeared to override "nature," because husbands were found no less involved as caregivers than wives (see Doll et al.). But these researchers expected the people they observed to do gender appropriately; the essentialist lens Doll et al. used in their analysis could not account for the dedication exhibited by some husband caregivers. The men were presented as heroes. And undaunted, the researchers proposed that mothers' caregiving exemplified the gold standard of family caregiving, since it was the essence of womanhood.

This unsophisticated perception of gender and caregiving was not an unusual one when family caregiving for older adults was initially investigated (cf., Montgomery, Gonyea, & Hooyman, 1985; Ungerson, 1983). Consider the opening of Jutras and Veilleux's (1991, pp. 2–3) literature review: "The fact that women are consistently more involved than men in different care-giving tasks toward their elderly relatives is consistent with their tendency to develop more intense and more intimate social relationships, to be more nurturant, to be more compassionate, and to make care for the fulfilling commitments a greater priority than work commitments." As this one example reveals, our understanding of informal caregiving will be abridged by the precepts of the separate spheres ideology and the presumption that gender roles are internalized as stable personality traits and predetermine behavior. Indeed, according to Kaye and Applegate (1994, p. 218–219), "conventional wisdom and stereotypical thinking have led us to assume that . . . men lack the inclination and capacity to meet the physical and emotional needs of another person."

Resulting perceptions. There are perceptual consequences arising from essentialist precepts. As W. I. Thomas' sociological axiom warns, "Once a situation is defined as real, it becomes real in its consequences." First, in that women are expected to be the caregivers, there is a propensity among researchers to disregard the husbands, adults sons, and sons-in-law that orchestrate and manage care. Men's caregiving can be made transparent when countless studies of caregivers impart the message that men comprise *only* 20% or 25% of the primary caregivers, and then the caregiving work men do is never discussed. Men's caregiving also is discounted when authors draw the conclusion that men's involvement in providing care is statistically less than women's involvement. For example, their active involvement is effectively dismissed when the sizeable number of hours per week caregiving men provide is couched in a gender comparative presentation such as "Women spend significantly more time caring than men—an average of 18.8 hours per week, in contrast with 15.5 hours per week for men" (National Alliance for Caregiving, 1997, p. 17). The observed difference of three hours is highlighted, rather than the fifteen hours of caregiving. Similarly, in a review article on elder husbands, Gregory, Peters, and Cameron (1990, p. 23) stated that "husbands as caregivers were more likely than wives to seek the help of formal providers and receive more informal support." The message is that men need and receive more outside assistance. Ironically, this article contradicts a national survey that showed husbands depended less on outside help than wives (cf., Stone et al., 1987).

Put simply, a comparative lens can always trivialize. The gender comparative lens has the tendency to snub many men's dedicated caregiving and many other men's attentive contributions. As Arber and Gilbert (1989, p. 80) observed:

> Although at least a third of carers of the frail elderly are men, caring conflicts with norms of masculinity and appears to break fundamental gender roles. One way in which the literature has addressed this problem has been to ignore it, and another has been to suggest that men carers are not really doing much caring because they obtain much more support than women from voluntary and statutory services and from informal carers living outside the household. This argument dismisses male carers as an artifact; men are not considered "real" carers who suffer the same social, emotional, and physical consequences which women carers have been demonstrated to suffer.

Second, men are not studied as *men*, but as members of a homogeneous class. The gender comparative lens narrows the range of masculinities exemplified by men caregivers into a gender stereotype. Although significant diversity exists, men are aggregated into the category "male caregivers," and the gender stereotype is the sole model of manhood imagined. The ethnic, sexuality, birth cohort, regional, religious, family history, and class differences crosscutting men's caregiving experiences are unintentionally homogenized. Adult sons and older husbands; White men and men of color; blue collar assembly line workers and financial planners who take up the responsibilities of caregiving are classified the same; they are "male." Ironically this categorical variable in multivariate analysis is very frequently coded "female," and thus even as a homogeneous class men caregivers are made invisible.

Finally, caregiving men do not fit the stereotype of sex-typed behavior and are defined as acting out-of-character *as men*. In a gendered society, everyone is expected to "do gender" appropriately, and when people fail to do so, they stand out. Men who are the caregivers for their wives, mothers, lovers, brothers, fathers, and friends should challenge gender stereotypes, but have they? For example, Bowers (1999) expected men caregivers to describe themselves as androgynous or feminine because of their caregiving; but she observed that the widowers who had been caregivers described themselves in more masculine terms than the non-caregiving widowers. Her expectation was that caregiving men would forfeit their masculine self-image. Another example: The precept of a single masculinity breeds an expectation that men and caregiving are incongruent. The incongruence is the expected "skill malfit," since there is an expected inadequacy in household management and nursing skills to perform as a caregiver (Allen, 1994), and an "identity malfit," since some men acknowledge discomfort in performing expressive or hands-on activities (McFarland & Sanders, 1999). Plainly, men who engage in caregiving may

not disturb researchers' gender expectations; caregiving men are expected to be "different" from caregiving women and most other men. Some
are portrayed as ordinary men motivated by obligation more than attachment, even when they are immersed in the caregiving role. Some are portrayed as extraordinary men, because they "step-up" to care for and
unequivocally care about the care-recipient. The so-called ordinary and
extraordinary *caregiving* men are mystifying, because they do and do not
adhere to the masculinity stereotype. However, are they so unusual?
Routinely found is that nearly one-half of spouse caregivers are men (e.g.,
Horowitz, 1985; Tennstedt, Crawford, & McKinlay, 1993) and their level of
involvement in caregiving (as defined by the amount, type, and style
of caregiving) is as equal to anyone else's involvement. Miller (1987),
Barusch and Spaid (1989), and Tennstedt, McKinlay, and Sullivan (1989)
have established that husbands perform no fewer caregiving tasks than
wife carers and are more likely to be the sole caregiver. Nonetheless, men
caregivers emerge as the atypical men, heroic.

STARTING PREMISE

There are many masculinities evident in our culture, in institutions, and
in relationships. There is, in effect, a matrix of masculinities that are influenced by social institutions and the larger stratification system (Connell,
1995; Hunter & Davis, 1992). Because these masculinities are experienced
through interaction and discourse, one man, the same man, in one day
can easily participate in different masculinities when he dresses and feeds
his infant daughter her breakfast, oversees an afternoon-long meeting,
plays racquetball, and prepares and feeds his stroke-handicapped father
his dinner. He does not follow a universal gender script across these settings. He cannot. The stereotypical standard does not assist him as he
actively parents or assists his own frail older parent.

   The matrix of masculinities organizing each man's social life is fashioned according to his culture and class, age, cohort experiences, and the
interactions he has with others. The matrix, also, subtly orchestrates
the man's initial approach to caregiving. Multiple motivations for caregiving are therefore possible. And multiple caregiving styles are possible.
For the men who are the primary caregivers for their wives or partners or
parents, the way they differentially "do caregiving" depends, for example, on their life stage (Archer & MacLean, 1993; Kaye & Applegate, 1994)
and employment demands (NAFC/AARP, 1997; Stone & Short, 1990),
access to and interaction with secondary caregivers (Matthews & Rosner,
1988), willingness to put self on hold (Hilton, Crawford, & Tarko, 2000),
and relationship with the care-recipient (Matthews, 1997). Risman (1998)

urges us to appreciate how the immediate structure of the caregiving setting is the most influential factor shaping men's caregiving. The setting and the relationship the caregiver has with his care-recipient influences the salience of his caring and his caregiving identity. If he is aware that his caregiving relationship requires him to be a particular type of caregiver and he values his relationship, he may become unconditionally committed to the caregiving identity and forfeit his paid work identity. He does caregiving and gender concurrently, and thus he actively constructs a new masculinity for himself, albeit one that entails caring for, nurturing, and a greater sense of connection to the care-recipient. In the documentary film *Grace* (New Day Films, 1990), this is exactly what the husband does over the course of caring for his Alzheimer's-effected wife. He forges an identity as Grace's caregiving *husband;* the husband role enlarges, and his caregiving motivation is his longing to extend his marriage as much as he can.

MEN'S STYLES OF CAREGIVING

The accumulated stock of knowledge regarding men and caregiving is, on close inspection, more detailed than many people might first expect. There are a number of qualitative studies that cogently describe the different ways husbands assist their wives (e.g., Fuller-Jonap & Haley, 1995; Harris, 1993, 1995; Hilton et al., 2000; Motenko, 1988). Harris (1998) detailed four different types of adult son caregiving styles, and earlier Matthews and Rosner (1988) identified some of the complex motivations behind the adult son's approach to caregiving. Other studies do not address the type of caregiver/care-recipient relations, rather they have begun to distinguish among men on the basis of participation in the labor market (Montgomery, 1992; Stoller, 1983), family position (Dwyer & Seccombe, 1991), and age and marital status (Marks, 1996). Collectively, this work dehomogenizes the collective called "male caregivers," helps deconstruct the breadwinner-caregiver divide (Derrida, 1981), and floats for recognition some of men's styles of caregiving.

What Men Do: The Spectrum of and Reasons for Care

Caregiving is a complex process involving a number of different kinds of work and a great deal of work. In broad terms there is both an instrumental and emotional dimension to caregiving. The dominant masculinity standards in American culture, or what is referred to as hegemonic masculinity (Connell, 1995), are believed to contribute to the expectation that men will "do caregiving" from an emotionally safe distance, whether the men are old or young, sole caregivers or secondary, rural African Americans or suburban Whites. These masculinity standards prescribe feeling rules that permit men to care *about* the care-recipient, to engage in caregiving as a labor of love; but, the same standards discourage men from becoming trapped by feelings of fear, anxiety, grief, or frustration as they care *for* the care-recipient. The feeling rules within contemporary manhood standards seem to nourish men's problem-solving style of coping (DeVries, Hamilton, Lovett, & Gallagher-Thompson, 1997), their attentiveness to their own need for respite and to control their emotional overload (Mac Rae, 1998; Motenko, 1988; Perkinson, 1995), their desire to control *their* experience of caregiving (Willoughby & Keating, 1991), and their genuine concern about the care-recipient's well-being (Hilton et al., 2000). It seems that men control their *felt experience* by maintaining a self outside the caregiving. For example, among HIV-negative gay men actively involved in caring for a lover or friend with AIDS, social coping increases positive affect, which resulted in less caregiving, stress-related physical symptoms (Billings, Folkman, Acree, & Moskowitz, 2000).

Men caring for their parents and wives typically are called upon to meet a wide range of caregiving needs, including emotional (Barusch & Spaid, 1989; Chang & White-Means, 1991; Kaye & Applegate, 1994; Kramer & Lambert, 1999; Miller & Kaufman, 1996; Morano, 1998; Neufeld & Harrison, 1998; Parsons, 1997; Siriopoulos, Brown, & Wright, 1999). Despite negative stereotypes, the evidence is that men do step up to provide whatever care is needed and will call in formal services to supplement their own caregiving. They invest themselves in their caregiving to provide quality care and comprehensive care. Hirsch and Newman (1995) report that it is not uncommon to find men involved in caregiving careers; in their small sample, more than one-third of the men were caring for one parent and had cared for a second person at some time. Studies show that when sons are the primary provider or sole caregiver, they do all that is necessary (Harris, 1998; Thompson, Tudiver, & Manson, 2000). By comparison, employed adult sons who have sisters may take advantage of patriarchal norms that privilege them; they "permit" their sisters to be primary caregivers and do more of the caring (Coward & Dwyer, 1990; Ingersoll-Dayton, Starrels, & Dowler, 1996; Matthews & Rosner, 1988; Stoller, 1983, 1990). However, maybe these sons' perceived diffidence to initiate caregiving or to get involved in the personal work of bathing, dressing, and toileting has less to do with their own traditionalism. It may be that the son is accommodating his mother's modesty needs and her preference for another woman to do the hands-on work of bathing and toileting (Lee, Dwyer, & Coward, 1993). Most studies of adult son–mother caregiving arrangements are based on the oldest women of the "Greatest Generation" (Brokaw, 1998) whose gender ideology was traditional and whose values underscored body modesty. Thus, perhaps, we have been observing cohort effects. Perhaps, also, the caregiving that sons engage in with their mothers or fathers has been designed to protect their mother's or father's autonomy (see Matthews, chap. 10). Sons "do caregiving" with their parents incrementally. As Thompson et al. (2000, p. 363) noticed, sons providing total care for their mothers "described it as a gradual process of taking over more and more activities," including diapering and bathing.

In sum, sons "do caregiving" in many masculine ways; typically, their daily lives remain orchestrated by their employment and the workplace culture that brands men as "unmasculine" if they take time off to caregive or talk about caregiving (Pleck, 1993); the men segment their lives, shifting selves as they begin work or begin caregiving, and struggle to prevent caregiving to "spill over" to affect another role. Employed sons are thus more likely to be secondary caregivers or part of a caregiving team; they seem to be fully part of a team and not likely to withdraw as caregiving demands escalate (Stoller, 1990). When needed, they "just do it" and cut back on their commitment to employment (Harris, 1998; Hirsch, 1996). Employed sons, however, are less likely than unemployed or marginally employed sons to be co-resident and managing a parent who needs several different, intense kinds of assistance (Campbell, 2000). In reality, employed sons incrementally commit to the caregiver role, and once they are caregivers they report their parent gets the best care available (cf., Archer & MacLean, 1993; Harris, 1998; Hirsch, 1996). Ironically, caregiving sons initially resist seeking help from formal support, perhaps because of the perceived dishonor in admitting the need for help and perhaps for valuing family privacy (Coe & Neufeld, 1999; Miller, 1987); they may later "give in" and use formal services, but at an initial perceived personal cost (see Coe & Neufeld). Thompson et al. (2000) suggest that sons' sparing use of formal support is initially associated with inadequate knowledge more than resistance to help-seeking; once valued services are identified there is no problem in using the service. This may be a key determinant to why Puerto Rican sons may be at higher risk for experiencing caregiving stress (Delgado & Tennstedt, 1997); they "go it alone" too long. Most sons approach caregiving from a gendered perspective, a "way of knowing," which defines caregiving in terms of the moral norm of "reciprocity" (Belenky, Clinchy, Goldberger, & Tarule, 1997; Delgado & Tennstedt, 1997; Neufeld & Harrison, 1998).

Chang and White-Means (1991) observed that caregiving husbands were more likely to provide hands-on personal care than nonspousal caregiving men. In this study husbands performed 65 hours a week of caregiving, on average. Barusch and Spaid (1989) reported that husbands performed many caregiving tasks, and these men were found to perform more tasks related to communication, mobility, hygiene, dressing, and feeding than a comparison sample of wives. Other studies have shown that

husbands provide care for a broader range of tasks and more hours of
assistance than other men caregivers; and, they are less likely to receive
help from secondary, informal caregivers, even though they are engaged
in providing care for someone who is more sick (cf., Kaye & Applegate,
1994; Stone et al., 1987; Tennstedt et al., 1989). Husbands in stable marriages who transitioned into the caregiving role, according to Kramer and
Lambert (1999), spent significantly more time doing household tasks than
non-caregiving husbands. They increased their hours per week on meal
preparation, dishes, cleaning, shopping, and laundry from approximately
7 to 17 as a result of caregiving. Their incipient immersion in caregiving,
however, was experienced as costly, compared to the lives of the husbands living with healthy wives. The men reported a decrease in emotional support from others and a decrease in their own happiness, as well
as an increase in expressed symptoms of depression. Spousal caregiving
is often not a choice (Wallsten, 2000), it is an unexpected career (Aneshensel,
Pearlin, Mullan, Zarit, & Whitlatch, 1995), and it may become a rewarding, satisfying career, however demanding. Miller and Kaufman (1996,
p. 196) understand, "The special nature of the spouse relationship, comprising love and responsibility between spouses, was offered frequently
as the main quality influencing caregiving. Caregiving was seen as part of
what spouses do for each other."

Because prospective studies of husband caregivers are rare, needed is
a better understanding of husbands' adaptation to each phase of caregiving—from the initial instrumental and housekeeping chores to the
hands-on physical, and, when necessary, to the wrenching decisions to
institutionalize. Kramer's (2000) longitudinal study of husbands caring
for wives with dementia reveals that the husbands who transitioned from
active caregiving to placing their spouse in a nursing home reported greater
depression, whereas the husbands who continued to care for their wives
at home seemed to adapt and reported less evidence of depression. The
husbands that institutionalized their wives were living with the sadness
and grief arising from the loss of their wives' presence and their career as
caregivers. But Bowers' (1999) study suggests that men who transitioned
into widowhood after having been a spouse's caregiver defined themselves as being in better psychological health than widows who had not
been caregivers. Caregiving is certainly taxing when compared to a matched
sample of non-caregivers (cf., Kramer & Lambert, 1999), and the emotion
work is men's special disadvantage (Miller & Kaufman, 1996); but are
husbands unhappy with their caregiving career, and is their reported psychological distress more with the "loss" of their marriages and married
selves as their wives become care-recipients instead of life partners?

Much like Hispanic husbands, it seems that White husbands are not
likely to use meal services to assist their caregiving; unlike Hispanics and

African Americans, White husbands are more likely to use in-home respite (Kosloski, Montgomery, & Karner, 1999). It also seems, caregiving inside the marital relationship, especially in late life, draws the spouses together interactively and affectively (Bleiszner & Shifflett, 1990; Chang & White-Means, 1991; Chappell & Kuehne, 1998; Fitting, Rabins, Lucas, & Eastham, 1986; Navon & Weinblatt, 1996; Thompson, 1993). Studies commonly find that husbands, when needed, are highly invested in the caregiver role, perhaps because caregiving becomes an opportunity structure to cross over and nurture as well as pay back for years of nurturing and support (Harris, 1993, 1995; Pruchno & Resch, 1989), or because caregiving provides a sense of continuity as "providers" as the husbands take up the responsibility to manage and control their wives' needs (cf., Miller, 1987; Sistler & Blanchard-Fields, 1993). Kaye and Applegate (1994) surmised that husbands reported their caregiving role was a labor of love, where caregiving became an extension and strengthening of their sense of devotion. Because they respond to the caregiving role as a new career, older husbands "do caregiving" differently than younger husbands or adult sons (cf., Archer & MacLean, 1993; Chang & White-Means, 1991; Hilton et al., 2000). They are more vigilant and invested and less likely to engage secondary caregivers or formal services. However, as Siriopoulos et al. (1999, p. 86) found, the age of the caregiving husband did not make a difference in the men's attitudes to the caregiving role. "They all cared for their wives in loving, supportive ways."

In general, husbands appear to accept caregiving as an extension of their marital vows and the constructed, ongoing reciprocity between spouses (Miller & Kaufman, 1996; Neufeld & Harrison, 1998). They enjoy the challenge of caregiving and approach caregiving with commitment and determination (Harris, 1993; Motenko, 1988; Mui, 1995). Men's approach often is "stoic" and, as a result, they minimally use formal services such as day care, respite help from secondary caregivers, or homemaker services (Coe & Neufeld, 1999; Kaye & Applegate, 1994). Husbands may resist outsider's solicitation to assist in a conscious effort to avert gnarled, conflicted interaction with friends and children who might want to approach caregiving differently (Barusch & Spaid, 1989; Carlson & Robertson, 1993); yet, they would like to receive more support than they do (Almberg, Jansson, Grafstrom, & Winblad, 1998; DeVries et al., 1997). They prefer psychoeducational interventions and information that describes specific caregiving problems (Garity, 1999; McFarland & Sanders, 1999); and, they are less inclined to try to keep family routines and activities intact and "normal," instead they relinquish earlier familial and gendered patterns and learn basic household and caregiving skills (Hilton et al., 2000).

The professional model. There is suggestive evidence that many men approach caregiving similar to the professional model of caregiving (cf., Fitting et al., 1986); that is, some men engage themselves in caregiving as if the responsibility was "work," and they take on a task-oriented, care management orientation as they provide care for the care-recipient. Caring refers to the emotional, physical, and mental work involved in looking after another. Caregiving husbands, sons, and gay lovers may not as likely perceive or discuss caregiving as "emotion work" (Hochschild, 1979; Mac Rae, 1998). The professional model emphasizes caregiver control (cf., Miller, 1987) and the completion of caregiving in the most efficacious manner with the least role engulfment (Skaff & Pearlin, 1992). Men who emulate the "professional" caregiver segment selves: On one hand, they are caregivers, fully engaged in the responsibilities and tasks of caregiving. They identify themselves as caregivers, and they "just do it" until the need to institutionalize the care-recipient dictates letting go (cf., Kramer, 2000). The ritualization of caregiving seems to provide a sense of constant activity (Navon & Weinblatt, 1996), some continuity of the man's sense of authority (Miller, 1987), and a meaningful distraction from workplace demands. Caregiving becomes an "unexpected career" (Aneshensel et al., 1995). On the other hand, as men, they never allow the greedy institution of caregiving to intrude so thoroughly that caring becomes the man's entire world. Men have a history of compartmentalizing. Thus, for example, husbands may experience a "calling" to become the sole caregiver of their long-term partner, but they "do caregiving" by compartmentalizing and by avoiding the experience of being swallowed by the caregiving situation. Their caregiving "work" is akin to the physician-surgeon who engages in the work of caregiving, intimately intrudes, yet is able to maintain another life outside the institution of medicine. As one study shows, husband caregivers do not show evidence of a reduction in social recreation activities as a result of taking on their caregiving, compared to non-caregiving husbands; and, they seek the company of others socially and spiritually by increasing their religious involvement as they experience less perceived encouragement and emotional support (Kramer & Lambert, 1999).

This management style is at times summarily dismissed as cold and uncaring. Meeting a care-recipient's needs via the recruitment of help from family members and professional services can be misperceived as cold when caregiving is tacitly defined by the gold standard of unconditional "mothering." However, some primary caregivers, particularly adults sons with their own families and employment demands (Jutras & Veilleux, 1991), serve as if they are a "case manager" and they coordinate care, in lieu of institutionalizing the care-recipient. These men orchestrate caregiving using lots of assistance; although they personally perform fewer chores than most older husband caregivers, they care about their parents' and friends' welfare and well-being rather than personally provide the care. Other men's management style demonstrates an effort to blend the gendered worlds of management and nurturing. Studies such as those by Motenko (1988), Harris (1993, 1995), Matthews (1997), Hirsch and Newman (1995), or Vinick (1984) reveal a model of caregiving that incorporates traditionally masculine, workplace values with an affective provision of care. The evidence to this combined management-nurturing approach is principally found among older husbands, and it is derived from in-depth, qualitative studies using small samples. These caring husbands are also caring *for* their wives.

Most often, studies examining caregiver distress find that men deeply engaged in the tasks of caregiving do not report significant distress or burden (e.g., Miller & Cafasso, 1992) as a result of their caregiving "work." The question is, why? There are at least two possibilities. One is that men's style of caring is truly less distressing, or it may be that men's true level of distress is poorly measured. First, perhaps it is the protective nature of the professional model that men emulate, or what Fitting et al. (1986) described as a managerial model; this caregiving style may well shelter caregiving men from symptoms of poor mental health and burnout (Braithwaite, 1996; Skaff & Pearlin, 1992). The managerial strategy and the professional model provide the men caregivers who use this strategy greater perceived control, the sense of being in charge, feelings of self-efficacy, the ability to choose to act or not act, and the opportunity to not become engulfed in the caregiving relationships (Sistler & Blanchard-Fields, 1993; Szabo & Strang, 1999; Wallhagen & Kagan, 1993; Willoughby & Keating, 1991). Men using a managerial approach seemingly engage in a prospective appraisal process as described by Lazarus and Folkman (1984). They manage caregiving by routinely evaluating their own skills against their ability to meet the care-recipient's needs. They report becoming more adept and tolerant (Miller & Kaufman, 1996). They do not experience dissonance with taking respite time for themselves (Motenko, 1988; Perkinson, 1995). They seem to avoid role engulfment by maintaining outside interests (Archer & MacLean, 1993; Corcoran, 1992; Miller, 1987) and, at times, by emotional withdrawal (Parks & Pilisuk, 1991). This cognitive and behavior distancing from the demands of caregiving may well assist men to temporarily forget the heavy responsibilities and thereby reduce the distress of caring *for*, as well as increase the perceived gains of caring *for* and *about*. In a longitudinal study of husbands caring for wives with dementia, Kramer (2000) observed that the group of husbands who continued to care for their wives in their homes experienced fewer symptoms of depression, even though the stressors associated with caregiving increased and resources remained stable. This set of husbands appeared to adapt over time.

The finding that men caregivers do not report significant distress could also be a research artifact that arises chiefly when men caregivers are compared to women, and thus the finding has nothing to do with the proposed protective nature of the management style. But Umberson, Chen, House, Hopkins, and Slaten's (1996, p. 852) conclusion about the nature of gender and caregiving is cautionary: "Contrary to much sociological theory, women do not seem to be more psychologically sensitive than men to the circumstances and quality of their [caregiving] relationships . . . This finding supports the structuralist position that similar social conditions elicit similar psychological reactions from individuals." Also as mentioned earlier, Kramer and Lambert (1999) found that older husbands who became caregivers within the five-year study period experienced greater depression and unhappiness than the comparison husbands whose spouse was not seriously ill. Because this is the only prospective study of men *becoming* caregivers to date, we must be cautious to not overgeneralize. But it is suggestive. One, this study examined one group of husbands' transitions to caregiving as well as the men's experiences in being caregivers. Caregiving is logically more psychologically, physically, and interpersonally demanding than not taking on the work of caregiving, and this is what Kramer and Lambert observed. Two, being the principal caregiver also serves as a painful reminder of the changed marriage. The experience of "becoming" a husband caregiver and no longer "being" only a husband is logically a distressing one, when compared to non-caregiving husbands, and this is what the study found. Three, caring for a wife with malignant cancer (which was the case for one-quarter of the caregiving husbands in Kramer and Lambert's study) would certainly be more depressing, on average, than living with a healthy wife. The point is, caregiving men do experience psychological costs, but their level of distress and general well-being may be protected by their style of caring and coping. It remains something that has not been studied thoroughly.

Caregiving does not exist in a vacuum, it is embedded in intimate personal relationships and entails emotion management. The professional model men seemingly emulate may be a successful strategy to manage the complex of feelings arising from both "doing caregiving" and "caring about."

The Meaning of Caregiving

Kaye and Applegate (1990, p. 146) reminded the research community that the meanings caregiving men give to their caring is poorly understood. Although a small number of studies have begun to outline the voices and lived experience of caregiving men, Kaye and Applegate's reminder remains salient. "What gives caregiving men's lives meaning?" is still uncertain. Some men seem to assume their caregiver responsibilities as a sense of fulfillment of unmet family needs (Pruchno & Resch, 1989); some men respond to their affection and feelings of interpersonal commitment (Fitting et al., 1986; Motenko, 1988); some seek to replace the gratifications and intrinsic rewards formerly found in work (Archer & MacLean, 1993; Corcoran, 1992; Vinick, 1984); some men consciously take the opportunity to experience nurturing (Hirsch, 1996; Kaye & Applegate, 1990); and, some men extend their work-related experiences of "taking control" into caregiving (Miller, 1987). Each of these explanations for why men are caregivers is an ad hoc explanation, and the meaning of caregiving for men has been given little a priori attention.

Carol Farran and her colleagues (1991, 1999) have begun to unravel the manner in which caregivers find meaning through the experience of caring. Her thesis is that both suffering and uplifts are managed by making choices. Underlying the action of making choices are the values held by the caregiver, and it is through action that caregivers find provisional meaning. Put differently, "doing caregiving" produces provisional meaning. For husbands, "doing caregiving" seems to be an extension of being a husband. Caregiving is a another pathway for intimacy-building; it is absolutely frightening and demoralizing (Parsons, 1997) at times, but it is a course of action that husbands "do."

In an important study, Parsons (1997) tried to explicate through depth interviewing the meaning of men's lived experiences as they cared for a parent or spouse with Alzheimer's disease. The first theme identified was "enduring." The men described how they worked hard as they toileted, washed, dressed, undressed, and medicated their spouse or parent, but it wasn't just the physical labor they endured. As Mac Rae (1998) also observed, it is the exhausting emotional labor of caring for, and the painful emotions of caring about that become a double-barrel blast of feelings. Another theme Parsons (1997) uncovered was the sense of loss (cf., Farran, Keane-Hagerty, Salloway, Kupferer, & Wilken, 1991; Harris, 1993, 1998). The men experienced and felt loss in many ways, from the absence of a marriage or parent-child relationship to the loss of relationships with other friends and family members as people stayed away. Most acutely felt was the loss of the person being cared for. "Caregiving, as the word suggests, is a giving of oneself, a giving of one's time, of one's effort. It is antithetical, therefore, to think that caregiving could be associated with taking something away, of withholding from the care recipient" (Parsons, 1997, p. 399). This "taking away" emerged as another troubling theme for the men. What the men experienced was the disease, not the care-recipient (cf., Gubrium, 1986). What they drew from it was a caregiving career; they were pioneers, and they learned about themselves. They thought that they had put themselves on hold; but they also recognized that they learned to be their wife's caregiver. As one husband in Miller and Kaufman's (1996, p. 197) study pointed out: "[Caregiving] depends on the person. If she were in a nursing home, I'd prefer a woman, but since she's here at home, I prefer to care for her." This man endures, feels loss, has to manage the emotional knots of "taking away" his wife's choices, engages in the emotion work of soothing the care-recipient's troubles, and becomes a caregiver.

EXIT THOUGHTS

Many men seemingly approach caregiving with a professional or managerial model, emphasizing caregiver control. The "professional" caregiver can be fully engaged in the tasks of caregiving or supervising the delivery of services by others. In both cases it appears that men are less engulfed by the emotions associated with providing care. This managerial-professional model seems to shelter men from undue suffering and caregiver burnout. Men endure and integrate their caregiving career into their daily lives. The managerial strategy provides greater perceived control, the sense of being in charge, feelings of self-efficacy, the ability to choose to act or not act, and less difficulty with taking respite time or asking for assistance without guilt. But is it understood by others?

What within-gender variations have been studied? Little is known about what determines the range of men's motivations to give care, or if the *meanings* men derived may systematically vary by class, religious background, marital intimacy, and so on. Does religious and spiritual involvement commonly shape the experience of men across ethnic backgrounds, or do Levkoff, Levy, and Weitzman's (1999) findings about the Irish American and African American caregivers carry over to also show ethnic variations in men's themes of alienation from religious groups, nonetheless their dependence on spirituality and prayer to cope. Rarely investigated are the ways different men interpret the caregiving experience.

FOR BETTER OR FOR WORSE/ Lynn Johnston

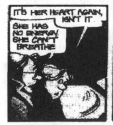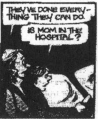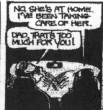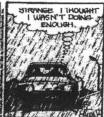

SOURCE: © 1991 Lynn Johnston Prod. Reprinted by permission of United Press Syndicate.

Comparison between adult sons with and without sisters (Matthews & Rosner, 1988) strongly suggests that men's experiences with caregiving are not uniform. When systematic variation among men is investigated, the prime basis for differentiating among men has been structural—for example, men's relationship to the care recipient (older husband vs. adult son). Very seldom have researchers set out to assess how styles of interaction, such as controlling or not, might differently shape the caregiving experiences of husbands or sons (Harris, 1993; Motenko, 1988) or how men's gendered lives relate to their style of caregiving (Hirsch & Newman, 1995). Are there different types of "managing" and "control" predictably associated with the quality of caregiving?

The salience of gender ideology. Masculinity scripts that exist in the culture may be less salient directives than previously thought for the men involved in caregiving. Risman (1998) would argue that it is the immediate social structural factors experienced at the personal level that determine men's involvement in caregiving, style of caregiving, and lived experience as caregivers. Umberson et al. (1996) studied men's and women's behavior across a range of relationships and surmised that there is little evidence that men are less emotionally sensitive to their quality of their relationships than women. Are the younger "Boomer" generation men, who have been more actively involved in parenting than the older generation, less likely to feel distance from caregiving? Kaye and Applegate (1994) found older caregiving husbands who are part of the "Greatest Generation" and who lived the breadwinner mandate, were a long way from being locked into the masculinity stereotype. When they described themselves in instrumental-affective terms, their self-descriptions indicated a blending of masculine-instrument and feminine-expressive traits. They saw themselves as self-sufficient, forceful, analytical, and competitive, as well as gentle, compassionate, loving, yielding, and warm. Kaye and Applegate (1990, 1994) observed that when traits were rank ordered, following "self-sufficient" the caregiving men perceived themselves in feminine terms, as gentle, compassionate, warm, and loving. These self-descriptions may be age related, rather than emergent from the context of the caregiving experience. Life course theories expect older men to explore their under-developed feminine side (Gutmann, 1987) and to focus less on "doing masculinity" (Erikson, 1963; Erikson, Kivnick, & Erikson, 1994; Levinson, Darrow, Klein, Levinson, & McKee, 1978). Whether the source is the opportunity structure of caregiving (cf., Risman, 1998) or age norms, the message is that many of the older men Kaye and Applegate studied crossed over the masculine-feminine divide; as "Greatest Generation" caregivers, they comfortably described themselves in "feminine" terms. Recently, Bowers (1999) observed that older widowers who had been caregivers before their wives died also described themselves in more "feminine" terms than widowers who had not been caregivers. Perhaps, the issue is us: Researchers, social service providers, clinicians, and the families and friends of men caregivers are socialized to view caregiving as "feminine" and we do not honor the fact that caring, compassion, empathy, and sensitivity are not traits specific to women. There certainly is wide variation in caregiving men's self-identity, reasons for caregiving, and styles of caring. This variation needs better documentation.

REFERENCES

Abel, E. K. (1990). Family care of the frail elderly. In E. K. Abel & M. K. Nelson (Eds.), *Circles of care: Work & identity in women's lives* (pp. 65–91). Albany, NY: SUNY Press.

Abel, E. K. (1995). "Man, woman, and chore boy": Transformations in the antagonistic demands of work and care on women in the 19th and 20th centuries. *The Milbank Quarterly, 73,* 187–211.

Administration on Aging. (1999). *Family caregiver fact sheet.* Washington, DC: U.S. Department of Health and Human Services.

Allen, S. M. (1994). Gender differences in spousal caregiving and unmet need for care. *Journal of Gerontology: Social Sciences, 49,* S187–S195.

Almberg, B., Jansson, W., Grafstrom, M., & Winblad, B. (1998). Differences between and within genders in caregiving strain: A comparison between caregivers of demented and non-caregivers of non-demented elderly people. *Journal of Advanced Nursing, 28,* 849–858.

Aneshensel, C. S., Pearlin, L. I., Mullan, J. T., Zarit, S. H., & Whitlatch, C. J. (1995). *Profiles in caregiving: The unexpected career.* New York: Academic Press.

Arber, S., & Gilbert, N. (1989). Transitions in caring: Gender, life course & the care of the elderly. In B. Bytheway, et al. (Eds.), *Becoming and being old: Sociological approaches to later life* (pp. 72–92). London: Sage.

Archer, C. K., & MacLean, M. J. (1993). Husbands and sons as caregivers of chronically ill elderly women. *Journal of Gerontological Social Work, 21*(1/2), 5–23.

Barusch, A. S., & Spaid, W. M. (1989). Gender differences in caregiving: Why do wives report greater burden? *The Gerontologist, 29,* 667–676.

Belenky, M. F., Clinchy, B. M., Goldberger, N. R., & Tarule, J. M. (1997). *Women's ways of knowing: The development of self, voice, and mind.* New York: Basic Books.

Billings, D. W., Folkman, S., Acree, M., & Moskowitz, J. T. (2000). Coping and physical health during caregiving: The roles of positive and negative affect. *Journal of Personality and Social Psychology, 79,* 131–142.

Bleiszner, R., & Shifflett, P. (1990). The effects of Alzheimer's disease on close relationships between patients and caregivers. *Family Relations, 39*, 57–62.

Bowers, S. P. (1999). Gender role identity and the caregiving experience of widowed men. *Sex Roles, 41*, 645–655.

Braithwaite, V. A. (1996). Understanding stress in informal caregiving: Is burden a problem of the individual or society? *Research on Aging, 18*, 139–174.

Brokaw, T. (1998). *The greatest generation.* New York: Random House.

Campbell, L. D. (2000). *Capturing the complexity of men's caregiving: The value of combining methodological approaches in the study of men's filial care.* Paper presented at the annual meeting of the Gerontological Society of America, Washington, DC.

Cancian, F. M., & Oliker, S. J. (2000). *Caring and gender.* Thousand Oaks, CA: Pine Forge Press.

Carlson, K. W., & Robertson, S. E. (1993). Husbands and wives of dementia patients: Burden and social support. *Canadian Journal of Rehabilitation, 6*, 163–173.

Chang, C. F., & White-Means, S. I. (1991). The men who care: An analysis of male primary caregivers who care for frail elderly at home. *Journal of Applied Gerontology, 10*, 343–358.

Chappell, N. L., & Kuehne, V. K. (1998). Congruence among husband and wife caregivers. *Journal of Aging Studies, 12*, 239–254.

Chodorow, N. (1978). *The reproduction of mothering: Psychoanalysis and the sociology of gender.* Berkeley: University of California Press.

Clinton, W. (1997, November 22). *National family caregivers week, 1997: A proclamation by the President of the United States of America.* Washington, DC: White House.

Coe, M., & Neufeld, A. (1999). Male caregivers' use of formal support. *Western Journal of Nursing Research, 21*, 568–588.

Connell, R. (1995). *Masculinities.* Berkeley: University of California Press.

Corcoran, M. A. (1992). Gender differences in dementia management plans of spousal caregivers. *American Journal of Occupational Therapy, 46*, 1006–1012.

Coward, R. T., & Dwyer, J. W. (1990). The association of gender, sibling network composition, and patterns of parent care by adult children. *Research on Aging, 12*, 158–181.

Delgado, M., & Tennstedt, S. (1997). Puerto Rican sons as primary caregivers of elderly parents. *Social Work, 42*, 125–134.

Derrida, J. (1981). *Dissemination.* Chicago: University of Chicago Press.

DeVries, H. M., Hamilton, D. W., Lovett, S., & Gallagher-Thompson, D. (1997). Patterns of coping preferences for male and female caregivers of frail older adults. *Psychology and Aging, 12*, 263–267.

Doll, W., Thompson, E. H., & Lefton, M. (1976). Beneath acceptance: Dimensions of family affect towards former mental patients. *Social Science and Medicine, 10*, 307–313.

Dwyer, J. W., & Seccombe, K. (1991). Elder care as family labor: The influence of gender and family position. *Journal of Family Issues, 12*, 229–247.

Erikson, E. (1963). *Childhood and society.* New York: Norton.

Erikson, E., Kivnick, H. Q., & Erikson, J. M. (1994). *Vital involvement in old age: The experience of old age in our time.* New York: Norton.

Farran, C. J., Keane-Hagerty, E., Salloway, S., Kupferer, S., & Wilken, C. S. (1991). Finding meaning: An alternative paradigm for Alzheimer's disease family caregivers. *The Gerontologist, 31*, 483–489.

Farran, C. J., Miller, B. H., Kaufman, J. E., Donner, E., & Fogg, L. (1999). Finding meaning through caregiving: Development of an instrument for family caregivers of persons with Alzheimer's disease. *Journal of Clinical Psychology, 55*, 1107–1125.

Finley, N. J. (1989). Theories of family labor as applied to gender differences in caregiving for elderly parents. *Journal of Marriage and the Family, 51*, 79–86.

Fitting, M., Rabins, P., Lucas, M. J., & Eastham, J. (1986). Caregivers for dementia patients: A comparison of husbands and wives. *The Gerontologist, 26*, 248–252.

Fredriksen, K. I. (1999). Family caregiving responsibilities among lesbians and gay men. *Social Work, 44*, 142–155.

Fuller-Jonap, F. A., & Haley, W. E. (1995). Mental and physical health of male caregivers of a spouse with Alzheimer's disease. *Journal of Aging and Health, 7*, 99–118.

Garity, J. (1999). Gender differences in learning style of Alzheimer family caregivers. *Home Healthcare Nurse, 17*, 37–44.

Gilligan, C. (1982). *In a different voice: Psychological theory and women's development.* Cambridge: Harvard University Press.

Gregory, D., Peters, N., & Cameron, C. F. (1990). Elderly male spouses as caregivers—toward an understanding of their experience. *Journal of Gerontological Nursing, 16*, 20–24.

Gubrium, J. (1986). *Oldtimers and Alzheimer's: The descriptive organization of senility.* Greenwich, CT: JAI.

Gutmann, D. (1987). *Reclaimed powers: Toward a new psychology of men and women in late life.* New York: Basic Books.

Harris, P. B. (1993). The misunderstood caregiver? A qualitative study of the male caregiver of Alzheimer's disease victims. *The Gerontologist, 33*, 551–556.

Harris, P. B. (1995). Differences among husbands caring for their wives with Alzheimer's disease: Qualitative findings and counseling implications. *Journal of Clinical Geropsychology, 1*, 97–106.

Harris, P. B. (1998). Listening to caregiving sons: Misunderstood realities. *The Gerontologist, 38*, 342–352.

Haug, M. (1994). Elderly patients, caregivers, and physicians: Theory and research on health care triads. *Journal of Health and Social Behavior, 35*, 1–12.

Hilton, B. A., Crawford, J. A., & Tarko, M. A. (2000). Men's perspective on individual and family coping with their wives' breast cancer and chemotherapy. *Western Journal of Nursing Research, 22*, 428–459.

Hirsch, C. (1996). Understanding the influence of gender role identity on the assumption of family caregiving by men. *International Journal of Aging and Human Development, 42*, 103–121.

Hirsch, C., & Newman, J. L. (1995). Microstructural and gender role influences on male caregivers. *Journal of Men's Studies, 3*, 309–333.

Hochschild, A. (1979). Emotion work, feelings rules, and social structure. *American Journal of Sociology, 85*, 551–575.

Hoffman, C., Rice, D., & Sung, H. (1996). Persons with chronic conditions: Their prevalence and costs. *Journal of the American Medical Association, 276*, 1473–1479.

Hooyman, N. R., & Gonyea, J. G. (1999). Feminist model of family care: Practice and policy directions. *Journal of Women and Aging, 11*, 149–169.

Horowitz, A. (1985). Sons and daughters as caregivers to older parents: Differences in role performance and consequences. *The Gerontologist, 25*, 612–617.

Hunter, A. G., & Davis, J. E. (1992). Constructing gender: An exploration of Afro-American men's conceptualization of manhood. *Gender & Society, 6*, 464–479.

Ingersoll-Dayton, B., Starrels, M. E., & Dowler, D. (1996). Caregiving for parents and parents-in-law: Is gender important? *The Gerontologist, 36*, 483–491.

Jutras, S., & Veilleux, F. (1991). Gender roles and care giving to the elderly: An empirical study. *Sex Roles, 25*, 1–18.

Kaye, L. W., & Applegate, J. S. (1990). *Men as caregivers to the elderly: Understanding and adding unrecognized family support.* Lexington, MA: Lexington Books.

Kaye, L. W., & Applegate, J. S. (1994). Older men and the family caregiving orientation. In E. Thompson (Ed.), *Older men's lives* (pp. 197–219). Thousand Oaks, CA: Sage.

Kennedy, J., & Walls, C. (1997). *A national profile of intrahousehold ADL/IADL assistants: Population estimates from the 1992 and 1993 surveys of income and program participation.* Department of Community Health, University of Illinois at Urbana Champaign.

Kimmel, M. (1997). *Manhood in America: A cultural history.* New York: Simon & Schuster.

Kingston, Maxine Hong. (1976). *China men.* New York: Alfred Knopf, pp. 3–5.

Kosloski, L., Montgomery, R. J. V., & Karner, T. X. (1999). Differences in perceived need for assistive services by culturally diverse caregivers of persons with dementia. *Journal of Applied Gerontology, 18,* 239–256.

Kramer, B. J. (2000). Husbands caring for wives with dementia: A longitudinal study of continuity and change. *Health & Social Work, 25,* 97–107.

Kramer, B. J., & Lambert, J. D. (1999). Caregiving as a life course transition among older husbands: A prospective study. *The Gerontologist, 39,* 658–667.

Lazarus, R. S., & Folkman, S. (1984). *Stress, appraisal, and coping.* New York: Springer.

Lee, G. R. (1992). Gender differences in family caregiving: A fact in search of a theory. In J. W. Dwyer & R. T. Coward (Eds.), *Gender, families, and elder care* (pp. 120–131). Newbury Park, CA: Sage.

Lee, G. R., Dwyer, J. W., & Coward, R. T. (1993). Gender differences in parent care: Demographic factors and same-gender preferences. *Journal of Gerontology; Social Sciences, 48,* S9–S16.

Levinson, D. J., Darrow, C. N., Klein, E. B., Levinson, M. H., & McKee, B. (1978). *The seasons of a man's life.* New York: Ballantine.

Levkoff, S., Levy, B., & Weitzman, P. F. (1999). Role of religion and ethnicity in the help seeking of family caregivers of elders with Alzheimer's disease and related disorders. *Journal of Cross Cultural Gerontology, 14,* 335–356.

Litwak, E. (1985). *Helping the elderly: The complementary roles of informal and formal systems.* New York: Guilford.

Mac Rae, H. (1998). Managing feelings: Caregiving as emotion work. *Research on Aging, 20,* 137–160.

Marks, N. F. (1996). Caregiving across the lifespan: National prevalence and predictors. *Family Relations, 45,* 27–36.

Matthews, S. H. (1997). *Older sons' relationships with very old parents.* Paper presented at the annual meeting of the Gerontological Society of America, Cincinnati.

Matthews, S. H., & Rosner, T. T. (1988). Shared filial responsibility: The family as the primary caregiver. *Journal of Marriage and the Family, 50,* 185–195.

McFarland, P. L., & Sanders, S. (1999). Male caregivers: Preparing men for nurturing roles. *American Journal of Alzheimer's Disease, 14,* 278–282.

Miller, B. (1987). Gender and control among spouses of the cognitively impaired: A research note. *The Gerontologist, 27,* 447–453.

Miller, B., & Cafasso, L. (1992). Gender differences in caregiving: Fact or artifact? *The Gerontologist, 32,* 498–507.

Miller, B., & Kaufman, J. E. (1996). Beyond gender stereotypes: Spouse caregivers of persons with dementia. *Journal of Aging Studies, 10,* 189–204.

Montgomery, R. J. V., Gonyea, J. G., & Hooyman, N. R. (1985). Caregiving and the experience of subjective and objective burden. *Family Relations, 34,* 19–26.

Montgomery, R. J. V. (1992). Gender differences in patterns of child-parent caregiving relationships. In J. W. Dwyer & R. T. Coward, (Eds.), *Gender, families, and elder care* (pp. 65–83). Newbury Park, CA: Sage.

Morano, C. (1998). Identifying the special needs of male caregivers. *Continuum, 18* (July/August), 8–13.

Motenko, A. K. (1988). Respite care and pride in caregiving: The experience of six older men caring for their disabled wives. In S. Reinharz & G. D. Rowles (Eds.), *Qualitative gerontology* (pp. 104–127). New York: Springer-Verlag.

Mui, A. C. (1995). Perceived health and functional status among spouse caregivers of frail older persons. *Journal of Aging and Health, 7,* 283–300.

Murray, S. B. (1996). We all love Charles: Men in child care and the social construction of gender. *Gender & Society, 10,* 368–385.

National Alliance for Caregiving and the American Association of Retired Persons. (1997, June). *Family caregiving in the U.S.: Findings from a national study.* Washington, DC.

National Family Caregivers Association. (2000, Oct.). *Caregiver survey— 2000.* Kensington, MD: NFCA.

Navon, L., & Weinblatt, N. (1996). "The show must go on": Behind the scenes of elderly spouse caregiving. *Journal of Aging Studies, 10,* 329–342.

Neufeld, A., & Harrison, M. J. (1998). Men as caregivers: Reciprocal relationships or obligation? *Journal of Advanced Nursing, 28,* 959–968.

Paine, Thomas. (1776). *Common sense.*

Parks, S. H., & Pilisuk, M. (1991). Caregiver burden: Gender and the psychological costs of caregiving. *American Journal of Orthopsychiatry, 61,* 501–509.

Parsons, K. (1997). The male experience of caregiving for a family member with Alzheimer's disease. *Qualitative Health Research, 7,* 391–407.

Perkinson, M. A. (1995). Socialization to the family caregiving role within a continuing care retirement community. *Medical Anthropology, 16,* 249–267.

Pleck, J. (1993). Are "family supportive" employer policies relevant to men? In J. C. Hood (Ed.), *Work, family, and masculinities* (pp. 217–237). Newbury Park, CA: Sage.

Pruchno, R. A., & Resch, N. L. (1989). Husbands and wives as caregivers: Antecedents of depression and burden. *The Gerontologist, 29,* 159–165.

Risman, B. (1998). *Gender vertigo.* New Haven, CT: Yale University Press.

Robinson, J. C. (1996). Decline in hospital utilization and cost inflation under managed care in California. *Journal of the American Medical Association, 276,* 1060–1064.

Robert Wood Johnson Foundation. (1996). *Chronic care in America: A 21st century challenge.* Princeton: The Robert Wood Johnson Foundation.

Shanas, E. (1979). The family as a social support system in old-age. *The Gerontologist, 19,* 169–174.

Siriopoulos, G., Brown, Y., & Wright, K. (1999). Caregivers of wives diagnosed with Alzheimer's disease: Husbands' perspectives. *American Journal of Alzheimer's Disease, 14,* 79–87.

Sistler, A. B., & Blanchard-Fields, F. (1993). Being in control: A note on differences between caregiving and noncaregiving spouses. *Journal of Psychology, 127,* 537–542.

Skaff, M. M., & Pearlin, L. I. (1992). Caregiving: Role engulfment and the loss of self. *The Gerontologist, 32,* 656–664.

Spillman, B. C., & Pezzin, L. E. (2000). Potential and active family caregivers: Changing networks and the "sandwich generation." *Milbank Memorial Fund Quarterly, 78,* 347–374.

Stoller, E. P. (1983). Parental caregiving by adult children. *Journal of Marriage and the Family, 45,* 851–858.

Stoller, E. P. (1990). Males as helpers: The role of sons, relatives, and friends. *The Gerontologist, 30,* 228–235.

Stone, R. I., & Short, P. F. (1990). The competing demands of employment and informal caregiving to disabled elders. *Medical Care, 28,* 513–526.

Stone, R. I., Cafferata, G. L., & Sangl, J. (1987). Caregivers of the frail elderly: A national profile. *The Gerontologist, 27,* 616–626.

Szabo, V., & Strang, V. R. (1999). Experiencing control in caregiving. *Image: Journal of Nursing Scholarship, 31,* 71–75.

Tennstedt, S. L., McKinlay, J. B., & Sullivan, L. M. (1989). Informal care for frail elders: The role of secondary caregivers. *The Gerontologist, 29,* 677–683.

Tennstedt, S. L., Crawford, S., & McKinlay, J. (1993). Determining the pattern of community care: Is coresidence more important than caregiver relationship? *Journal of Gerontology: Social Sciences, 48,* S74–S83.

Tennstedt, S. L. (1999, March 29). *Family caregiving in an aging society.* Paper presented at the U.S. Administration on Aging Symposium: Longevity in the New American century. Baltimore, MD.

Thompson, B., Tudiver, F., & Manson, J. (2000). Sons as sole caregivers for their elderly parents. *Canadian Family Physician, 46,* 360–365.

Thompson, E. H. (2000). The gendered caregiving of husbands and sons. In E. Markson & L. Hollins (Eds.), *Intersections of Aging: Readings in Social Gerontology* (pp. 333–344). Los Angeles: Roxbury.

Thompson, L. (1993). Conceptualizing gender in marriage: The case of marital care. *Journal of Marriage and the Family, 55,* 557–569.

Umberson, D., Chen, M. D., House, J. S., Hopkins, K., & Slaten, E. (1996). The effect of social relationships on psychological well-being: Are men and women really so different. *American Sociological Review, 61,* 837–857.

Ungerson, C. (1983). Why do women care? In J. Finch & D. Groves (Eds.), *A labour of love: Women, work and caring.* London: Routledge & Kegan Paul.

Vinick, B. H. (1984). Elderly men as caretakers of wives. *Journal of Geriatric Psychiatry, 17,* 61–68.

Wagner, D. L. (1997, June). *Comparative analysis of caregiver data for caregivers to the elderly, 1987 and 1997.* Bethesda, MD: National Alliance for Caregiving.

Walker, A. J. (1992). Conceptual perspectives on gender and family caregiving. In J. W. Dwyer & R. T. Coward (Eds.), *Gender, families, and elder care* (pp. 34–46). Newbury Park, CA: Sage.

Wallhagen, M. I., & Kagan, S. H. (1993). Staying within bounds: Perceived control and the experience of elderly caregivers. *Journal of Aging Studies, 7,* 197–213.

Wallsten, S. S. (2000). Effects of caregiving, gender, and race on the health, mutuality, and social supports of older couples. *Journal of Aging and Health, 12,* 90–111.

Willoughby, J., & Keating, N. (1991). Being in control: The process of caring for a relative with Alzheimer's disease. *Qualitative Health Research, 1,* 27–50.

Wilson, V. (1990). The consequences of elderly wives caring for disabled husbands: Implications for practice. *Social Work, 35,* 417–421.

Conceptual, Theoretical, and Methodological Insights

II

Theoretical Perspectives on Caregiving Men[1]

3

Eleanor Palo Stoller

Almost a decade ago, Gary Lee (1992) pointed out that the facts of women's dominance in caregiving were well established empirically but poorly understood theoretically. Social gerontologists and family study scholars have responded to Lee's theoretical challenge, but the majority of efforts to explain family care to frail older relatives still poses the question, "Why do *women* care?" Researchers have applied a number of conceptual frameworks to understanding men's infrequent appearance as the unpaid providers of long-term care, but they have failed to address the broader questions, "How do we explain the division of family labor among men and women in caring for frail older relatives?" and "Why do some men 'choose' to be primary caregivers?"

Theoretical explanations of the gendered division of labor in family care for older relatives often imply an essentialist framework, in which gender differences are treated as transcultural and transhistorical and in which differences of degree are converted into differences of kind (Chafetz, 1997). Many studies have overlooked or marginalized family care provided by male relatives, despite an accumulation of studies suggesting that as many as one-third of family caregivers are men (Kaye & Applegate, 1990; Strawbridge, Wallhagen, Shema, & Kaplan, 1997). Indeed, one of the most intriguing findings in Logan and Spitze's (1997) *Family Ties* is the relatively small number of gender differences in family and neighborhood networks.

The earliest studies of elder caregiving, begun in the late 1970s, rarely introduced gender into the analysis, focusing instead on seemingly gender-neutral categories like family, older parent, and adult child. Consistent with

[1] I would like to thank Edward H. Thompson, Jr., Holy Cross College, and Adam Perzynski, Case Western Reserve University, for their comments on an earlier draft of this chapter.

the debunking tendency of social science research, these early investigators challenged the stereotype of family abandonment of the elders by uncovering the empirical reality that most long-term care was provided by informal rather than formal sources (Shanas, 1979; Brody, 1981). Investigators conducting these early studies emphasized the distinction between formal sources of care such as nursing homes or social service agencies and informal assistance provided by relatives or friends. These early studies demonstrated that the majority of family caregivers were spouses (most often wives caring for husbands) and adult children (most often daughters caring for their older mothers).

The next generation of studies, building on empirical findings of women's prominence in providing family care for older relatives, adopted a "women's issues" approach. This perspective, which relies on women's voices, emphasized the physical labor, emotional strains, and social isolation that often accompanies caring for a frail, older relative or a spouse recovering from a myocardial infarction. Researchers documented the dimensions and distribution of caregiver burden.

A third generation of studies moved toward explaining the empirical generalizations that women provide more care—and a greater variety of care—than do men and that women experience greater caregiver burden than do men. This chapter engages in the ongoing project of developing a theoretical framework for understanding the gendered work of elder care. Elder caregiving is viewed as an instance of unpaid social production, and the latter portion of the chapter integrates findings from research on the gendered division of domestic labor in families. The larger part of this chapter reviews what different theoretical perspectives have taught us about men's caregiving. The review begins with individual-level explanations linking gender and family care for frail older adults to early childhood experiences. I then explore institutional and interactional approaches. The chapter concludes with my application of Risman's conceptualization of gender as a structure reflecting the intersection of individual, institutional, and interactional within the province of men's elder caregiving. My objective is to show that elder caregiving can be understood within a life course perspective that bridges research on caregiving across the life course.

INDIVIDUAL-LEVEL EXPLANATIONS

Socialization Theories

The earliest and most widely employed explanations of the gender division of family care of older relatives emphasized socialization. Reflecting structural functionalist arguments, some sociologists have linked caregiving with the "expressive" nature of women's roles and their "specialization" within the private, or domestic, sphere (Dressel & Clark, 1990). From this perspective, caring for an ill or disabled spouse is seen as more "unnatural" for men and more inconsistent with their other family roles, particularly breadwinning. As Pruchno & Resch (1989, p. 159) suggest, "it may be expected that . . . women would view caregiving as a continuation of earlier responsibilities, whereas men, socialized to focus on the external world, would view [these] demands as foreign." Often we describe men as less accomplished caregivers, because they are oriented to market work and have less experience with household work (Allen, 1994). When they do contribute to care, their efforts presumably involve male stereotypic tasks (e.g., yardwork, household repairs, and financial management) or to support the primary caregiving efforts of their wives or sisters. By arguing that gender is learned, these explanations reject biological for social definitions of gender (Andersen, 1997).

Criticism of this dualistic approach has demonstrated the inappropriateness of using dichotomies such as men's instrumentality versus women's expressiveness or men's role in the public sphere versus women's role in the private sphere in attempting to understand the division of domestic labor. The distinction between public and private spheres emerged with the doctrine of separate spheres that described a separation of work and family life (Reskin & Padavic, 1994). Coltrane (1996, p. 25) explains:

> According to [this] view, it is a man's duty to serve his family by being a breadwinner and protector, whereas a woman's duty is to be a good wife and mother. More than any other cultural belief, this idealized notion of separate spheres for mothers and fathers shapes what it means to be a man or a woman in our society.

But the doctrine of separate spheres—of a separation of public and private domains—has proved a false dichotomy. The notion of "dual spheres" ignores how social production blurs the boundaries between public and private. It ignores the fact that poor and working-class families have always had women engaged in some form of productive activity in the public sector, such as working for wages, taking in boarders, or selling items produced in the home, as well as had men participating in family care when women worked either side-by-side with them or outside the home. As noted by Hochschild (1997), sometimes husbands and wives do separate shifts in their paid work in order to do the family work. Furthermore, as discussed below, the ideology of separate spheres also masks the extent to which work and family have become gendered institutions. The "ideal worker norm" that emerged with industrialization assumes the existence of backup support provided by unpaid domestic labor. Market work is organized around "the ideal of a worker who works full-time and overtime and takes little or no time off for childbearing or childrearing [or caregiving for frail elders]" (Williams, 2000, p. 1). Williams' notion of the ideal worker norm parallels Acker's (1990) conception of the disembodied worker.

Reliance on socialization in explaining men's and women's unequal contributions to caring for frail elders suffers from the same limitations as does socialization as an explanation for other gender differences (Andersen, 1997). First, this approach is not a causal theory, because it fails to explain the structural origins of the allocation of family care for frail elders. It emphasizes learned behavior and internalization of cultural norms, but it does not explain how these so-called gender roles developed. Second, socialization explanations tend to underemphasize the significance of gender in the institutional framework of society. Focusing on the internalization of gender roles, we forget how institutional arrangements channel the "choices" that men and women make about the division of both paid work in the economy and unpaid work within the informal economy and the family (Williams, 2000). Third, socialization explanations focus on and therefore tend to exaggerate differences between the sexes. As a result, the wide variation that exists among women and among men is overlooked. Socialization encourages us to focus on differences in central tendency between men and women and to ignore overlap in the corresponding distributions. Women do provide more care and a greater range of family care for frail, older relatives than do men (Allen, 1994; Coward & Dwyer, 1990). But, as the research reviewed in other chapters demonstrates, higher averages in hours and scope of assistance does not mean that men do not care for older relatives in need of support. Finally, an emphasis on socialization underplays the importance of adult experiences, the demands of current situations, and location on intersecting hierarchies such as race-ethnicity, social class, and partner preference. These factors assume central importance in the institutional and interactional perspectives described below.

Psychoanalytic and Gender Feminism

Grounded in a reinterpretation of Freud's theory of personality development, psychoanalytic feminism focuses on psychosexual development and emphasizes differences between the sexes in connectedness and independence (Gilligan, 1982). Gender feminism (sometimes called cultural feminism) emphasizes psychosocial or psychomoral development (Tong, 1998). Women, this perspective tells us, speak and think in a voice different from men's, reflecting differences in their need for connection and empathy (Belenky, Clinchy, Goldberger, & Tarule, 1986). Popularizers of this perspective ascribe virtues of compassion, patience, and empathy to women, in sharp contrast to the competitiveness and emotional aloofness ascribed to men (Tavris, 1992).

Theorists working within this perspective emphasize men's lower levels of attachment to care recipients. They stress the greater emotional significance of caring in women's lives, arguing that internalization of an injunction to care and concern for others rather than the self is a central element of feminine identity (Gilligan, 1982). Women's capacity for empathy and intimacy, which contrasts with men's separateness and more rigid ego boundaries, is said to be rooted in the asymmetrical structure of parenting, a social and cultural arrangement in which women perform most of the work associated with "mothering" (Chodorow, 1978). According to this framework, caregiving, whether for young children, ill spouses, or frail elders, is more attuned with women's sense of connection with others; men's experiences of emotional distance and independence places them in foreign territories when they initiate caregiving. Not encouraged to internalize the injunction to care means that most men can negotiate away their caregiving responsibility for a dependent parent or child more easily than they might walk away from a poorly paid job (Hooyman & Gonyea, 1995). Thus, men's alleged lesser emotional ties to family members both motivate the avoidance of caregiving and help blunt the distress of caregiving. This perspective is used to explain the fact that men caregivers report lower levels of burden than women caregivers, a gendered pattern that Miller and Cafasso (1992) reported in their meta-analytic review of the caregiving literature on gender differences. Men, these theorists explain, appear better able to distance themselves from the care recipient, focusing primarily on economic responsibilities and concrete assistance. For example, husband caregivers are less likely than wife caregivers to feel guilty about not doing enough or to feel personal responsibility for their wives' well-being (Stoller, 1992).

Psychoanalytic and gender feminism explains the underrepresentation of men as family caregivers as a response to a cultural imperative that caregiving is feminine and more in sync with a personality characterized by connectedness and commitment to other people. This cultural imperative reflects the consequences of the infant's primary attachment to a mother. Critics point out that psychoanalytic and gender feminist theories assume a family consists of two heterosexual adults in which the woman is the primary parent (Lorber, 1994). Bordering on essentialist accounts, these explanations fail to address the diversity both of family structures and of men's and women's enactments of family responsibilities. Critics of this perspective claim also that too much attention is focused on "the inner dynamics of the psyche and not enough on the external permutations of society as the primary source of women's oppression" (Tong, 1989, p. 157). These psychological accounts also obscure the material aspect of caring; that is, they mask the labor-intensive, physically demanding, and emotionally stressful nature of the caring role. Most important, essentialist arguments do not explain variation in the distribution of care responsibilities across all families. They fail to explain why some men provide care to their frail older relatives and some women do not. They fail to explain why affluent women sometimes delegate family care responsibilities to formal providers. They fail to explain why African American families have exhibited less rigidity than European American families in sharing domestic tasks and responsibility for earning a living, or why African American elders are able to draw on a broader range of helpers than are European American elders.

Both personality explanations like psychoanalytic or gender feminism and explanations grounded in socialization generally assume a continuity of behavior and preferences across the life course—an assumption that has been challenged by recent studies of the gender division of household labor. These studies emphasize the adaptability of men's and women's behavior, thereby countering the assumption that adult behavior conforms to the imprint of early socialization. For example, in her study *No Man's Land*, Gerson (1994) observed that the developmental paths men anticipate in their childhood were poor predictors of their actual life patterns as breadwinners and involved parents. One-third of the men she interviewed had increased their family involvement over the course of their lives, despite earlier expectations to become primary breadwinners or to remain single and childless. Gerson attributes their greater family involvement to their adult experiences. At home, they were committed to women who espoused egalitarian gender roles. At work, they were either disillusioned with traditional male occupations or attracted to lucrative but more intrinsically rewarding careers. In her earlier book *Hard Choices*, Gerson (1985) found a similar adaptability among women. Once again, she found that the life patterns anticipated in childhood were poor predictors of actual life patterns among the women she studied. Shifts from anticipated "traditional" domestic to actual nondomestic life patterns were triggered by instability in marriage, expanded workplace opportunities, economic squeeze within the household, and negative experiences with domesticity. Shifts from anticipated nondomestic to actual domestic life patterns were equally triggered by limited workplace opportunities, geographic mobility, and the husband's career. Scott Coltrane's (1996) study *Family Man* also identified predictors of shared parenting in two-earner families. Cautionary tales of rarely present fathers reflect the impact of childhood socialization, but his other explanatory factors emphasize adult experiences, including a new cultural imagery of fatherhood, comparable education, earnings, as well as employment responsibilities of husband and wife, delayed childrearing, and loose-knit cosmopolitan social networks. Jean Potuchek (1997) studied identification with breadwinning responsibilities in two-earner couples, identifying both "pushes" and "pulls" toward negotiated redefinitions. Husbands who did not earn enough income to adequately meet financial needs of the family often found themselves sharing breadwinner identities with their wives. Men married to women whose career success had increased the salience of work identity or to women whose high earnings were central to the family's lifestyle also encountered pressures to move toward co-breadwinner family definitions. Finally, Risman (1998, p. 154) concluded that, although men are capable of mothering, most men undertake mothering work only when they do not have wives to do it for them. Furthermore, the fathers in her study, who became primary caretakers because of deceased or deserting wives, thought of themselves as having personality traits traditionally labeled as feminine. She concludes, "the contexts faced in adulthood are stronger explanations for life choices than gender socialization."

INSTITUTIONAL EXPLANATIONS

Institutional explanations attribute gender differences in behavior to the fact that women and men occupy different positions in families and in work organizations (Risman, 1998). The emphasis of theorists working with these perspectives is on the ways in which gendered institutions constrain choices regarding both market work and family labor for men and for women.

The Family Division of Labor and Rational Choice

One institutional approach to explaining men's involvement in family care emphasizes household decisions regarding the allocation of family time and financial resources. Gerontologists and family study scholars working within this tradition often draw on a rational choice perspective, which defines family members as purposive actors who undertake behaviors that are consistent with their preference hierarchies (Ritzer, 2000). However, the "actor" is often defined as the family unit rather than individual family members. Family care arrangements are conceptualized as the outcome of a decision-making process (Soldo, Wolf, & Agree, 1990). Researchers hypothesize that families face an array of possible caregiving or helping arrangements, which are constrained by personal, familial, and financial resources of the care recipient and by resources within the environment (e.g., availability and accessibility of formal services). From the perspective of the older relative, needs for assistance and preferences regarding the sources of this assistance influence the ways in which elders configure caregiving arrangements from available alternatives. Family caregivers, in turn, balance the older person's needs and preferences for care against constraints on their own ability or willingness to provide that care, including opportunity costs and constraints of competing institutions such as paid work. Thus, rational choice theorists argue that preference and need influence selection of possible care arrangements (opportunities), contingent upon available resources (Stoller & Cutler, 1992).

One strain of this research emphasizes the *competing time demands* accruing from other social roles, arguing that men assume fewer unpaid responsibilities in the home because they are more likely to be employed in the labor market and more likely to be employed full-time. This explanation may appear to fit the experiences of single-earner couples. However, it is inconsistent with data on the division of domestic labor in dual-earner households. On one hand, women who are employed full-time typically retain responsibility for domestic work, whether they perform the tasks themselves or supervise the work of others. A number of studies have found that employed women provide as many hours of care as do those who are not employed outside the home. By comparison, most men's involvement in caregiving is suppressed by multiple factors, not just competing time demands. Their greater earnings relative to their wives, social disapproval by peers, and employer resistance to men's restructuring their work to facilitate greater involvement in family labor are three social forces that act upon men's "choices" to become actively involved in family labor (Hochschild, 1997).

Another approach drawing on a rational choice framework emphasizes *specialization of tasks*. A specialization-of-tasks perspective suggests that men's relatively higher wages in the labor market means that their opportunity costs for specializing in unpaid domestic labor are greater than for women. According to this perspective, the gender division of household labor emerges from joint efforts to maximize the well-being of the family unit rather than from negotiations among individuals who differ in their access to resources. This approach stresses the importance of resources obtained outside the household (e.g., education and income) in family negotiations regarding the division of labor (Ross, 1987), but it fails to address the ways in which the organization of work, particularly the ideal worker norm, perpetuates a gender gap in caregiving and social incentives for men's breadwinning over caregiving (Cancian & Oliker, 2000).

Once again, empirical research on both household labor and family caregiving challenges these explanations. Hochschild (1989) failed to find any direct relationship between human capital factors (e.g., education, occupational status, and wages or salaries) and the distribution of household labor. Indeed, she argues that men who earn less than their wives generally shoulder less of the unpaid domestic work as a balancing strategy—a way of compensating for the threat their lower salary presents to their self-esteem. To some extent, this explanation becomes a tautology: Men do less domestic work because they earn more than women in the labor market, but one reason they earn more is that they have—and are perceived by their employers as having—greater responsibility for bread-winning and lesser responsibility for unpaid family work. Socialist feminists address this dilemma by arguing that the cultural assignment of unpaid domestic production to women constrains labor market choices of both women and men.

Socialist Feminism and Neo-Marxist Theories

Emphasizing the interplay of gender with social relations of production and reproduction, socialist feminists begin by taking the standpoint of women and asking who controls and who benefits from women's labor (Calasanti, 1992). These theorists differ from orthodox Marxism by empha-sizing the importance of the nonwaged labor that maintains and repro-duces the workforce (Chafetz, 1997). From this perspective, the relative truancy of men as family caregivers is neither a reflection of their "natural" detachment from other people nor the result of preferences internalized through socialization. Rather, it emerges from the cultural assignment of unpaid domestic production to women that emerged historically from the relationship between capitalism and patriarchy. With industrialization, men were recruited as paid laborers into factory production and expected to leave family labor to women. Women were assigned the unpaid domes-tic labor, including care of dependent family members. Women's entry into the paid labor force has yet to bring about a change in this division of productive activity. Even when women enter the paid workforce, few men take up the responsibility for domestic production (Hochschild, 1989). These caregiving arrangements are reinforced by patterns of occu-pational segregation and wage discrimination, which in turn channel the "choices" men and women make in allocating paid work and unpaid domestic labor within the family.

This inequitable division of family labor is also reinforced by an ideol-ogy that has defined caring as women's natural expression of their attach-ment to others and stresses the primacy of family responsibilities for women. As Williams (2000, p. 23) argues, the gender structure she calls domesticity "not only bifurcated the work of adults into a women's sphere of the home and men's market work out of it; it justified that reor-ganization through new descriptions of the 'true natures' of men and women." Socialist feminists thus recognize the internalized motivations emphasized by socialization theorists and psychoanalytic feminists, but they interpret them as unessential and part of a belief system that justifies structural inequalities based on gender.

Given this intersection of structural realities and ideological forces, men who are excluded from family labor seldom feel that they had a choice. This perspective challenges arguments that men "choose" to specialize in market work and that women, when they are employed, seek positions that accommodate their domestic responsibilities Women's overrepresentation as elder caregivers reflects these constraints on choice. Men's decision to care—or not to care—is overdetermined: It emerges from the structural constraints men experience in the public sector; the limited availability of public services; a constricted sense of responsibility among men in the family; internalization of an ideology that includes an injunction for women to care; and a complex interplay of power between the generations and the sexes (Aronson, 1992; Lewis & Meredith, 1988).

Just as psychoanalytic accounts can be criticized for masking the material dimensions of caregiving, socialist feminism may be criticized for obscuring the social connections that are integral to the experience of providing care (Abel & Nelson, 1990; Walker, 1992). Institutional explanations emphasize the impact of structures on behavior, either constraining behavior or making it possible (Risman, 1998). But they tend to minimize the role of men and women in creating and producing these structures. Risman critiques structural analyses of gender as overly deterministic. She argues that structural conditions channel possible action but do not preordain outcomes.

INTERACTIONAL EXPLANATIONS: CONSIDERING SOCIAL CONTEXT

Ethnomethodological Approaches: Doing Gender

While recognizing that socialization shapes gendered selves and that social structure channels potential actions, gender theorists increasingly focus on contextual and interactional explanations of gender-linked behaviors. From this perspective, gender is not a property of individuals—it is not *what we are*. Rather, gender is *what we do* in interaction with others. Ridgeway and Smith-Lovin (1999, p. 214) summarize this approach by describing gender as an "adverb rather than a noun." Gender is "something that modifies the ways that role behaviors are enacted." Following Schutz, these actions are seen as routine and relatively unreflective (Ritzer, 2000). Candace West and Don Zimmerman (1987) first applied this ethnomethodological approach to gender in their article titled "Doing

Gender." They conceptualized gender as a routine accomplishment embedded in everyday interaction. Because the social scripts for many tasks are associated with gender, people constantly recreate gender differences and (re)produce gender inequality as they perform these tasks (Chafetz, 1997). For example, within families, men "do gender" by assuming responsibility for breadwinning, even if their wives earn wages or salaries (DeVault, 1991). Women "do gender" by keeping the house clean and by feeding the family. When men participate in domestic production, their contributions are often limited to particular types of tasks and are seen as "helping."

When we do gender, we have historically both created and reaffirmed differences between men and women. Lorber (1998) argues that we find it difficult to stop "doing gender" this way, because it is part of our identity. "In a social order based on gender divisions, everyone always 'does gender' almost all the time. . . . Indeed it is this pervasiveness that leads so many people to believe that gendering is biological and therefore natural" (Lorber, 1998, p. 161). If we fail to do gender as it is conventionally defined, we as individuals are called to account for our character (West & Zimmerman, 1987). It is for this reason that criticisms of caregiving standards may have a less negative impact on men than on women but that loss of a job is often more devastating personally for men than for women. For this reason, both researchers and employers perceive men who are primary caregivers as acting out-of-character. To the extent that nurturing and meeting the emotional and physical needs of others is one way in which women can "do gender," the lived experience of caring for older relatives encompasses different meanings for women and for men. Husbands caring for frail wives can concentrate on companionship, ignoring dirty dishes or delegating personal care tasks to hired workers without risking criticism from others for failing to "do gender" appropriately.

Complicating our analysis of family caregiving is the fact that the instrumental and nurturing activities of caregiving produce gender and family simultaneously (DeVault, 1991). The reciprocal exchange of assistance between older parents and their adult children can also be conceptualized as "doing generation" (Treas, 1999). How do these intersecting structures guide individual action when these structures intrude in various combinations? Studies of "doing gender" and "doing family" in transgender relationships focus on parents with dependent children in the household. Social gerontologists have been slow to adopt an ethnomethodological approach to explaining family care of older relatives, so we have little empirical evidence of the complications that arise when we mix cohorts and generations. Will negotiated redefinitions of gender between husbands and wives apply in their relationships with aging parents—relationships in which gender and family were performed in a different time and a different place? Will definitions of "doing family" encourage new definitions of gender among siblings when a geographically proximate son and geographically distant sister devise strategies for caring for their older widowed mother? Indeed, as Ridgeway and Smith-Lovin point out (1999), we need a better understanding of the way gender combines with other identities-roles-statuses and shapes the way they are performed.

Role Theory and Self-Concepts

Role theory reminds us that roles vary in salience, not only across individuals but also across contexts for the same individual. People's behavior is shaped by the most salient roles for each individual in a particular setting (Ridgeway & Smith-Lovin, 1999). From this perspective, gender is a background identity that modifies other identities which are often more salient in the setting than is gender itself (Ridgeway & Smith-Lovin). Stets and Burke (1996) argue that gender can be viewed as a "master identity," because it is invoked across a range of interactional and institutional contexts.

Rather than the static construction implied by socialization and psychoanalytic feminist theories, this perspective conceptualizes the self as both multifaceted and dynamic, as "simultaneously a social construction and a social constructor of experience, actively selecting among various interpretations; claiming, elaborating and personalizing some of them while ignoring, contesting, or rearranging others" (Herzog & Markus, 1999, p. 228).

The experience of providing care to frail older relatives depends, therefore, on the frameworks an individual invokes to lend structure and meaning to caregiving tasks. Gender has a greater influence on behavior when tasks are stereotypically gendered (Ridgeway & Smith-Lovin, 1999). These predictions are consistent with empirical findings that men provide less assistance than women when older people require assistance with daily household chores and personal care, yet men provide the majority of assistance with yard work and household repairs (Kramer & Kipnis, 1995). The interpretative frameworks that people invoke shape not only what they are motivated to do, but also the meanings and emotions associated with those behaviors (Herzog & Markus, 1999).

Gender is but one facet of a caregiver's identity. Men caregivers can also be husbands or sons. They may be employed workers in settings that vary in the flexibility of work responsibilities and the organizational culture. Sons are members of sibling networks that vary in size and the geographic proximity of sisters and brothers. Ethnic or religious heritage provides cues for family values and norms. Social class structures the distribution of resources to hire market substitutes for domestic labor, geographic region can determine the availability and acceptability of formal services, and neighborhood characteristics can influence both structure and process within informal networks (Logan & Spitze, 1997). These other facets of identity can mediate the impact of gender on men's and women's performance of the caregiver role.

The centrality of gender identity in people's self structures also varies across individuals and contexts. Ridgeway and Smith-Lovin (1999) argue that the salience of gender identity reflects both personal biography and structural context. They predict that behavior is shaped by the most salient role in a setting and that gender differences in behavior are minimized when men and women occupy similar formal roles. Herzog and Markus (1999) cite studies indicating that gender differences are minimized when men and women occupy positions of equal status and equal power. As we saw above, Risman (1988) reports that men who find themselves primary caretakers for a child exhibit both behaviors and personality traits usually associated with mothers. To assume that being male or female is the primary predictor of both the willingness to provide family care and the consequences of providing that assistance is to overlook the importance of context in people's lives. As Herzog and Markus note (1999, p. 234), "people are responsive to the requirements of their various sociocultural environments and typically create selves in ways that resonate with what is valued in those environments."

TOWARD AN INCLUSIVE APPROACH TO GENDER AND FAMILY CARE OF ELDERS

This review of the literature on gender and caregiving suggests several guideposts for theory development. First, it supports Thompson's (2000) conclusion that comparing men to women in terms of the amount and types of caregiving tasks provided has institutionalized the use of a single, feminine yardstick to measure caregiving. Viewing men caregivers through the lens of women's experiences can undermine our ability to understand the lived experience of men who care for older partners or parents. The hegemony of the feminine yardstick that has been used has become so unnoticed that it constrains imagination and understanding. Only when we cease measuring men against the experiences of women can we begin to query men about why they care in the variety of ways they do and about the impact of providing that care on their daily lives. Perhaps men do experience less burden than women when they care for older relatives. Or, perhaps instruments cannot capture men's experience of burden based on the experience of women caregivers.

Second, social gerontologists have been slow to incorporate the concept of gender as a social construction—as a property of social systems rather than an individual attribute. Especially in quantitative analyses, gender is too often treated as a fixed property of individuals rather than a property of the social structures within which women and men forge identities and through which they realize their life chances (Hess, 1980). Theoretical efforts to understanding family care of older relatives have focused almost exclusively on the question of "Why do women care?" Too often this question is interpreted as ". . . and why don't men?" The growing evidence that men in certain conditions provide varying levels of care necessitates broadening our focus to reexamine the assumptions we make about the gendered division of elder care within family networks.

Sociologists studying work and family are struggling with similar issues, and social gerontology could benefit from integrating studies of elder caregiving within a life course perspective on unpaid social production. Toward this goal, I will conclude the chapter by using the multilevel framework developed by Barbara Risman (1998) as the next step toward answering the question: "Why do men and women care in the ways that they do?"

In her recent book *Gender Vertigo*, Barbara Risman (1989) conceptualizes gender as a structure that reflects the intersection of the individual, the interactional, and the institutional levels of analysis. The individual level refers to the emergence of gendered selves, through socialization or the emergence of personality. The interactional level incorporates the insights of ethnomethodologists regarding "doing gender" or "doing family." The institutional component would include a sex-segregated labor force, the wage gap between men and women, hegemonic definitions of full-time employment, and the lack of available, accessible, and high-quality respite or home care for frail elders. As a social structure, gender organizes our lives, but individuals participate in creating, reinforcing, and changing that structure as they interact and negotiate opportunities and constraints (West & Zimmerman, 1987; Lorber, 1994). Risman argues that although all three levels of gender structure push men and women toward gendered lives and gendered choices, contextual and interactional factors are the most immediate and strongest explanations of patterns of family care.

Risman's multilevel approach helps us understand why men and women make the choices that they do—why many women and some men "choose" to provide care to frail older relatives. Risman explains that we can best understand these gendered choices as "social constructions based on institutionally constrained opportunities and the limited availability of nongendered cognitive images" (p. 105). She provides us with a framework for moving beyond comparisons of men and women to understanding both cross-sectional variation and longitudinal change. As she concludes, "Gendered displays—as natural as they feel—are socially defined . . . Strategies for 'doing gender' change when institutional or situational changes require" them to change (Risman, 1998, pp. 156 & 160).

Risman's (1998) approach to gender and Williams' (2000) discussion of domesticity as structures provide important alternatives to explanations that assume men freely choose to specialize in paid market work and choose to avoid unpaid family labor. Both theorists focus on families caring for young children rather than families providing support for frail elders. Theories surrounding elder care should include studies of family care at different places in the life course, but integrating these two strains of research demands sensitivity to life course issues. A life course perspective directs our attention to the powerful connection between individual lives and the historical context in which these lives unfold (O'Rand, 1998). The parents of young children in current studies of work-family balance represent a different cohort than either the middle-aged caregivers of frail older parents or the older caregivers of seriously ill spouses. These three cohorts live with different expectations regarding family arrangements and different opportunity structures with respect to paid work. Variation in historical experience refracts through the intersections of gender, race or ethnicity, and social class. Nevertheless, even cross-sectional comparisons of contemporary studies of family labor suggest guideposts for theory development. Family care as an obligation has different meanings for men and for women. Older and younger generations within families negotiated definitions of family responsibilities within different historical periods. Although husbands and wives or sons and daughters may employ a rhetoric of choice and while some theoretical perspectives accent the rhetoric of choice, the decision to assume a caregiver role is channeled by the gender-based division of domestic labor, by family scripts for "doing gender," by an implicitly gendered workplace, and by the marginalization of unpaid work. Theories that encompass both institutional and interaction dimensions and that ground these dimensions in an historical context will enrich our understanding of the ways in which current changes in both work and family will shape the experience of elder care in the coming decades.

REFERENCES

Abel, E., & Nelson, M. (1990). Circles of care: An introductory essay. In E. Abel & M. Nelson (Eds.), *Circles of care: Work and identity in women's lives* (pp. 65–91). Albany, NY: SUNY Press.

Acker, J. (1990) Hierarchies, jobs, bodies: A theory of gendered organizations. *Gender and Society, 4,* 139–158.

Allen, S. (1994). Gender differences in spousal caregiving and unmet need for care. *Journal of Gerontology, 49,* S187–S195.

Andersen, M. (1997). *Thinking about women: Sociological perspectives on sex and gender* (5th ed.). New York: Macmillan.

Aronson, J. (1992). Women's sense of responsibility for the care of old people: But who else is going to do it? *Gender and Society, 6,* 8–29.

Belenky, M., Clinchy, B., Goldberger, N., & Tarule, J. (1986). *Women's ways of knowing· The development of self, voice and mind.* New York: Basic Books.

Brody, E. M. (1981). Women in the middle and family help to older people. *The Gerontologist, 21,* 471–479.

Calasanti, T. (1992). Theorizing about gender and aging: Beginning with women's voices. *The Gerontologist, 3,* 280–282.

Cancian, F. M., & Oliker, S. J. (2000). *Caring and gender.* Thousand Oaks, CA: Pine Forge.

Chafetz, J. S. (1997). Feminist theory and sociology: Underutilized contributions for mainstream theory. *Annual Review of Sociology, 23,* 197–120.

Chodorow, N. (1978). *The reproduction of mothering; psychoanalysis and the sociology of gender.* Berkeley: University of California Press.

Coltrane, S. (1996). *Family man.* New York: Oxford University Press.

Coward, R. T., & Dwyer, J. W. (1990). The association of gender, sibling network composition, and patterns of parent care by adult children. *Research on Aging, 12,* 158–181.

DeVault, M. (1991). *Feeding the family.* Chicago: University of Chicago Press.

Dressel, P., & Clark, A. (1990). A critical look at family care. *Journal of Marriage and the Family, 52,* 769–782.

Gerson, K. (1985). *Hard choices: How women decide about work, career and motherhood.* Berkeley: University of California Press.

Gerson, K. (1994). *No man's land: Men's changing commitment to work and family.* New York: Basic Books.

Gilligan, C. (1982). *In a different voice.* Cambridge, MA: Harvard University Press.

Herzog, A., & Markus, H. (1999) The self-concept in life span and aging research. In V. L. Bengtson & K. W. Schaie (Eds.), *Handbook of theories of aging* (pp. 227–252). New York: Springer.

Hess, Beth (1980). Beyond dichotomy: Drawing distinctions and embracing differences. *Sociological Forum, 5,* 75–93.

Hochschild, A. (1989). *The second shift: Working parents and the revolution at home.* New York: Viking Penguin.

Hochschild, A. (1997). *The time bind: When work becomes home and home becomes work.* New York: Henry Holt.

Hooyman, N., & Gonyea, J. (1995). *Feminist perspectives on family care: Policies for gender justice.* Thousand Oaks, CA: Sage.

Kaye, L., & Applegate, J. (1990). *Men as elder caregivers to the elderly.* Lexington, MA: Lexington Books.

Kramer, B. J., & Kipnis, S. (1995). Eldercare and work-role conflict: Toward an understanding of gender differences in caregiver burden. *The Gerontologist, 35* (3), 340–348.

Lee, G. R. (1992). Gender differences in family caregiving: A fact in search of a theory. In J. W. Dwyer & R. T. Coward (Eds.), *Gender, families, and elder care* (pp. 120–131). Newbury Park, CA: Sage.

Lewis, J., & Meredith, B. (1988). *Daughters who care: Daughters caring for mothers at home.* London: Routledge & Kegan Paul.

Logan, J., & Spitze, G. (1997). *Family ties.* Pittsburgh, PA: Temple University Press.

Lorber, J. (1994). *Paradoxes of gender.* New Haven: CT: Yale University Press.

Lorber, J. (1998). *Gender inequality: Feminist theories and politics.* Los Angeles: Roxbury.

Miller, B., & Cafasso, L. (1992). Gender differences in caregiving: Fact or artifact? *The Gerontologist, 32,* 498–507.

O'Rand, A. (1998). The craft of life course studies. In J. Giele & G. H. Elder, Jr. (Eds.), *Methods of life course research: Qualitative and quantitative approaches* (pp. 52–74). Thousand Oaks, CA: Sage.

Potuchek, J. (1997). *Who supports the family: Gender and breadwinning in dual-earner marriages.* Palo Alto, CA: Stanford University Press.

Pruchno, R. A., & Resch, N. L. (1989). Husbands and wives as caregivers: Antecedents of depression and burden. *The Gerontologist, 29,* 159–165.

Reskin, B., & Padavic, I. (1994). *Men and women at work.* Thousand Oaks, CA: Pine Forge.

Ridgeway, C. L., & Smith-Lovin, L. (1999). The gender system and interaction. *Annual Review of Sociology, 25,* 191–216.

Risman, B. (1998). *Gender vertigo.* New Haven, CT: Yale University Press.

Ritzer, G. (2000). *Modern sociological theory* (5th ed.). Boston: McGraw Hill.

Ross, C. (1987). The division of labor at home. *Social Forces, 65,* 816–833.

Shanas, E. (1979). The family as a social support system in old age. *The Gerontologist, 19,* 169–174.

Soldo, B., Wolf, D., & Agree, E. (1990). Family households and care arrangements of frail older women: A structural analysis. *Journal of Gerontology, 45* (6), S238–S249.

Stets, J. E., & Burke, P. J. (1996) Gender, control and interaction. *Social Psychology Quarterly, 59,* 193–220.

Stoller, E. P. (1992). Husbands as caregivers. In J. W. Dwyer & R. T. Coward (Eds.), *Gender, families, and elder care.* Newbury Park, CA: Sage.

Stoller, E. P., & Cutler, S. J. (1992). The impact of gender on configurations of care among elderly couples. *Research on Aging, 14* (3), 313–330.

Strawbridge, W. J., Wallhagen, M. I., Shema, S. J., & Kaplan, G. A. (1997). New burdens or more of the same? Comparing grandparent, spouse, and adult-child caregivers. *The Gerontologist, 37,* 505–510.

Tavris, C. (1992). *The mismeasure of women.* New York: Touchstone Books.

Thompson, E. (2000). Gendered caregiving of husbands and sons. In E. Markson & L. Hollis (Eds.), *Aging in the twenty-first century: Issues and inequalities in social gerontology* (pp. 333–344). Los Angeles: Roxbury.

Tong, R. P. (1989). *Feminist thought.* Boulder, CO: Westview.

Tong, R. P. (1998). *Feminist thought, A more comprehensive introduction.* Boulder, CO: Westview.

Treas, J. (1999). *Author meets critic: John Logan and Glenna Spitze's Family Ties.* Presentation at the American Sociological Association, Chicago, IL.

Walker, A. J. (1992). Conceptual perspectives on gender and family caregiving. In J. W. Dwyer & R. T. Coward (Eds.), *Gender, families, and elder care* (pp. 34–46). Newbury Park, CA: Sage.

West, C., & Zimmerman, D. (1987). Doing gender. *Gender and Society, 1,* 125–151.

Williams, J. (2000) *Unbending gender: Why family and work conflict and what to do about it.* New York: Oxford University Press.

Methodological Issues in Research on Men Caregivers

4

Jamila Bookwala
Judith L. Newman
Richard Schulz

Male family caregivers—that is, men who provide ongoing care to parents, spouses, and partners—comprise a sizable proportion of caregivers nationally. According to recent estimates, approximately 25% of family caregivers are men (National Alliance for Caregiving and American Association for Retired Persons, 1997). Given this substantial number of male caregivers, researchers and practitioners have attempted to develop a better understanding of the experience of caregiving men. As a result, several studies based exclusively on male caregivers have examined the nature and context of men's caregiving experiences. To date, however, there has been little attempt to evaluate the methodological strengths and limitations of this growing body of literature. The goal of this chapter is to describe and assess the research methodology employed by studies of caregiving men.

In 1992, Horowitz articulated the pressing need for methodologically rigorous studies on the demands and outcomes of caregiving among men. She criticized the existing research on male caregiving for its reliance on volunteer samples, the small sizes of samples, and the use of cross-sectional design. In this chapter, we evaluate the methodology of empirical studies that were based exclusively on male caregivers published around and since Horowitz's (1992) article to determine the overall advancement in the scientific study of male caregiving. Empirical studies on male caregivers published during and after 1990 were identified by searching the *PsychInfo* and *Current Contents* electronic databases using the following keywords: caregiver and caregiving in combination with male, men, husband, son, or brother. We reviewed a total of 19 studies, focusing on the following dimensions of research methodology: the study's sample (its type, size and composition, recruitment strategy, response rate, and characteristics), its methods (design, procedure, and measures), and the data analytic techniques that were employed.

We have organized this chapter to first provide details on the methodological characteristics of reviewed studies (see Table 4.1, p. 72).[1] In tabular form, we present information about the sample, methods, and data analytic techniques employed by each study. Based on the tabled information, we discuss the strengths and limitations of the studies of male caregivers. This is followed by a discussion of the specific methodological challenges that the field of male caregiving research continues to face. We conclude with a brief overview of the methodology of studies that have examined gender differences in the caregiving experience. Although these studies have played a vital role in developing the current knowledge base about male caregivers, there has been little commentary on their methodological strengths and limitations.

STUDIES OF MALE CAREGIVERS

Methodological Strengths

Since the beginning of the last decade, there has been a surge in the number of studies focused exclusively on the experience of male family caregivers. In the simplest sense, the rapid increase in this body of literature in and of itself represents a strength of the research in this area. It is an index of the growing awareness among scientists, practitioners, and policymakers of the need for a clearer understanding of the male experience of caregiving—not merely as a deviation from the female normative caregiving experience, but instead as comprising a set of demands and outcomes that are possibly unique to the male caregiver. The steadily increasing body of literature on the experiences of male caregivers is rich in depth and variety. For example, researchers have studied male caregivers within the context of a wide variety of care recipient illnesses. As in the caregiving field at large, dementia and related cognitive impairment were the most common care recipient illness (Coe & Neufeld, 1999; Fuller-Jonap & Haley, 1995; Harris & Long, 1999; Kaye & Applegate, 1990; Kirsi, Hervonen, & Jylha, 2000; Kramer, 1997; Mathew, Mattocks, & Slatt,

---

[1] Given the current focus on research methodology, only one published report relevant to male caregiving was included when multiple published reports based on a single data set were reviewed. Thus, Table 4.1 represents a sample of published reports on male caregivers, not an exhaustive tabulation of articles that have been published in this area.

1990; Parsons, 1997). Other researchers have studied male caregivers of persons with mental illness (e.g., Archer & MacLean, 1993; Mays & Lund, 1999), functional or other impairment (e.g., Archer & MacLean, 1993; Campbell & Martin-Matthews, 2000), arthritis and stroke (Harris & Long, 1999), and AIDS (e.g., Cooke, Gourlay, Collette, Boccellari, Chesney, & Folkman, 1998; Folkman, Chesney, Cooke, Boccellari, & Collette, 1994; Wight, 2000). Kramer and Lambert (1999) in a single study included caregivers of care recipients with a wide range of illnesses, including cancer and heart disease.

Concomitant with an increase in the sheer number of studies based exclusively on male caregivers, there has been an increased sophistication in the quality of research being conducted. A sample of studies have included male non-caregivers as the comparison group for male caregivers (e.g., Folkman et al., 1994; Fuller-Jonap & Haley, 1995; Kramer & Lambert, 1999; Mathew et al., 1990). For example, Folkman and her colleagues (1994) compared male caregivers of persons with AIDS who were HIV+ with those who were HIV− and also compared both these groups to HIV+ male non-caregivers who resided with a healthy gay partner. In this way, Folkman et al. (1994) were able to distinguish the detrimental effects of caregiving to persons with AIDS from the stressful impact of being a caregiver who is also HIV+. Mathew and colleagues compared the experiences of male primary caregivers of a relative with dementia who lived at home with those of men who also considered themselves to be "primary" caregivers (albeit not involved in day-to-day caregiving activities) of a relative with dementia whom they had recently placed in a nursing home. Although research comparing male and female caregivers on the stressors and outcomes related to caregiving typically indicates that male caregivers experience fewer caregiving demands and adverse effects compared to female caregivers (e.g., Bookwala & Schulz, 2000; see also Yee & Schulz, 2000), directly comparing male caregivers with male non-caregivers provides a more accurate understanding of the potential impact of caregiving on the health of male caregivers relative to the general male population. Hence, studies of male caregivers that include male non-caregivers as a comparison group represent an important advancement in our understanding of the male caregiving experience.

The vast majority of studies that have focused exclusively on male caregivers have been qualitative studies aimed at augmenting current understanding about the uniqueness of the male caregiving experience (e.g., Campbell & Martin-Matthews, 2000; Coe & Neufeld, 1999; Harris & Long, 1999; Hirsch & Newman, 1995; Kirsi et al., 2000; Mathew et al., 1990; Matthews & Heidorn, 1998; Mays & Lund, 1999; McFarland & Sanders, 1999; Parsons, 1997; Siriopoulos, Brown, & Wright, 1999). These studies have provided rich and valuable data about the specific nature of male

TABLE 4.1 Summary of Study Methodology Used in Empirical Studies (1990–)

Authors	Sample	Methods & Analytic Approach
Archer & MacLean, 1993	*Type:* non-random. *Size & composition:* 6 male CGs (3 husbands, 3 sons) of 6 chronically ill (visually impaired or mentally ill) women. *Recruitment:* from local support groups for the visually impaired or a mental illness hospital out-patient department; response rate: information not provided. *Characteristics:* Age range = 52 to 71 years.	*Design:* qualitative, cross-sectional. *Procedure:* in-depth, semi-structured, open-ended interviews lasting approximately 2 hours in length conducted in the CG's home. *Measures:* questions formulated to elicit information from the male CGs about their individual perceptions of the caregiving role (e.g., changes in their relationships, their levels of satisfaction, their experiences of stress and isolation). *Analytic approach:* content analysis.
Campbell & Martin-Matthews, 2000	*Type:* non-random. *Size & composition:* n = 772 men who provided care to at least one parent/parent-in-law 65 years of age or older. *Recruitment:* selected from large survey of Canadian employees from different provinces in Canada; response rate: no information provided. *Characteristics: M* age = 45 years; 57% of men provided care to only one relative (range = 1–4); majority are married, have children, have siblings.	*Design:* quantitative, cross-sectional. *Procedure:* no information provided. *Measures:* existing measure of caregiving involvement; developed measures of commitment to care, legitimate excuses, and caring by default. *Analytic approach:* secondary data analysis; correlations, multiple regressions.

Coe & Neufeld, 1999

Type: non-random.
Size & composition: 24 male CGs who assumed primary responsibility, without remuneration, for the care of a cognitively impaired adult older than 60 years, who spoke and read English, resided in an urban area (but not necessarily with CG), and had a phone.
Recruitment: secondary analyses of volunteer data, little detail provided; response rate: no information provided.
Characteristics: Only ranges provided, age of CGs ranged from 33 to 87, with more than 70% being older than 60, retired and caring for their wives. Education ranged from < high school to college graduate, < $20,000 yearly income to > $40,000, and < 2 years of caregiving to >11 years.

Design: qualitative, longitudinal.
Procedure: In depth information was acquired through 2 to 3 guided interactive interviews, ranging in length from 1 to 2 hours, over 18 months.
Measures: No information provided regarding interview used in original study of formal support system. Seven CGs engaged in focus group discussions to elaborate perceptions.
Analytic approach: Content analysis used in grounded theory included constant comparisons, attention to negative cases, generation of concepts and linkages. Used coding, memoing, and diagramming to help identify themes and links.

Cooke et al., 1998

Type: non-random.
Size & composition: n = 140 bereaved caregiving partners of men with AIDS.
Recruitment: via ads in print and electronic media; response rate: no information provided.
Characteristics: M age = 38.9 years; 90% White; median education level of some college; approximately one-third CGs seropositive for HIV; care recipient's diagnosis of AIDS approximately 2 years old.

Design: quantitative, prospective.
Procedure: in-person interviews conducted at four different data collection points (baseline, last bimonthly interview before care recipient's death, within 2 weeks following care recipient's death, and 3 months after care recipient's death).
Measures: medication administered to hasten death and existing measures of caregiver distress, social support, coping, burden, positive meaning of caregiving, couple adjustment.

(continued)

TABLE 4.1 Summary of Study Methodology Used in Empirical Studies (1990–) (*Continued*)

Authors	Sample	Methods & Analytic Approach
Cooke et al., 1998 (*cont.*)		*Analytic approach:* analysis of variance, Chi-square test, analysis of covariance, repeated measures ANOVA.
Folkman et al., 1994	*Type:* non-random. *Size & composition:* 82 HIV+ male CGs, 162 HIV– male CGs coresiding with a gay partner with AIDS who requires assistance on 2 or more ADLs and 61 HIV+ male noncaregivers residing with a healthy gay partner. *Recruitment:* ads in gay press, PSA's, referrals from clinics and related organizations, and annual mailings to residents in San Francisco area; response rate: 71%. *Characteristics:* for HIV+ CGs, HIV– CGs and HIV+ non-CGs, demographics are as follows: White, 79%, 93%, and 88%, respectively; Education, ≥ college, 36%, 50%+, and 50%+, respectively; Age, 37.5 years, 39.2 years, and 37.7 years, respectively; Length of relationship, 6.4 years, 6.3 years, and 5.2 years, respectively; the majority of each group were employed full-time.	*Design:* quantitative and cross-sectional. *Procedure:* in-person interviews in home or researcher's office after initial office visit during which HIV test occurred. *Measures:* mix of existing Likert rating scales (e.g., to assess depression, perceived support, quality of relationship); health assessments (physical symptoms and CD4 levels) and new or modified assessments of stressors (e.g., losses, hassles, burden, coping styles). *Analytic approach:* Chi-square tests, MANOVAs, correlations, hierarchical regression analyses.

Fuller-Jonap & Haley, 1995

Type: non-random for CG sample.
Size & composition: CGs = 52 husbands who coresided with & provided primary care to wives showing signs of dementia, spoke English, were ≥ 65 years old; Comparison group = 53 husbands meeting same conditions, whose wives were free of any condition requiring caregiving.
Recruitment: CGs from phone contacts after being identified by research center, announcements in ADRDA newsletters in 2 large cities, day care centers, support groups; controls randomly selected from computer generated list of volunteers, senior centers; response rate: CGs—30 of 31 agreed to participate; Controls—42 of 57 agreed.
Characteristics: All White and majority earn within $10,000 to $40,000; CGs: *M* age = 74.5 years; *M* education = 12.4 years; *M* length of marriage = 48.2 years; *M* spousal age = 73.1 years, moderately to severely demented wife and about 4.5 years since diagnosis.

Design: quantitative, cross-sectional.
Procedure: interview.
Measures: existing scales measuring functional ability, gender role identity, mental health, physical health, psychotropic medications taken over the past month, number of physician visits in the past year, and a self-rated health measure.
Analytic approach: Chi-square, Fisher Exact, MANOVA, ANOVA, correlations, *t* tests.

Harris & Long, 1999

Type: non-random.
Size & composition: American samples—*n* = 15 husbands & *n* = 15 sons providing care to a family member whose primary diagnosis

Design: qualitative and cross-sectional.
Procedure: in-depth unstructured interviews (lasting 1.5–2.5 hours).
Measures: interviews covered 4 major

(continued)

TABLE 4.1 Summary of Study Methodology Used in Empirical Studies (1990–) (*Continued*)

Authors	Sample	Methods & Analytic Approach
Harris & Long, 1999 (*cont.*)	was dementia; Japanese samples—*n* = 10 husbands & *n* = 5 sons for a family member with dementia or severe physical impairments caused by stroke or arthritis. *Recruitment:* American samples—via newspaper ads, staff referrals, review of calls to local Alzheimer's disease help line; Japanese samples—via staff & agency referrals; response rate: no information provided. *Characteristics:* American samples—*husbands* had *M* age = 71 years; diverse occupations; varying levels of education; lived with care recipient or had placed her in nursing home; *M* caregiving duration = 5 years; *sons* had *M* age = 50 years; majority were college graduates; predominantly middle-class; varying birth order; varied living arrangements with regard to care recipient; *M* caregiving duration = 3.5 years. Japanese samples—*husbands* had *M* age = 75 years; diverse occupations; varied educational levels; varied living arrangements; *M* caregiving duration = 4.5 years; *sons* had *M* age = 56 years; all university graduates; all living with care recipient; all eldest sons; *M* caregiving duration = 5 years.	topics—caregiver role, stress and coping, marital and family relationships, meaning and motivation. Exact wording varied from interview to interview. Pretested with 2 American male CGs. *Analytic approach:* content analysis.

Hirsch & Newman, 1995

Type: non-random.
Size & composition: 32 males providing 50% or more of the care for an elderly ill relative or friend suffering from moderate to severe impairment on IADLs due to chronic disease or Alzheimer's disease.
Recruitment: newspapers, announcements at a small college, social and health agencies with target population; response rate: no information provided.
Characteristics: M age = 52.75 years (range = 21–79), majority provide care for mother (34%) or wife (22%), 60% had some college experience, 80% lived with recipient and others lived closeby, 56% considered themselves of European ethnic background; majority were Catholic and Protestant.

Design: partly quantitative, cross-sectional.
Procedure: one-to one-and-a-half-hour long interview in the home.
Measures: sociodemographics, presence of siblings, financial resources, history of caregiving roles and reasons for becoming a caregiver, sex roles, single self-rated health item.
Analytic approach: Kruskal-Wallis one-way ANOVA, Chi-square; alpha set at .15 given exploratory nature of study. Case descriptions.

Kaye & Applegate, 1990

Type: non-random.
Size & composition: 148 male CGs, typically providing care to a wife over 70 years of age diagnosed with Alzheimer's disease or a related disorder.
Recruitment: 2 male members of a national sample of caregiver support groups who had maintained membership in the group for the longest time; response rate: 64.6%.

Design: quantitative, cross-sectional.
Procedure: mail surveys.
Measures: abbreviated versions of existing assessments of sex role orientation, caregiver burden, frequency of, perceived expertise at performing, and satisfaction with caregiving tasks.
Analytic approach: correlations, *t* tests.

(continued)

TABLE 4.1 Summary of Study Methodology Used in Empirical Studies (1990–) (Continued)

Authors	Sample	Methods & Analytic Approach
Kaye & Applegate, 1990 (cont.)	*Characteristics:* M age = 67.8 years, 70.2% married and living with their spouse, 95.8% white, 72.8% retired or unemployed, 94.4% with at least a high school education, 44% with annual income between $20,000 & $50,000, 64.7% resided with care recipient.	
Kirsi et al., 2000	*Type:* non-random. *Size & composition:* n = 15 husbands who were giving or who had given care to spouse with dementia; subgroup of larger (n = 159) CGs. *Recruitment:* via local Alzheimer's disease association; response rate: for overall study, 12.8%. *Characteristics:* no information provided.	*Design:* qualitative, cross-sectional. *Procedure:* mailed letters of request to members of local Alzheimer's disease association appealing for a story. *Measures:* stories described a close one suffering (or who had suffered) from dementia—"the whole story with all its twists and turns, authentically and in detail without hiding your feelings." *Analytic approach:* discourse analysis.
Kramer, 1997	*Type:* non-random. *Size & composition:* n = 74 husbands caring for wife with dementia. *Recruitment:* via community agencies, geriatric evaluation services, ads; response rate: no information provided. *Characteristics:* M age = 72 years; 81% had high school or better education; 78% retired; 100% White; median income = $20,000–29,000; M caregiving duration = 52 months.	*Design:* primarily quantitative, cross-sectional. *Procedure:* in-person interviews lasting approximately 90 mins. *Measures:* existing measures of care recipient characteristics (e.g., memory & behavior problems), caregiver resources (e.g., satisfaction with social participation), caregiver appraisal (e.g., strain). *Analytic approach:* hierarchical multiple regressions.

Kramer & Lambert, 1999

Type: random.
Size & composition: n = 26 husbands who transitioned into caregiving between T1 & T2 (5 years later) caring for wives with varying illnesses (e.g., cancer, heart disease); n = 262 non-caregiving husbands at T1 & T2 served as controls.
Recruitment: selected from larger nationally representative survey; response rate: national survey had response rates of 75% at T1, 82% of T1 respondents at T2; 61% overall.
Characteristics: CG group had M age = 68.1 years; M years of education = 11.1 years; M income = $29,740; 23% non-Caucasian; 23% employed; Control group had M age = 64.7 years; M years of education = 11.6; M income = $39,780; 17% non-Caucasian; 50% employed. Two groups differed significantly in age, income, employment status.

Design: quantitative, prospective.
Procedure: in-person interviews and sensitive information through self-administered questionnaires.
Measures: existing measures of functional impairment of spouse, household tasks, psychological well-being; additional questions assessing social integration, marital relationship.
Analytic approach: analysis of covariance.

Mathew et al., 1990

Type: non-random.
Size & composition: Group 1—n = 12 male CGs caring for demented elderly relative at home, considered themselves primary CG, & actively involved in patient's daily care. *Group 2—n* = 8 comparison group, male who had placed demented relative in nursing home, considered themselves primary CG, but not typically involved in patient's daily care. All participants had to have been in their role for at least 4 mos.

Design: partly qualitative, cross-sectional.
Procedure: in-person interview.
Measures: questionnaire designed to gather descriptive information; included two existing scales (e.g., burden interview, activities of daily living).
Analytic approach: percentages, t tests, descriptions of responses to open-ended questions.

(continued)

TABLE 4.1 Summary of Study Methodology Used in Empirical Studies (1990–) (Continued)

Authors	Sample	Methods & Analytic Approach
Mathew et al., 1990 (cont.)	*Recruitment:* referrals via local support groups; response rate: 71.4%. *Characteristics: Group 1*—83% White; M age = 59.3 years; 75% married; 50% caring for spouse, 42% for mother, 8% other; 58% employed; education range: < high school—college degrees. *Group 2*—100% white; M age = 65.7 years; 62% caring for spouse; 37% for mother/other relative; 37% employed; 50% college educated.	
Matthews & Heidorn, 1998	*Type:* non-random. *Size & composition:* 49 pairs of brothers (with no sisters) who had at least one non-institutionalized parent aged 74 or older. *Recruitment:* via parent referrals and a registry of elders; response rate: information not provided. *Characteristics: M* age = 50.5 years; 98% White; 87.7% married; 73.5% had at least one child; nearly 50% had graduate or professional training; all coded in highest three occupational status categories.	*Design:* qualitative, cross-sectional. *Procedure:* approximately one-hour long in-person or phone interview (depending on residence of caregiver) developed as a "guided conversation." *Measures:* 18 questions regarding the caregiving situation (e.g., a description of the current situation with parent(s); division of filial responsibilities). *Analytic approach:* qualitative data analysis.

Mays & Lund, 1999

Type: non-random.
Size & composition: $n = 10$ male CGs of mentally ill family for at least 2 years.
Recruitment: via local community mental health centers and local chapter of the Alliance for the Mentally Ill; response rate: 100%.
Characteristics: 50% husbands, 50% fathers; 80% White; M age = 59.9 years; range of education = GED–PhD; range of yearly income: $10,000–>$ 50,000; 50% attended mental health support group at least once, all saw social worker on occasion, and almost all had little assistance with caregiving responsibilities.

Design: qualitative, cross-sectional.
Procedure: in-depth, audiotaped interviews (1–1.5 hours) in CG home or other agreed upon location.
Measures: 22 questions designed for study, related to psychosocial, physical, financial, and crisis management issues, role affirmation in male CGs, dominant areas of concern for CGs. Content validity established by review and approval of 2 mental health practitioners. Piloted on 2 nonparticipating male CGs.
Analytic approach: content analysis to identify concepts and themes in data using the constant-comparison method that relies on transcribed interviews, observational field notes, demographic sheets, researcher memos, and participant checks for credibility during debriefing.

McFarland & Sanders, 1999

Type: non-random.
Size & composition: male caregivers who were sons, husbands, or sons-in-law; no other information provided.
Recruitment: no information provided; response rate: no information provided.
Characteristics: age range from 33–70, living in the South Central Pennsylvania Alzheimer's Association Chapter service area.

Design: qualitative, three data points.
Procedure: focus groups that met on three separate occasions.
Measures: exploration of the differences between male and female caregivers and assessment of the unique needs of male CGs.
Analytic approach: content analysis.

(continued)

TABLE 4.1 Summary of Study Methodology Used in Empirical Studies (1990–) (Continued)

Authors	Sample	Methods & Analytic Approach
Parsons, 1997	*Type:* non-random. *Size & composition:* n = 8 (5 husbands, 3 sons) who were primary caregivers to a parent or spouse with Alzheimer's disease. *Recruitment:* no information provided; response rate: no information provided. *Characteristics:* all middle-aged to elderly men, 5 of whose care recipients were deceased, 2 had placed them in a nursing home, and 1 was providing ongoing care.	*Design:* qualitative, two-wave data collection (second phase intended to clarify T1 responses, further explore omitted areas). *Procedure:* in-person interviews lasting 30–75 minutes each. *Measures:* participants asked to describe their phenomenological experience of caregiving. *Analytic approach:* content analysis using the selective reading approach.
Siriopoulos et al., 1999	*Type:* non-random. *Size & composition:* n = 8 husband CGs, 6 caring for spouse at home and 2 at institutional settings. All had role of primary full-time CG for wife. *Recruitment:* no information provided; response rate: no information provided. *Characteristics:* all White, Anglo-Saxon Protestants; age range = 64–92 years; range of education = 5th grade–PhD; years of caregiving = <1–10.	*Design:* qualitative, using naturalistic inquiry and phenomenological research methods; two-wave data collection. *Procedure:* 2 in-depth semistructured interviews (lasting 45 minutes–2 hours) with each CG, supplemented by field notes and reflective journal. *Measures:* guiding questions to look into the experiences and needs of husbands caring for wives with Alzheimer's disease (content unspecified). *Analytic approach:* Giorgi's method of qualitative data analysis involving a search for meaningful units that lead to guiding themes regarding the experiences and needs of husband CGs.

Wight, 2000

Type: non-random.
Size & composition: n = 642 CGs providing assistance with activities of daily living to a friend, partner, or family member living with HIV.
Recruitment: via mass media announcements, community-based AIDS organizations, other health- and gay-related sources; response rate: no information provided.
Characteristics: M age = 38.9 years; 79% White; 59% lover/partner of care recipient; 41% CGs HIV+; 26% HIV symptomatic; M years of education = 14.98; M annual income = $27,650; M caregiving duration = 1.78 years.

Design: quantitative, longitudinal.
Procedure: 3 in-person interviews lasting approximately 2 hours each conducted at 7-month intervals.
Measures: self-rated health, CD4 counts, HIV-related symptoms, AIDS-related dispositions, gay acceptance; existing measures of personal and instrumental activities of daily living, role overload, financial worry, depression.
Analytic approach: multiple regressions.

Note. CG = caregiver.

caregiving. For example, using an established content analytic method of qualitative data analysis, Siriopoulos et al. identified five guiding themes regarding the experiences and needs of caregiving husbands. These themes center around the quality of the previous relationship with the ill spouse, the sense of loss, caregiving burden, coping and support methods, and the effects of Alzheimer's disease. Harris and Long used qualitative data analytic techniques to collect information on what motivated men to become involved in elder care, what tasks they undertook, what influence caregiving had on their family and work lives, and how others had reacted to their adoption of the caregiving role. Some of the qualitative studies on male caregiving have enhanced their methodological robustness by pilot testing their in-depth interview protocols (e.g., Harris & Long; Mays & Lund) or engaging groups of participants in focus group discussions to obtain greater elaboration on male caregivers' perceptions (e.g., Coe & Neufeld; McFarland & Sanders). Mays and Lund also attempted to establish the content validity of their qualitative interview measure (including a series of questions on the psychosocial, physical, financial, crisis management, and role affirmation areas of concern for male caregivers) through consultations with two mental health practitioners.

The quantitative studies on male caregivers (Cooke et al., 1998; Folkman et al., 1994; Fuller-Jonap & Haley, 1995; Kramer, 1997; Kramer & Lambert, 1999; Wight, 2000), although few in number, have several methodological strengths. Typically, these studies have employed well-established measures to assess caregiving variables such as care recipient impairment, caregiving burden and strain, and caregiver mental health. It remains to be determined, however, if the development of these measures with the female caregiver as the target are sensitive to capturing the male caregiving experience. Some researchers also have included an assessment of caregivers' physical health. For example, Folkman and her colleagues as well as Wight have used lymphocyte counts (CD4/CD8 cells) to assess the immunological status of male caregivers, and Fuller-Jonap and colleagues have assessed male caregivers' medication use and physician visits as indices of physical health status. The quantitative studies of male caregivers also are characterized by the use of multivariate statistical analyses on their data, including analysis of covariance, multivariate analysis of variance, and hierarchical regression analysis.

Methodological Limitations

Despite the several methodological advances discussed above that are evident in research based exclusively on male caregivers, there are a considerable number of shortcomings that continue to characterize this area of research. Most of the studies—quantitative and qualitative—employ fairly small sample sizes, ranging from 6 to approximately 100 male caregivers (e.g., Archer & MacLean, 1993; Coe & Neufeld, 1999; Fuller-Jonap & Haley, 1995; Harris & Long, 1999; Hirsch & Newman, 1995; Kramer, 1997; Mathew et al., 1990; Mays & Lund, 1999; Parsons, 1997; Siriopoulos et al., 1999). The reliance on small sample sizes of male caregivers is especially problematic in the case of quantitative research because the statistical power to identify even modest effect sizes is seriously compromised in such studies. Small sample sizes also compel researchers to rely on simple data analytic techniques over more sophisticated multivariate procedures.

In addition, with one exception (Kramer & Lambert, 1999), all the studies we reviewed were based on nonprobability samples. Typically, male caregivers were recruited via local Alzheimer's disease diagnostic and support centers, community and social service agencies, other support groups, and physician's offices. Caregiving men recruited through such means may represent a unique group that is either comfortable with seeking community-level assistance or experiences caregiving strain that is sufficiently severe to prompt seeking out external assistance. As a result, the caregiving experience of such male caregiver volunteers may be qualitatively different from that of male caregivers who are less comfortable reaching out to local agencies for support or those who prefer to cope more privately with the strains of caregiving. Hence, the generalizability of findings based on male volunteers who are recruited using nonprobability sampling techniques to the population of male caregivers at large may be seriously limited. In addition, the general paucity of male caregiver participants or the difficulty in making contact with them has forced some researchers to treat a heterogeneous group of caregivers as though homogeneous. For example, some researchers (e.g., Mathew et al., 1990; Siriopoulos et al., 1999) combine prevailing caregivers and caregivers of recently institutionalized care recipients into one group. Because ongoing caregivers are likely to be coping with stressors that are quite distinct from those of caregivers who have relinquished their role, combining such disparate types of caregivers is likely to further confound the conclusions reached about the experiences of the male caregiver.

Research with male caregivers also tends to favor simple over sophisticated research methodologies. With only a few exceptions (e.g., Coe & Neufeld, 1999; Cooke et al., 1998; Kramer & Lambert, 1999; Siriopoulos et al., 1999; Wight, 2000), the studies with male caregivers that we reviewed were cross-sectional in design. Most researchers also have preferred a single form of data collection, relying partly or completely on in-person interviews (e.g., Archer & MacLean, 1993; Coe & Neufeld, 1999; Cooke et al., 1998; Folkman et al., 1994; Fuller-Jonap & Haley, 1995; Harris & Long, 1999; Hirsch & Newman, 1995; Kramer, 1997; Kramer & Lambert,

1999; Mathew et al., 1990; Matthews & Heidorn, 1998; Mays & Lund, 1999; Parsons, 1997; Wight, 2000). Other less commonly used data collection techniques include mailed surveys (Kaye & Applegate, 1990) and phone interviews (see Matthews & Heidorn). However, the use of more complex research methodologies involving daily or weekly diaries, multiple daily assessments (e.g., through the use of beepers), or direct observational techniques to assess the experience of male caregivers is absent. In addition, several studies that we reviewed favored the use of measures of care giving variables (e.g., of caregiver burden, caregiver well-being) that were developed by researchers expressly for the study being conducted over the use of existing, validated measures of these variables (see Archer & MacLean; Harris & Long; Matthews & Heidorn). This has compromised the consistency of findings in the field of male caregiving research and may further bring into question the validity of the conclusions about male caregivers' experiences. With few exceptions (see Folkman et al.; Fuller-Jonap & Haley; Kaye & Applegate; Kramer & Lambert; Mathew et al.; Mays & Lund), studies of male caregivers also have failed to provide data on the response rate for participant recruitment. It is unclear from the published reports, however, whether researchers had access to but excluded this information or whether they failed to record this information at the outset. Response rates, if available and reported, however, could provide important information about the limits of the external validity of findings based on volunteer samples of male caregivers.

Recommendations for Methodological Advancement

In view of the limitations evident in the studies of male caregivers described above, several recommendations can be made for future research. We reiterate Horowitz's (1992) call for the use of larger samples of male caregivers. Ideally, these larger samples should be selected using random, probability sampling techniques that can augment the representativeness of the samples to the larger population of male caregivers or render them comparable to the general male population (e.g., in terms of sociodemographic variables). Large probability-based samples also would permit the application of more sophisticated data analyses to enhance current understanding of the experiences of the male caregiver. One approach for achieving this goal would be to examine the data from male caregivers that are a part of existing data sets of large-scale national or multisite studies of caregiving (e.g., Campbell & Martin-Matthews, 2000; Kramer & Lambert, 1999) that are now available for secondary data analyses through various agencies, such as the National Institutes of Health.

It also is important that researchers expand their research on male caregivers to using panel or longitudinal designs. This is important for several reasons. Using data collected at multiple time points would provide information on the long-term associations between caregiving stressors and outcomes for male caregivers. Such data also would permit researchers to uncover possible causal links among the wide range of caregiving demands among male caregivers on the one hand and their mental and physical health on the other. In addition, researchers could use data generated from panel studies to examine the caregiving trajectory among male caregivers with regard to changes in caregiving demands and their association with exit and reentry into the caregiving role or the decision to institutionalize the care recipient. An alternate research design to cross-sectional methodology that also could provide valuable information about male caregiving involves obtaining multiple assessments over a short period of time (e.g., several daily or weekly assessments of caregiver demands and outcomes). Such data can provide important insights into the extent of intraindividual variability over the short term in the experiences of male caregivers.

Based on our review, we also concluded that there remains a pressing need to develop research goals with an explanatory focus. Most of the studies we reviewed explored and described the specific caregiving demands and needs among male caregivers. However, we believe that the field of male caregiving research is ready to extend itself beyond this descriptive level. Researchers must increasingly focus their efforts on conducting theory-driven research to test theoretically derived hypotheses. The ultimate goal of such research would be to develop a caregiving stress-outcome model that is specific to male caregivers, one that identifies and explains the similarities and differences in the caregiving experiences of men and women.

We are not suggesting, however, that qualitative (or descriptive) research should come to a halt. On the contrary, there continues to be a need for more qualitative research that can further enhance our understanding of who among potential male caregivers takes on the caregiving role and why, what factors facilitate such role occupation, and the circumstances under which male caregivers transition in and out of the caregiving role. Qualitative research also can provide valuable data on issues that remain largely unexplored with male caregivers. What types of formal services are most needed by male caregivers? At what points in the caregiving trajectory are their stressors most severe? What kinds of social support do they most require? These and similar questions would be best answered at this point by well-designed qualitative studies.

Finally, we urge researchers to design intervention research specifically for male caregivers. To date, caregiving intervention research is heavily biased in favor of female caregivers. Given the substantial proportion of male caregivers nationwide, however, it is important to begin to design and test intervention protocols that are uniquely tailored for them. For example, special skills training seminars that teach male caregivers to assist with basic activities of daily living such as bathing and cooking meals for the care recipient may be useful in lowering their levels of strain. Support group participation also may be valuable for male caregivers as a means to exchange information or develop supportive relationships with other male caregivers. However, given men's reluctance to participate in support groups, Yee and Schulz (2000) suggest that the use of terms such as "forum" or "seminar" in place of "support group" may be more favorable for the recruitment of male caregivers in intervention research.

Challenges to Methodological Advancement

We recognize that the recommendations we have made for further methodological advancement are especially challenging to carry out in the field of male caregiving research for several reasons. In general, it remains difficult to identify and recruit caregiving men for research purposes (Yee & Schulz, 2000). Given the stronger association of caregiving with female gender roles, male caregivers may not associate the label of "caregiver" to themselves despite their involvement in parental or spousal care. As a result, they may be less likely to respond to advertisements and community announcements calling for caregivers for research purposes. Spouses and parents who are cared for by a male relative (husband or adult son) also are more apt to guard their caregiver from researchers' attempts to recruit them for their studies. In addition to these obstacles, men are generally less likely to participate in scientific research than are women. All of these factors present powerful obstacles to the scientific study of the experience of the male caregiver.

Recruitment of a diversity of male caregivers also remains a significant methodological challenge. For example, little research has directly compared the experiences of caregiving husbands with the experiences of other male caregivers such as sons or brothers (Harris & Long, 1999). As in other fields of research, the comparison of male caregivers based on sociodemographic variables (e.g., co-residing vs. non–co-residing caregivers, Caucasian vs. African American and other non-Caucasian caregivers) also requires attention. For example, it is yet unknown whether Caucasian and African American men differ in their willingness to take on the caregiving role or in their readiness to relinquish it. Or, whether they differ in the types of assistance they provide or the amount of formal and informal support they have available to them in carrying out their caregiving activities. Comparisons of the caregiving experiences of primary, secondary, and potential male caregivers also are lacking in the literature. Such research may be especially important, however, in distinguishing levels of male caregivers' responsibility because men are more likely to receive assistance from others in carrying out their caregiving activities (Yee & Schulz, 2000). Cross-cultural comparisons of male caregivers are also rare, with Harris and Long's comparison of American and Japanese caregiving husbands and sons providing the sole exception.

Once male caregivers are recruited in a study, other methodological questions emerge that deserve attention. Namely, to what extent are male respondents comfortable detailing the demands made on them as caregivers? Are they open to discussing the stressors associated with their caregiving role with a relative stranger, especially an interviewer of the opposite sex? Are measures used to assess the caregiving stressors and outcomes with female caregivers suitable for use with male caregivers? Are attrition rates high for male caregivers in panel or longitudinal studies because of the types of questions asked, the length of the interview, or the long-term commitment required? Clearly, these are important questions for researchers to consider with no unequivocal answers available at present.

CAREGIVING STUDIES ON GENDER DIFFERENCES

Numerous studies have compared male caregivers to female caregivers in terms of caregiving activities, demands, or outcomes, and as such they also represent an important source of information about men's experience as caregivers. Although these studies have tended to treat the female caregiver as the norm and have examined the experience of male caregivers as a deviation from the female normative experience, they have shed considerable light on the caregiving experiences of men.

Methodological Strengths

Overall, caregiving studies on gender differences that have been published since 1990 are characterized by several methodological strengths. As in the case of studies based exclusively on male caregivers, several studies have compared the health outcomes of male caregivers with those of female caregivers and male non-caregivers (e.g., Irwin et al., 1997; Scanlan, Vitaliano, Ochs, Savage, & Borson, 1998; Wright, 1991). As a case in point, Scanlan et al. included male and female comparison groups for their male and female caregivers, respectively, matching caregiver and comparison groups on the sociodemographic variables of age, gender, and kinship to the care recipient. These studies have enabled us to understand the extent to which the experiences of male caregivers vary from those of female caregivers as well as men not involved in caregiving.

Another methodological strength of several recent studies on gender differences in caregiving is their incorporation of relatively objective measures of physical health indicators. For example, researchers have compared male caregivers with female caregivers or male noncaregivers on immunological assays (Scanlan et al., 1998), physiological measures (Irwin et al., 1997; Lutzky & Knight, 1994), and information obtained from medical records (see Scanlan et al.). Others have extended their assessment of caregivers' physical health to include measures of medication use (see Scanlan et al.) and health behaviors (Gallant & Connell, 1998; Scanlan et al.). In addition, a strength of many studies with regard to caregivers' mental health (e.g., Bookwala & Schulz, 2000; Borden & Berlin, 1990; Collins & Jones, 1997; Fuller-Jonap & Haley, 1995; Gallant & Connell, 1998; Hinrichsen, 1991; Irwin et al., 1997; Lutzky & Knight, 1994; Parks & Pilisuk, 1991; Sparks, Farran, Donner, & Keane-Hagerty, 1998; Williamson & Schulz, 1990) is their use of existing, well-established measures such as the Center for Epidemiological Studies—Depression (CES-D) scale (Radloff, 1977) and the Beck Depression Inventory (BDI; Beck, Ward, Mendelson, Mock, & Erbaugh, 1961). Other researchers (e.g., Scanlan et al.) have used the Hamilton Depression Rating Scale that provides an interviewer-rated continuous index of depressive symptoms (HDRS; Hamilton, 1967).

More recent caregiving studies on gender differences are also increasingly using sophisticated statistical analyses. Multivariate analyses are commonly used by researchers (e.g., Bookwala & Schulz, 2000; Borden & Berlin, 1990; Crawford, Bond, & Balshaw, 1994; DeVries, Hamilton, Lovett, & Gallagher-Thompson, 1997; Gallant & Connell, 1998; Hinrichsen, 1991; Ingersoll-Dayton, Starrels, & Dowler, 1996; Kramer & Kipnis, 1995; Lee, Dwyer, & Coward, 1993; Lutzky & Knight, 1994; Mui, 1995; Parks & Pilisuk, 1991; Pushkar-Gold, Franz, Reis, & Senneville, 1994; Scanlan et al., 1998; Sparks et al., 1998), including such techniques as multivariate analyses of variance, multivariate logit modeling, multiple regression, path analysis, and structural equation modeling. Some researchers (e.g., Bookwala & Schulz; Gallant & Connell; Lutzky & Knight) have extended their analysis from a descriptive or predictive level to a potentially explanatory one in which pathways linking different components of the caregiving experience are simultaneously tested. For example, Bookwala and Schulz have examined gender differences and similarities in the caregiving process—that is, differences and similarities in the interrelationships between primary stressors, secondary stressors, and caregivers' mental health between male and female elderly spouse caregivers. However, their reliance on cross-sectional data limits the ability of these studies to identify causal relationships among the different components of the caregiving experience.

Methodological Limitations

Despite the above-mentioned strengths that characterize caregiving studies of gender differences, there also are several methodological shortcomings that we cannot overlook. One important shortcoming is that, like
studies based exclusively on male caregivers, these studies also have used
fairly small-sized nonprobability samples (e.g., Archer & MacLean, 1993;
Borden & Berlin, 1990; Calderon & Tennstedt, 1998; Collins & Jones, 1997;
Crawford et al., 1994; DeVries et al., 1997; Irwin et al., 1997; Lutzky &
Knight, 1994; Pushkar-Gold et al., 1994; Sparks et al., 1998; Wright, 1991).
Fewer studies have included sample sizes of male caregivers that are in
excess of 100 (e.g., Bookwala & Schulz, 2000; Chang & White-Means, 1991;
Gallant & Connell, 1998; Ingersoll-Dayton et al., 1996; Lee et al., 1993;
Mui, 1995; Turner, Catania, & Gagnon, 1994). In addition, relatively few
studies are based on samples of caregivers drawn randomly—for example, through random digit dialing techniques—or drawn from larger
population-based randomly selected samples (e.g., Bookwala & Schulz;
Calderon & Tennstedt; Chang & White-Means; Crawford et al.; Kramer
& Kipnis; Lee et al.; Mui; Turner et al.). Finally, with only a few exceptions (e.g., Scanlan et al., 1998; Williamson & Schulz, 1990), studies of
gender differences in caregiving continue to be cross-sectional in design.
However, some of the studies have analyzed data from the first wave of
a multiwave study (e.g., Bookwala & Schulz; Chang & White-Means;
Crawford et al.; Hinrichsen; Irwin et al.; Mui). As subsequent waves of
data become available from large scale caregiving studies, one can
expect this trend to change and analyses of longitudinal data to become
more common.

Methodological Challenges

As is the case with studies that include only male caregivers, special
methodological challenges are relevant to caregiving studies of gender
differences. Perhaps most significant among these is the potential reporting bias that may characterize male caregivers' responses (Horowitz,
1992). Several studies document significant gender differences in caregiver health outcomes such as psychological well-being, with men reporting
fewer detrimental health effects than women (see Yee & Schulz, 2000).
However, it remains unclear to what extent these gender differences represent true differences or tendencies among men to underreport, for example, symptoms of depression or anxiety. In addition, as pointed out earlier,
the use of measures that have been developed, tested, or used primarily
with female caregivers may not be sensitive to the caregiving experiences
of men, undermining the validity of such measures when used with this

group. Hence, researchers are urged to examine the content of scales that they use to measure caregiving variables with men to ensure their appropriateness for use with this segment of the caregiving population.

Another challenge researchers encounter when examining gender differences is the recruitment of approximately equal numbers of male and female caregivers. In general, the proportion of male caregivers in a sample is substantially smaller than that of female caregivers (e.g., Borden & Berlin, 1990; Chang & White-Means, 1991; DeVries et al., 1997; Ford, Goode, Barrett, Harrell, & Haley, 1997; Kramer & Kipnis, 1995; Lee et al., 1993; Miller & Kaufman, 1996; Mui, 1995; Parks & Pilisuk, 1991; Pushkar-Gold et al., 1994; Sparks et al., 1998; Williamson & Schulz, 1990). Vastly unequal cell sizes can pose a significant problem for certain statistical analyses, making the direct comparison of male and female caregivers difficult. Hence, researchers interested in statistically examining gender differences in caregiving are encouraged to oversample male caregivers to yield approximately equal numbers of caregiving men and women.

The road ahead for studies of gender differences in caregiving is quite similar to that of studies based on male caregivers exclusively. It is important to include large samples of male and female caregivers to study gender differences so that more sophisticated data analyses may be applied. Ideally, these larger samples should be selected using random, probability sampling techniques that can enhance the representativeness of the male and female samples to the larger population of caregiving men and women. Researchers also must begin to favor panel or longitudinal designs over cross-sectional designs to determine possible gender differences in causal pathways linking various caregiving variables. This would permit researchers to shift their research goals from being descriptive to being more explanatory in nature.

CONCLUSION

In sum, our review of studies based exclusively on male caregivers indicates that important methodological advancements are evident in the area of male caregiving research. These advancements include the wide variety of care recipient illnesses represented, the use of male non-caregivers as a comparison group, the design of qualitative studies to gain insight into the unique aspects of male caregiving, and the use of existing measures of caregiving variables and outcomes in quantitative research. Methodological shortcomings that persist in the field include the use of small, nonprobability-based samples, the preponderance of cross-sectional studies that use simple research methodologies, and failure to report response rates of participant recruitment. Likewise, the body of literature on gender differences in caregiving is characterized by both methodological strengths (e.g., the use of male non-caregiver comparison groups, assessment of caregivers' physical health, the use of sophisticated analytic strategies) and shortcomings (e.g., reliance on small, nonprobability samples; underrepresentation of longitudinal research; lack of data on potential reporting biases in male caregivers or the validity of existing scales to measure caregiving variables for use with men). To further advance the knowledge base on male caregiving, researchers are encouraged to use larger, probability-based samples of male caregivers; recruit from among diverse groups of caregiving men to permit between-group comparisons that are based on sociodemographic variables, kinship ties, or caregiving involvement; and continue to investigate the potentially unique experiences of the male caregiver that may be linked to their being male or taking on the relatively unfamiliar role as caregiver.

REFERENCES

Archer, C. K., & MacLean, M. J. (1993). Husbands and sons as caregivers of chronically-ill elderly women. *Journal of Gerontological Social Work, 21*, 5–23.

Beck, A. T., Ward, C. H., Mendelson, M., Mock, J., & Erbaugh, J. (1961). An inventory for measuring depression. *Archives of General Psychiatry, 4*, 561–571.

Bookwala, J., & Schulz, R. (2000). A comparison of primary stressors, secondary stressors, and depressive symptoms between elderly caregiving husbands and wives: The Caregiver Health Effects Study. *Psychology and Aging, 15*, 607–616.

Borden, W., & Berlin, S. (1990). Gender, coping, and psychological well-being in spouses of older adults with chronic dementia. *American Journal of Orthopsychiatry, 60*, 603–610.

Calderon, V., & Tennstedt, S. L. (1998). Ethnic differences in the expression of caregiver burden: Results of a qualitative study. *Journal of Gerontological Social Work, 30*, 159–178.

Campbell, L. D., & Martin-Matthews, A. (2000). Caring sons: Exploring men's involvement in filial care. *Canadian Journal of Aging, 19*, 57–79.

Chang, C. F., & White-Means, S. I. (1991). The men who care: An analysis of male primary caregivers who care for frail elderly at home. *The Journal of Applied Gerontology, 10*, 343–358.

Coe, M., & Neufeld, A. (1999). Male caregivers' use of formal support. *Western Journal of Nursing Research, 21*, 568–588.

Collins, C., & Jones, R. (1997). Emotional distress and morbidity in dementia carers: A matched comparison of husbands and wives. *International Journal of Geriatric Psychiatry, 12*, 1168–1173.

Cooke, M., Gourlay, L., Collette, L., Boccellari, A., Chesney, M. A., & Folkman, S. (1998). Informal caregivers and the intention to hasten AIDS-related death. *Archives of Internal Medicine, 158,* 69–75.

Crawford, L. M., Bond, J. B., & Balshaw, R. F. (1994). Factors affecting sons' and daughters' caregiving to older parents. *Canadian Journal on Aging, 13,* 454–469.

DeVries, H. M., Hamilton, D. W., Lovett, S., & Gallagher-Thompson, D. (1997). Patterns of coping preferences for male and female caregivers of frail older adults. *Psychology and Aging, 12,* 263–267.

Folkman, S., Chesney, M. A., Cooke, M., Boccellari, A., & Collette, L. (1994). Caregiver burden in HIV-positive and HIV-negative partners of men with AIDS. *Journal of Consulting and Clinical Psychology, 62,* 746–756.

Ford, G. R., Goode, K. T., Barrett, J. J., Harrell, L. E., & Haley, W. H. (1997). Gender roles and caregiving stress: An examination of subjective appraisals of specific primary stressors in Alzheimer's caregivers. *Aging and Mental Health, 1,* 158–165.

Fuller-Jonap, F., & Haley, W. E. (1995). Mental and physical health of male caregivers of a spouse with Alzheimer's disease. *Journal of Aging and Health, 7,* 99–118.

Gallant, M. P., & Connell, C. M. (1998). The stress process among dementia spouse caregivers: Are caregivers at risk for negative health behavior change? *Research on Aging, 20,* 267–297.

Hamilton, M. (1967). Development of a rating scale for primary depressive illness. *British Journal of Social and Clinical Psychology, 6,* 278–296.

Harris, P. B., & Long, S. O. (1999). Husbands and sons in the United States and Japan: Cultural expectations and caregiving experiences. *Journal of Aging Studies, 13,* 241–267.

Hinrichsen, G. A. (1991). Adjustment of caregivers to depressed older adults. *Psychology & Aging, 6,* 631–639.

Hirsch, C., & Newman, J. L. (1995). Microstructural and gender role influences on male caregivers. *The Journal of Men's Studies, 3,* 309–333.

Horowitz, A. (1992). Methodological issues in the study of gender within family caregiving relationships. In J. W. Dwyer & R. T. Coward (Eds.), *Gender, families, and elder care* (pp. 132–150). Newbury Park, CA: Sage.

Ingersoll-Dayton, B., Starrels, M. E., & Dowler, D. (1996). Caregiving for parents and parents-in-law: Is gender important? *The Gerontologist, 36,* 483–491.

Irwin, M. Hauger, R., Patterson, T. L., Semple, S., Ziegler, M., & Grant, I. (1997). Alzheimer caregiver stress: Basal natural killer cell activity, pituitary-adrenal cortical function, and sympathetic tone. *Annals of Behavioral Medicine, 19,* 83–90.

Kaye, L. W., & Applegate, J. S. (1990). Men as elder caregivers: A response to changing families. *American Journal of Orthopsychiatry, 60,* 86–95.

Kirsi, T., Hervonen, A., & Jylha, M. (2000). A man's gotta do what a man's gotta do: Husbands as caregivers to their demented wives: A discourse analytic approach. *Journal of Aging Studies, 14,* 153–169.

Kramer, B. J. (1997). Differential predictors of strain and gain among husbands caring for wives with dementia. *The Gerontologist, 37,* 239–249.

Kramer, B. J., & Kipnis, S. (1995). Eldercare and work-role conflict: Toward an understanding of gender differences in caregiver burden. *The Gerontologist, 35,* 340–348.

Kramer, B. J., & Lambert, J. D. (1999). Caregiving as a life course transition among older husbands: A prospective study. *The Gerontologist, 39,* 658–667.

Lee, G. R., Dwyer, J. W., & Coward, R. T. (1993). Gender differences in parent care: Demographic factors and same-gender preferences. *Journal of Gerontology: Social Sciences, 48,* S9–S16.

Lutzky, S. M., & Knight, B. G. (1994). Explaining gender differences in caregiver distress: The roles of emotional attentiveness and coping styles. *Psychology and Aging, 9,* 513–519.

Mathew, L. J., Mattocks, K., & Slatt, L. M. (1990). Exploring the roles of men caring for demented relatives. *Journal of Gerontological Nursing, 16,* 20–25.

Matthews, S. H., & Heidorn, J. (1998). Meeting filial responsibilities in brothers-only sibling groups. *Journal of Gerontology: Social Sciences, 53,* S278–S286.

Mays, G. D., & Lund, C. H. (1999). Male caregivers of mentally ill relatives. *Perspectives in Psychiatric Care, 35,* 19–28.

McFarland, P. L., & Sanders, S. (1999). Male caregivers: Preparing men for nurturing roles. *American Journal of Alzheimer's Disease, 14,* 278–282.

Miller, B., & Kaufman, J. (1996). Beyond gender stereotypes: Spouse caregivers of persons with dementia. *Journal of Aging Studies, 10,* 189–204.

Mui, A. C. (1995). Caring for frail elderly parents: A comparison of adult sons and daughters. *The Gerontologist, 35,* 86–93.

National Alliance for Caregiving and the American Association for Retired Persons. (1997). *Family caregiving in the U.S.: Findings from a national survey. Final report.* Bethesda, MD: National Alliance for Caregiving.

Parks, S. H., & Pilisuk, M. (1991). Caregiver burden: Gender and the psychological costs of caregiving. *American Journal of Orthopsychiatry, 61,* 501–509.

Parsons, K. (1997). The male experience of caregiving for a family member with Alzheimer's disease. *Qualitative Health Research, 7,* 391–407.

Pushkar-Gold, D. P., Franz, E., Reis, M., & Senneville, C. (1994). The influence of emotional awareness and expressiveness on care-giving burden and health complaints in women and men. *Sex Roles, 31,* 205–224.

Radloff, L. S. (1977). The CES-D scale: A self-report depression scale for research in the general population. *Applied Psychological Measurement, 1,* 385–401.

Scanlan, J. M., Vitaliano, P. P., Ochs, H., Savage, M. V., & Borson, S. (1998). CD4 and CD8 counts are associated with interactions of gender and psychosocial stress. *Psychosomatic Medicine, 60,* 644–653.

Siriopoulos, G., Brown, Y., & Wright, K. (1999). Caregivers of wives diagnosed with Alzheimer's disease: Husbands' perspectives. *American Journal of Alzheimer's Disease, 14,* 79–87.

Sparks, M. B., Farran, C. J., Donner, E., & Keane-Hagerty, E. (1998). Wives, husbands, and daughters of dementia patients: Predictors of caregivers' mental and physical health. *Scholarly Inquiry for Nursing Practice: An International Journal, 12,* 221–234.

Turner, H. A., Catania, J. A., & Gagnon, J. (1994). The prevalence of informal caregiving to persons with AIDS in the United States: Caregiver characteristics and their implications. *Social Science and Medicine, 38,* 1543–1552.

Wight, R. G. (2000). Precursive depression among HIV infected AIDS caregivers over time. *Social Science and Medicine, 51,* 759–770.

Williamson, G. W., & Schulz, R. (1990). Relationship orientation, quality of prior relationship, and distress among caregivers of Alzheimer's patients. *Psychology and Aging, 4,* 502–509.

Wright, L. K. (1991). The impact of Alzheimer's disease on the marital relationship. *The Gerontologist, 31,* 224–237.

Yee, J. L., & Schulz, R. (2000). Gender differences in caregiving: A critical review. *The Gerontologist, 40,* 147–164.

Research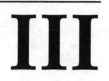

Psychosocial Challenges and Rewards Experienced by Caregiving Men: A Review of the Literature and an Empirical Case Example

5

Elizabeth H. Carpenter
Baila H. Miller

Providing assistance to an intimate who is living with the challenges posed by a chronic illness necessitates psychosocial adjustments and adaptation on the part of both the care-receiver and the caregiver. That some participants in this endeavor appear to adapt to the inherent demands of the process with low levels of psychosocial disturbance while others sustain clinical levels of *dis*tress has long been a focus of study in the informal caregiving literature. A substantial body of literature has documented lower levels of depression (Pruchno & Resch, 1989), less subjective burden or strain (Horowitz, 1985), fewer role conflicts (Cafferata & Stone, 1989; Young & Kahana, 1989), and higher levels of life satisfaction (Barusch & Spaid, 1989; Gallagher, Rose, Rivera, Lovett, & Thompson, 1989) among male caregivers relative to female caregivers. Replicated across diverse disease contexts such as heart surgery (Young & Kahana, 1989), cancer (Blood, Simpson, Dineen, Kauffman, & Raimondi, 1994), clinical depression (Hinrichsen, 1991), and dementia (Horowitz, 1985; Kramer & Kipnis, 1995; Stoller, 1990), early findings suggested that because male caregivers appeared to experience less psychosocial distress than female caregivers, gender may moderate the outcomes of caregiving stress.

Recent studies, however, have challenged these early findings (Schulz, O'Brien, Bookwala, & Fleissner, 1995). Attempting to disentangle the psychosocial effects of caregiving within subgroups, studies of spousal caregivers have shown that men sustain similar levels of caregiving burden as women (Jutras & Veilleux, 1991; Miller 1991), similar levels of depressive affect (Lutzky & Knight, 1994), and higher levels of hostility and work-family conflict (Marks, 1998). Similarly, studies of filial caregivers indicate that adult sons experience similar levels of stress and burden as adult daughters (Coward & Dwyer, 1990; Montgomery & Kamo, 1989), similar levels of emotional strain (Mui, 1995), but more difficulty combining work and family responsibilities (Starrels, Ingersoll-Daylon, Dowler, & Neal, 1997). The contrast between these findings and earlier findings (e.g., Collins & Jones, 1997; Horowitz, 1985; Montgomery & Kamo, 1989) high-lights the necessity of disentangling the effects exerted by methodological or reporting biases from "true" effects exerted by sex and gender (Kaye & Applegate, 1995).

Past studies in the caregiving literature that yielded findings on male caregivers possessed a wide range of conceptual and methodological challenges. Conceptual frameworks that once guided such research efforts have limited explanatory power relative to the diversity of psychosocial experiences *within* male caregivers as a distinct subgroup of caregivers (Applegate, 1997; Walker, 1992). Methodological issues such as sample underrepresentativeness, gender-bias of self-report instruments (Ford, Goode, Barrett, Harrell, & Haley, 1997; Stommel et al., 1993) and the time-boundedness of cross-sectional designs, have limited the generalizability of the findings. Thus, researchers have been unable to capture the dynamic processes underlying the male caregiver's experience that may be separate from, albeit related to, the feminine norms that have dominated the caregiving literature (Horowitz, 1992; Matthews & Heidorn, 1998). Furthermore, many caregiving studies that compared the male experience with the female experience failed to take into account a range of factors beyond gender that may be associated with the psychosocial adaptation of male caregivers. Such factors include racial-cultural-ethnic norms (Ikels, 1983), disease unpredictability or debilitation-disfigurement (Folkman, Chesney, & Christopher-Richards, 1994), or age (Fitting, Rabins, Lucas, & Eastham, 1986). Without such information, it is difficult to determine whether the outcomes experienced by male caregivers are due to their gender or to these other factors which covary with psychosocial adaptation (Dwyer & Coward, 1991). In short, deficiencies in the literature have hindered our understanding of the psychosocial challenges and rewards of male caregivers (see Applegate, 1997).

As noted in chapter 1, obtaining a better understanding of these dynamics is important due to an increasing number of men who may be called upon to serve as caregivers in the future, and because male caregivers may have unique challenges. Because men caregivers initially have a more physiological response to psychosocial stress (Scanlon, Vitaliano, Ochs,

Savage, & Borson, 1998), with psychosocial reactions presenting at a more distal point in a male caregiver's career (Williamson & Schulz, 1990), it is important to consider the extent to which the experience of caregiving may place men at greater risk for detrimental impacts not captured in the psychometric instruments used in much of the current caregiving research. Of particular concern are older male caregivers who tend to downplay their health problems and burden when responding to surveys or interviews (Fuller-Jonap & Haley, 1995; Horowitz, 1992; Kaye & Applegate, 1995; Vinick, 1984). Under the proscriptions of internalized gender attitudes to "tough it out" or to not "go public" with problems (Applegate & Kaye, 1993), these older male caregivers may inadvertently contribute to their own mental and physical decline through physiologically stress-induced reactions such as increased cardiovascular-immunological dysfunction (Eisler, 1995; Vitaliano, Russo, & Niaura, 1995).

The purpose of this chapter is to critically review the published literature that examines the psychosocial challenges and rewards experienced by men caregivers. The organizational framework for this review, which has informed much of the current literature on the psychosocial consequences of caregiving, is the stress process model originally developed by Pearlin, Lieberman, Menaghan and Mullan in 1981 (Aneshensel, Pearlin, Mullan, Zarit, & Whitlatch, 1995). This model views the caregiving process as comprised of three conceptual components: (a) stressors (primary and secondary), (b) moderating resources (e.g., social supports and coping strategies), and (c) outcomes (e.g., psychosocial adaptation or well-being), all of which are embedded in contextual factors such as race, sex-gender, socioeconomic status, and kin relationships (see Aneshensel et al.). This review summarizes the methodological approaches used; identifies the contextual factors, stressors, resources, and outcomes that have been studied; and synthesizes the findings concerning how contextual variables, stressors, and resources influence outcomes among male caregivers. Additionally, we provide data from a study on spouse caregivers of persons with dementia to explore the effects of racial variation on caregiving distress and adaptation within male caregivers. As noted below, few studies have examined contextual differences such as race among male caregivers.

LITERATURE REVIEW

Research abstracts that included the words male caregivers plus various descriptive terms for psychosocial adaptation (e.g., caregiver strain, burden, depression, psychological costs, caregiver gains, well-being, coping, appraisal, or role conflict) were identified through a computer search of the 1978–1999 databases of *Ageline, Medline, Social Work Abstracts, Social Science Abstracts, Social Sciences Citation Index, PsychInfo, PsycLit,* and *AIDSLine.* Reflecting the relative dearth of studies focused specifically on the male caregiving experience, *AIDSLine, Social Science Citation Index (1992–1996),* and *PsycInfo* produced 0 abstracts while *Ageline* produced a total of 18 relevant abstracts. Manual searches of the reference lists of these studies also were conducted to ensure an adequate depth and breadth of search. Focusing specifically on published research, studies were then selected that addressed aspects of the psychosocial experience of male caregivers who were actively engaged in providing assistance to noninstitutionalized care-receivers. Although two studies had mixed samples of active and bereaved caregivers and institutionalized and noninstitutionalized care-receivers (Parson, 1997; Siriopoulos, Browne, & Wright, 1999), we decided to include these studies in the analysis in the interests of capturing as much information as possible about the male caregivers' experience.

Application of these selection criteria resulted in a final sample of 18 studies published in professional journals and books between 1988 and 1999. A broader search on gender, gender by relationship, and various psychosocial outcomes such as depression or life satisfaction yielded a far more robust set of findings on psychosocial differences between male and female caregivers. We chose, however, to heed the advice in the literature to focus specifically on the phenomenological and subjective experience of caregiving from *within* the male perspective (Kaye & Applegate, 1995). Thus, we selected only those studies that identified male caregivers as the unit of analysis.

Most studies focused on the experience of men caring for elders with dementia; one study, however, focused on male caregivers of persons with AIDS (Folkman et al., 1994). The majority of caregivers represented in the samples were Caucasian, 55 years or older, and had the minimum of a high school diploma. The largest subgroup of male caregivers studied consisted of spousal-partnered caregivers, while sons-siblings made up the second largest category. (Only a few of the studies identified fathers, brothers, or in-laws as distinct subgroups.) Among spousal caregivers, most were retired and co-resided with the care-receiver. Few studies identified the degree of caregiver involvement or the breadth of the caregiving network in any systematic way.

Most studies utilized small convenience samples and were therefore subject to selection bias. Sample sizes ranged from 6 to 288. Many of the respondents were recruited through community service agencies such as the Alzheimer's Disease and Related Disorders Association, the Association on Aging, or home health agencies. Other respondents were recruited through the media (newspaper ads, public service announcements), from support groups, or through care receivers who were receiving services from clinics or hospitals. Only two studies used national samples (Kaye & Applegate, 1990a; Kramer & Lambert, 1999). All of the care receivers were adults living with some form of (a) mental disorder, such as clinical depression; (b) cognitive impairment, such as dementia; or (c) physical impairment that required assistance with ADL or IADL tasks.

Ten of the 18 studies comprising the male caregiving literature were qualitative, although three studies (Folkman et al., 1994; Hirsch, 1996; Kaye & Applegate, 1990) incorporated both qualitative and quantitative methods. In adopting qualitative approaches, researchers sought to capture men's lived experience of the caregiving role as they perceived it. This emphasis reflected calls in the caregiving literature for ". . . less documentation of specific gender differences in isolated components of caregiving and more attention to the role that gender plays in assigning meaning to the caregiving experience" (Miller & Cafasso, 1992, p. 506) and ". . . for more research that [is] designed to capture the intersubjective phenomenology of male caregiving" (Kaye & Applegate, 1990a, p. 146).

Of the qualitative studies, three used content analysis to identify common themes in case studies (Archer & MacLean, 1993; Harris, 1993; Harris, 1998), two used the constant comparison method to identify emergent concepts in the data that could be used in subsequent studies to develop theory (Coe & Neufeld, 1999; Mays & Lund, 1999), two used narrative analysis (Folkman et al., 1994; Matthews & Heidorn, 1998), two used phenomenological analysis to capture the meaning of the male caregiver's experience (Parson, 1997; Siriopoulos et al., 1999), and one did not specify the methodological approach used in data analysis (Motenko, 1988). Given the diversity of these analytic techniques, the interpretation of these findings is limited to a report of only those themes that appear to be substantively consistent across studies. The five quantitative studies focused on patterns of association between (a) background-contextual variables (e.g., caregiver and care-receiver characteristics such as gender identity or the kinship relationship between caregiver and care-receiver); (b) stressor variables (e.g., illness related variables); (c) resource variables (e.g., social service utilization, coping, and social involvement); and (d) outcome variables (e.g., subjective burden, strain, depression, or life satisfaction).

RESEARCH THEMES

The Relevance of Context

The major contextual-background variables studied were age, quality of relationship, and education. All of these were found to play a role in male caregiver's psychosocial well-being. Qualitative studies indicated that younger men had more "difficulties" in the caregiving role (Mays & Lund, 1999) and communicated particular "psychological stress" when having to choose between work responsibilities and caregiving responsibilities (Folkman et al., 1994). Men with enduring and affectionate relationships with their care-receiver expressed lower levels of burden and higher levels of satisfaction (Kaye & Applegate, 1990a; Montenko, 1988). Furthermore, male caregivers who described themselves in terms of androgynous gender traits expressed lower levels of burden and higher levels of competence in the caregiving role (Applegate & Kaye, 1993). One quantitative study found that education had a negative effect on men's satisfaction with caregiving while duration of caregiving had a positive effect on men's experience of strain (Kramer, 1997). [Both these findings have been confirmed in the caregiving literature with other caregiver populations (Miller, 1989; Picot, Youngblut, & Zeller, 1997; Zarit, Todd, & Zarit, 1986)]. In short, male caregivers' education, age, years of experience in the caregiving role, relationship with the care-receiver, and gender identity contribute to male caregiver's psychosocial well-being, both negatively (burden or strain) and positively (competence and satisfaction). Although these contextual variables suggest important sources of intergroup heterogeneity among male caregivers that need further investigation, they represent a limited set of relevant male caregiving contexts. Little is known about the extent to which race, religion, socioeconomic status, and other contextual factors affect caregiving strains and rewards among male caregivers.

According to the reviewed qualitative studies, however, age and length–quality of relationship appear to be especially relevant. These attributes may be confounded with the relationship of the male caregiver to the care-receiver (e.g., husband or son). For instance, younger male caregivers with fewer years of caregiving expressed more difficulty with staying in the caregiving role than did older caregivers with more years in the caregiver role (Mays & Lund, 1999). Similarly, young male caregivers expressed intense psychological stress when having to choose between work responsibilities and caregiving responsibilities (Folkman et al., 1994). Folkman et al. reported that the quality of the relationship with the care-receiver (i.e., having a loving relationship) was important to male caregivers' ability to endure the disease course. Three other qualitative studies (Kaye & Applegate, 1990a, 1999b; Motenko, 1988; Parson, 1997) echoed this theme. As summarized by Motenko (1988), "The present caregiving relationship was rooted in the [past] relationship . . . In this way, the past is part of the present and infuses meaning into caregiving . . . [Caregiving] perpetuates a relationship that continues to hold valuable meaning for the caregiver" (p. 111).

Gender as a contextual factor was examined only in terms of sex-roles, rather than other current interpretive frameworks such as feminist theory. Three studies used the Bem's Sex Role Inventory (BSRI) to determine if male caregivers endorsed particular degrees of masculine, feminine, androgynous, or undifferentiated characteristics (Fuller-Jonap & Haley, 1995; Hirsh, 1996; Kaye & Applegate, 1990a). Male caregivers were no more likely to endorse one sex-role characteristic over another when compared to a group of male non-caregivers (see Fuller-Jonap & Haley). A factor analysis of a modified BSRI that produced two subscales—an instrumental (male-oriented) subscale and an affective (feminine-oriented) subscale—indicated that male caregivers used both instrumental and affective terms to describe themselves (Kaye & Applegate, 1990a, 1990b). Men who rated themselves higher on affective-feminine traits experienced lower levels of caregiver burden and a greater sense of competence (Kaye & Applegate, 1990a). Surprisingly, men who described themselves in instrumental-masculine terms experienced higher levels of satisfaction in performing hands-on caregiving tasks than did men who described themselves in affective terms (Kaye & Applegate, 1990a).

Stressor Variables

Illness-Related Variables

As noted, most of the illness variables studied related to care of persons with cognitive impairments. Two quantitative studies (Kramer, 1997; Mathew, Mattocks, & Slatt, 1990) reported that men who cared for individuals with illness-associated memory-behavior problems experienced high levels of strain. Qualitative studies elaborated upon this association between illness characteristics and strain. Men described the vigilance required to keep care-receivers from wandering as "being locked in one's own house" (Parson, 1997) or as being "tied down" (Siriopoulos et al., 1999). Other caregivers described feelings of intensified loneliness, powerlessness, or loss of control as the disease progressed from one stage to another (Folkman et al., 1994; Harris, 1995; Parson, 1997) or, a "sensory deprivation" once the disease robbed care-receivers of their ability to communicate (Motenko, 1988). Sons described the process of observing their father's physical and mental decline as emotional strain (Hirsch, 1996), while other male caregivers described an intensifying awareness of "psychological vulnerability" as they viewed the care-receiver's disease progression as a forecast of their own future (see Folkman et al. and Kaye & Applegate, 1994). Furthermore, many men expressed profound grief and loss in watching the steady deterioration of a loved one (see Parson, Folkman et al., and Siriopoulos et al.) (Harris, 1993, 1995; Kaye & Applegate, 1990a). As the care-receiver's health deteriorated, the caregivers grieved for "someone they once knew, someone they no longer recognized, and who no longer recognized them" (see Parson, 1997, p. 399).

In addition to identifying the physical and cognitive deterioration of one's loved one as a stressor, a psychosocial deterioration related to the progression of disease among persons with dementia was also identified by male caregivers as a stressor. This psychosocial deterioration was variously described as "shifting responsibilities" (Folkman et al., 1994) and as "taking away" (Parson, 1997). Male caregivers noted increased stress when their assumption of increasing responsibility for the care-receiver's health necessitated an invasion of that person's rights or privacy (see Folkman et al.). Parson echoed this theme by describing the distress male caregivers experienced when they had to "take away" from the care-receiver:

> As care-receivers became progressively worse . . . caregivers were forced in a number of situations to take away from the care-receiver . . . In removing tangible objects (e.g., sons taking away their fathers' car keys), caregivers felt they were taking away care-receivers' dignity [as well as caregivers] trust of the care-receiver . . . In the midst of trying to serve what was left of the person . . . the very things that mattered to [the care-receiver's self-definition] had to be taken away. (pp. 398–400)

This "taking away" induced stress because it was antithetical to the notion of caregiving as an act of giving of oneself (see Parson, 1997).

In short, such factors related to care-receivers' illness as behavior problems, physical deterioration, or psychosocial decline, contributed to men's negative psychosocial well-being in the form of strain or burden, loss and grief, and an intensified awareness of their own physical-psychosocial vulnerability. The conflict between providing good care as the disease progressed and respecting the care-receivers' autonomy contributed to increased levels of distress in male caregivers. It is worth noting, however, that many of the reports regarding this latter type of illness-related stressor were made within the context of male caregivers assisting male care-receivers (e.g., sons assisting fathers or male caregivers assisting men with AIDS). This observation suggests that psychological transference or identification processes may be worthy of future study. In addition, the predominant focus on studies of persons with dementia needs to be expanded to include more studies on male caregivers' adaptive capacities to other forms of physical disability.

Type of Caregiver Involvement

Another stressor, the amount and type of caregiving tasks, may represent nontypical activities for many males. Only one quantitative study (Mathew et al., 1990) reported a relationship between the type of tasks performed (e.g., toileting) and male caregivers' negative psychosocial well-being (described as a challenge). Two qualitative studies (Kaye & Applegate, 1995; Parson, 1997) reported that male caregivers described the process of providing hands-on personal care as the one caregiving activity in which men felt the least competent, the most stress, and the most dissatisfaction. These tasks were particularly taxing emotionally for sons (see Parson). However, in contrast to caregiving literature that focuses predominantly on the negative effects of caregiver involvement, Kaye and Applegate (1990b) described how men saw ". . . the most salient task [of their involvement] as providing dimensions of social support, especially companionship and emotional sustenance" (p. 93). In this arena, male caregivers found the most gratification.

Once again, the range of stressor variables studied among male caregivers was limited. Other stressors, such as degree of patient's functional difficulties, type of emotional and cognitive impairment, or disease state were not examined. Based on the studies reviewed however, two stressor variables (i.e., illness-related variables and type of caregiver involvement) played a role in male caregiver's psychosocial well-being. Regarding illness-related variables, quantitative studies found that memory-behavior problems had a positive effect on men's sense of strain (Kramer, 1997; Mathew et al., 1990). Qualitative studies found that the overall disease progression was emotionally straining and instilled a sense of psychological vulnerability while the process of providing hands-on care was viewed as emotionally taxing and dissatisfying. Qualitative studies also indicated, however, the presence of a positive association between caregiver well-being and affective tasks such as providing companionship or "emotional sustenance." Thus, instruments used to study the role of stressors in male caregivers' psychosocial well-being should include not only a summation of types of stressors (e.g., care receiver functional needs or behavior problems), but also a subjective assessment of these stressors (i.e., how challenging, ubiquitous, or rewarding they are) in order to better assess the effect of stressors on outcomes.

Resource Variables

Social and personal resource variables examined in studies of male caregivers were primarily informal and formal social supports, as well as coping styles.

Informal Supports

Three quantitative studies examined some aspects of informal support or social life. Drawing upon a national probability sample, Kramer and Lambert (1999) documented detrimental changes in the social integration of husbands who entered the caregiving role. They reported that older husbands who transitioned into the caregiving role reported a greater decline in their emotional support and marital happiness, and were more likely to report that their marriages were in trouble than husbands who lived with well spouses. In terms of relationships between informal support and burden, Kaye and Applegate (1990a) reported that, although there was no relationship between the frequency of help provided by family members and caregiver burden, men who perceived that their families held them in positive esteem as caregivers experienced lower levels of burden (Kaye & Applegate, 1990a). Another study documented that satisfaction with social participation was differentially predictive of negative and positive outcomes. This resource variable was negatively correlated with strain but positively correlated with caregiver gain (Kramer, 1997).

Qualitative studies (Archer & MacLean, 1993; Kaye & Applegate, 1990a; Parson, 1997) echoed these themes regarding the salience of male caregiver's perception of informal support. They described the sense of abandonment and social isolation that men experienced when family and friends did not appear to appreciate the problems men faced in caregiving. For instance, when informal assistance was not offered by family and friends in the form of physical (i.e., respite) or emotional support, male caregivers described increased conflicts with other family members (see Parson), increased feelings of bewilderment and loss (see Archer & MacLean), or increased sense of social isolation when contact with friends and family members declined as their wives' conditions deteriorated (Harris, 1993, 1995).

On the other hand, qualitative studies also reported the positive effects male caregivers experienced when informal emotional support was forthcoming. For instance, caregiving sons who confided in their wives described lower levels of burden or stress (Harris, 1998), while male caregivers who received positive feedback from family or other important referents described this support as critical to their ability to sustain the enactment of a non-normative role (Hirsch, 1996). In addition, the level of perceived reciprocity between the male caregiver and the care receiver, particularly in the areas of emotional support, concern, and affection, appeared to effect male caregiver's overall resiliency (Kaye & Applegate, 1990a, 1990b).

In summary, the perception of informal support indicated both positive and negative effects on psychosocial well-being (i.e., the presence of positive informal supports decreased caregiver burden while negative informal supports increased burden). These findings support other studies in the caregiving literature in which informal supports have been found to play an ameliorative role in caregiver burden and strain (Biegel, Sales, & Schulz, 1991). Yet only limited dimensions of informal support were examined in these studies. The qualitative studies focused more on personal relationships, whereas the quantitative studies focused on social integration and participation.

Formal Social Supports

A quantitative study (Kaye & Applegate, 1990a) found that men's feelings of burden increased in association with outside community service assistance, but because these studies were cross-sectional, the direction of effect cannot be established. Qualitative studies reporting on male caregiver's resistance to formal social supports described the use of formal supports as a sign of dishonor, as a violation of their own sense of pride as well as their family's privacy (Coe & Neufeld, 1999). They tended to use formal supports only as a "support of last resort" in times of crisis or when caregiving demands exceeded caregivers' abilities (Coe & Neufeld). Furthermore, when male caregivers did use formal supports, they did not describe it in terms of relief or respite from caregiving, but in terms that emphasized its status as a concession (Motenko, 1988; Coe & Neufeld).

Men's resistance to formal social supports may vary by race, cohort, kinship status, or disease progression. Male caregivers who were part of a brothers-only sibling network of informal caregivers viewed the use of formal services as an acceptable solution to problems that undermined their parents' independence (Matthews & Heidorn, 1998). Older male spousal caregivers, however, tended to view formal supports adversarially, as reflecting negatively on their abilities to live up to their marital commitments (Motenko, 1988), and thereby inducing stress (Kaye & Applegate, 1994). Men's resistance to formal supports also varied with the progression of the disease. When a care-receiver's disease shifted into a new stage, some male caregivers exhibited a greater amount of stress that induced, in turn, a greater willingness to explore different options to caregiving, including increased formal supports (Harris, 1995).

In short, male caregivers' attitudes toward (and use of) formal supports reflected an ambivalence that was apparent in both positive and negative effects on men's psychosocial well-being. It is difficult to determine, however, if this ambivalence was due to possible cohort effects or to variability in disease progression. Furthermore, as these findings suggest, the effects of social supports (both informal and formal) on male caregiver's psychosocial well-being may not be mutually exclusive categories (either positive or negative) but degrees of both (positive and negative outcomes at the same time). If the latter is a more accurate representation, then future research on the role that social supports play in male caregivers' psychosocial well-being would be well served by using dynamic, process-oriented methodologies.

Coping

A number of coping mechanisms have been identified in the caregiving literature. Only a few were examined in these studies of male caregivers, such an instrumental behavioral orientation (Kaye & Applegate, 1995) and the use of emotion-focused strategies (i.e., wishful thinking, denial, suppressed feeling, self-blame and avoidance), versus problem-focused strategies (Kramer, 1997). Kramer reported that emotion-focused coping was a predictor of strain, whereas problem-focused coping was a predictor of gain among older husbands caring for wives with dementia.

To determine how male caregivers coped with the internal cognitive dissonance that sometimes occurs when performing a non-normative role (i.e., a female-defined caregiving role), Hirsch (1996) employed Bem's Sex Role Inventory in a study of 32 male caregivers. He found that male caregivers who adopted multiple alternative ideologies (i.e., a masculine identity coupled with androgynous gender proscriptions, religious beliefs, and ethnic-familial norms) experienced less cognitive dissonance or greater cognitive valence when having to act in "non-normative manners regarding gendered behaviors . . ." (Hirsch, 1996, p. 115). This adoption of alternate ideologies was identified as a salient coping strategy in qualitative studies as well. For instance, son caregivers described their religious convictions as an important source of solace and support (Harris, 1998).

Qualitative studies reported expressions such as "rational feeling" (Kaye & Applegate, 1990a), "realistic" or "action oriented" (Mays & Lund, 1999), and "problem-solving" (Harris, 1998) when describing other coping strategies men employed to overcome the stress associated with the caregiving experience. Some men described their coping strategy as intensified "determination" when confronted by feelings of ineptitude in providing personal care (Kaye & Applegate, 1990a). Sons used a range of strategies described as "present-focused" or "problem solving" when trying to gain control of a caregiving crisis: ". . . rather than focusing on past problems that had been solved or on problems that might occur in the future . . . [sons] focused on the immediate situation [and] solved the problems . . . [in an attempt] to return their parents to a state in which they were as independent from sons as soon as possible" (Matthews & Heidorn, 1998, pp. S281–S284). Several men used terms such as "being firm, consistent, and patient" to describe their approach to crisis management rather than terms such as "nurturing" or "supportive" often used to describe female caregivers (see Mays & Lund). Male caregivers, however, did not appear to experience such instrumental coping strategies as necessarily exclusive of emotional expressivity. Those who initiated affectionate behavior toward their care receivers expressed less stress and burden (Kaye & Applegate, 1995). Such reports challenge popular notions of male caregivers as emotionally distant and detached (Applegate & Kaye, 1993).

Another coping strategy identified in the qualitative studies was a technique loosely described as "recognizing one's limitations" or as "taking care of yourself" (Mays & Lund, 1999; Motenko, 1988). Many male caregivers seemed to purposefully establish boundaries between their caregiving responsibilities and taking time to foster interests outside the home in order to regain or maintain energy (Archer & MacLean, 1993). This recognition of limitations seemed most common in male caregivers who approached caregiving by employing skills and patterns of behavior acquired through their working careers (Harris, 1995, 1998). Establishing routines and setting up schedules as well as plans of action enabled these male caregivers not only to assert a modicum of control over a disease that was constantly changing, but also to establish a new (or to continue an ongoing) work identity (Harris, 1995). In short, male caregivers who employed proactive coping strategies, such as problem-focused coping, appeared to experience more competence and less inadequacy in the role that, in turn, appeared to preserve a sense of self esteem (Kaye & Applegate, 1990a) and to increase their sense of caregiver gain (Kramer, 1997).

In summary, social support (informal and formal) and coping were found to play an important role in moderating the impact of stressors on male caregivers' psychosocial outcomes. Male caregivers who perceived family members and friends to be supportive of their caregiving efforts (informal support) reported less social isolation and burden. Formal supports, however, appeared to have both negative and positive effects. Younger male caregivers reported less stress as formal support increased while older male caregivers reported more stress. As summarized by Kramer (1997), however, of all the contextual and resource variables examined in the caregiving literature, social support was the strongest predictor of caregiver strain and gain. In addition, male caregivers who employed emotion-focused coping strategies reported higher levels of stress whereas men who employed "rational feeling" strategies reported less stress. These findings have been supported elsewhere in the caregiving-coping literature and do not represent factors that are necessarily unique to male caregivers.

Psychosocial Outcomes

Negative Well-Being

In general, male caregivers to people with Alzheimer's disease or AIDS had poorer mental health and experienced more depressive symptomatology than comparison groups of male non-caregivers (Folkman et al., 1994; Fuller-Jonap & Haley, 1995), but few of the male caregiver studies, in general, made such comparisons. Of the studies that did employ a matched comparison group, male caregivers showed a trend toward higher levels of psychoticism, reported more respiratory problems, more difficulty sleeping and taking regular exercise, and a trend toward using over-the-counter medicines more frequently than male non-caregivers (Fuller-Jonap & Haley). Furthermore, husbands who became caregivers reported increased depression and decreased happiness counteracting the more "benign experience of male caregiving that is frequently conveyed in gender comparative studies" (Kramer & Lambert, 1999, p. 666).

Qualitative studies echoed these themes of depression and burden. Male caregivers described themselves as going through "some kind of depression" or of having a "feeling of confinement" (Mays & Lund, 1999, p. 25). Several contributing factors were identified in male caregivers' narrative accounts. These included the pain of assimilating the shifts from periods of stability to periods of overt illness progression, fatigue, the powerlessness of dealing with a virtually uncontrollable disease, and conflicts experienced between work responsibilities and caregiving responsibilities (Folkman et al., 1994). The conflict between work and caregiving was also expressed in relation to increased levels of burden (Kaye & Applegate, 1990a). Other factors contributing to the sense of burden included co-residence with the care-receiver, poor to moderate caregiver health, and fear of what the future held for the care-receiver (Kaye & Applegate, 1990a). However, an equally salient outcome of caregiving that was reported above, but that has received less attention in the caregiving literature, in general, was the profound sense of loss and grief (Folkman et al., 1994; Harris, 1993, 1995; Kaye & Applegate, 1990a; Parson, 1997; Siriopoulos et al., 1999) and the psychological vulnerability (Folkman et al.; Kaye & Applegate, 1994) that caregivers experienced as the illness-related stressors increased.

In summary, male caregivers experienced a range of difficult outcomes (i.e., depression, hostility, burden or strain, grief and profound social isolation). Yet many of these studies indicated that while men found aspects of caregiving to be frustrating, trying, or irritating, they did not experience caregiving as emotionally debilitating. Rather, "Reinhard (1994) describes the negative outcomes of caregiving as arising more from a relentless sense of responsibility than from threats to one's psychosocial sense of well-being" (cited in Mays & Lund, 1999, p. 26). Future studies on male caregivers may benefit from using instruments that emphasize expressions of compromised psychosocial functioning that may not be immediately apparent but that may contribute to the development of ongoing difficulties at a more distal point in caregivers' careers (e.g., instruments measuring grief or complicated mourning).

Positive Well-Being

The psychosocial rewards from caregiving were conceptualized variously as caregiver gain or satisfaction (Kramer, 1997; Mathew et al., 1990).

Significant predictors of gain were found to include education, satisfaction with social participation, and problem-focused coping (see Kramer). Although these predictors of gain shared some similarities with predictors of strain (i.e., satisfaction with social participation and caregiver health), they were not affected by other predictors of strain (i.e., care-receiver characteristics); therefore, ". . . predictors of caregiver gain should not be presumed to be the same as the predictors of strain" (Kramer, p. 247).

Qualitative studies echoed the themes of satisfaction and intense gratification when summarizing the positive aspects of caregiving that male caregivers experienced (Archer & MacLean, 1993; Folkman et al., 1994; Harris, 1998; Kaye & Applegate, 1990a). The men in one study unanimously described caregiving as immensely gratifying and satisfying (see Archer & MacLean) while elsewhere male caregivers expressed gratification in mastering challenges to their personal competence (Kaye & Applegate, 1990a, 1990b). Male caregivers reported the gratification in being able to "pay back" the care-receiver for the care they had received from the care-receiver (Harris, 1998; Motenko, 1988; Parson, 1997). As Parson reported, caregiving was "the final act of gratitude," a "balancing of the symbolic exchange" (pp. 401–402).

Another theme echoing throughout many of the qualitative studies was the sense of personal growth or purposefulness associated with the caregiving experience (Harris, 1998; Motenko, 1988). Caregiving gave husbands, many of whom were retired, an ongoing role to play in society, thereby instilling a sense of security, belonging, and continuity (Motenko). Other men who were providing assistance to an intimate living with mental illness expressed pride in the accomplishment of their role (Mays & Lund, 1999). One man described caregiving as ". . . something a real man [does]" stating that it was ". . . good to know that a man can take care of someone and be proud of it" (Mays & Lund, p. 25). These themes were echoed in Motenko, Harris (1995), and Kaye and Applegate (1990a) as well.

In short, these statements contrast sharply with traditional stereotypes of men as non-nurturing or as preferring to keep their emotional distance (Archer & MacLean, 1993). As Folkman et al. (1994) summarized, caregiving provided men the opportunity to "create meaning out of horror . . . to convey dignity in a situation in which a person who is ill might otherwise feel mortified or humiliated . . . to experience competence in difficult circumstances . . ." (pp. 47–49).

This review of male caregiver literature using a stress process framework reveals many gaps in research on this topic—especially when compared to the voluminous literature on female caregivers or on gender differences in caregiving. Because most of the studies were qualitative and used small samples, many sources of heterogeneity among male caregivers remain unexplored or insufficiently examined. In addition, the uniqueness of male

caregiving experiences is difficult to identify because there is little concomitant interpretive theory in the reviewed literature of specific male
role attributes that could illuminate uniqueness but also identify the
important sources of heterogeneity that are worthy of further study.
Much of this literature is descriptive in nature, meeting the aim of providing insight into men's caregiving experiences, but provides little in
terms of explanation of patterns identified. The following empirical
example also does not contribute to theoretical explanation but does
provide an example of a source of heterogeneity among male caregivers
not studied previously.

EMPIRICAL CASE EXAMPLE

As noted, one of the major findings identified in the foregoing literature
review on male caregivers is the lack of empirical attention to race and
cultural factors within male caregivers. Drawing on responses from male
spouse caregivers interviewed in a National Institute of Aging study of
spouse caregivers of persons with dementia, we explored the association
between a selection of many of the concepts identified above with stress
process theory and caregiver depression and satisfaction. For purposes of
this case example, race was viewed as a socially constructed category that
represents ways in which American society distributes a variety of resources.
We can assume that race differences in marital status, living arrangements, mortality, and morbidity influence the probability of African
American and Caucasian men becoming caregivers. Thus, lower marital
rates within the African American community lower the likelihood that
older men will be caregivers. These demographic differences, however,
do not tell us much about variation in caregiving challenges and rewards
among African American and Caucasian married men who are caring for
a spouse with dementia.

Consistent with the stress process model highlighted in this review, we
examine stressors (caregiver's self-reported health, behavior problem upset,
and task distress), and resources (social support and caregiver mastery) as
predictors of caregiver outcomes, that is, caregiver depression, role strain,
and satisfaction. This is a cross-sectional analysis, and thus we cannot
represent the process adequately. Depression, role strain, and caregiver
satisfaction are imperfect outcome measures because they can be easily
confounded with predictor variables that are measured at the same time.
Nevertheless, we attempted to test two hypotheses:

1. Mean values on male caregiver depression, role strain, and satisfaction will vary by race.

Many prior studies show that African American female caregivers are less depressed than Caucasian caregivers. African American caregivers have reported lower levels of perceived burden, caregiving intrusion, and depression (Hinrichsen & Ramirez, 1992; Lawton, Rajagopal, Brody, & Kleban, 1992; Mintzer & Macera, 1992). Although most of these studies involved primarily female caregivers, there is no clear reason to anticipate different cultural processes among male caregivers. However, there is less evidence to assume racial differences in caregiver satisfaction.

2. The extent of racial differences in male caregiver depression, role strain, and satisfaction will diminish after stressors and resources are taken into account.

Many reasons have been suggested for the findings of less depression among African Americans. The most common is that older African Americans appear to have broad, active networks of support and assistance (Chatters, Taylor, & Jackson, 1986; Taylor, 1988), although some recent studies have questioned this advantage in support, noting demographic changes in African American communities (Silverstein & Waite, 1993; Smerglia, Deimling, & Barresi, 1988). Furthermore, the extent to which racial differences in social supports impact the experience of caregiver satisfaction has been rarely studied.

Sample

The data were from an NIA-supported study of the influence of race and gender on spouse caregivers of persons with dementia. In-home structured interviews were performed, with the interviewer and respondent matched by race. Selection criteria for respondents included: (a) English-speaking spouse caregivers of persons over age 60 with a diagnosis of some form of dementia, and (b) co-residence of the impaired person and the spouse caregiver. Although based on a convenience sample, African Americans and males were oversampled relative to their proportion in the caregiving population at a rate of approximately 1.75 to 1, an approach designed to insure orthogonality of race and gender and reasonable cell sizes. Our final sample size was 215, which included 22 African American males, 56 Caucasian males, 55 African American females, and 82 Caucasian females. This analysis is based only on the 78 male caregivers. Because of the lower marital rates among African Americans, this sample may be less representative of African American caregivers compared to Caucasians. For a fuller description of the sample design, see Miller, Campbell, Farran, Kaufman, and Davis (1995) and Miller and Kaufman (1996). As in other studies of caregivers, the sample does not represent an easily definable universe (Lawton et al., 1992).

Sample characteristics were similar to those of other studies of spouse caregivers (Pruchno & Potashnik, 1989). The mean age of spouse caregivers was 74.7. Average education level was 13.1 years and average years married was 43.6. Fifty-four percent of the sample were Protestant, 27% were Catholic, and 18.6% were Jewish or other religions. African American caregivers were almost three years younger than Caucasian spouse caregivers and had been married seven years less, on the average. Race differences also occurred in religious identification and income level. African Americans were significantly more likely to be in the lower income brackets and to be Protestant than their Caucasian counterparts. There were relatively few differences in caregiving attributes among the husband caregivers in this sample when compared to the wife caregivers. The differences that did exist were as follows: Husbands cared for wives with somewhat higher numbers of ADL limitations, expressed higher levels of task distress, and had fewer helpers.

Measures

As noted above, measures were selected to present facets of the stress process model. Because we were concerned about the number of predictors for multivariate analysis, we performed preliminary bivariate analyses of the relationship of a wider variety of predictors on depression, role strain, and satisfaction. Only variables with significant correlations were retained for a more parsimonious model. Although not a significant correlate, we retained income in our trimmed model, to confirm that any race effects found were not confounded by socioeconomic status differentials.

Context variables included race (1 = African American, 0 = Caucasian) and income. Income was coded in 16 categories (1 = under $3,000; 16 = $50,000 or more). Income information was missing for 40 persons. We imputed values using a two-step procedure. First we determined through a regression analysis that race, sex, impaired spouse education, and caregiver education predicted 33% of the variance in income. We summed spouse and caregiver education to represent the couple's educational level and created 4 categories of education. Frequency distributions of income for each of 16 subgroups of race by gender by education were developed. The modal income within each subgroup was then assigned to the missing cases for that subgroup. The imputed income variable and the original income variable had similar means, medians, and standard deviations. The mean and median annual income of this sample is within the $20,000–24,000 range.

Stressor variables included caregivers' self-report of physical health, the number of spouse's limitations in physical activities of daily living (PADL), behavior problem upset, and task distress. Caregiver's physical health was measured by a self-report rating from 1 (poor) to 4 (excellent), mean of 2.8 (SD = 0.9). Seven PADL limitations of mobility, eating, dressing, grooming, bed mobility, bathing, and toileting were coded 0 or 1 and summed. The mean level of spouse PADL impairment for male caregivers was 4.2 (SD = 2.8; range 0–7) with an internal consistency reliability of .95.

Behavior problem upset refers to caregiver reactions to the disruptive behaviors exhibited by people who have dementia. Such disruptive behaviors include emotional lability (irritability or volatile outbursts); management problems (wandering, destroying property, or aggressiveness); behavioral changes (hoarding or hiding things, misplacing or losing objects, starting but not completing tasks); and cognitive problems (forgetfulness or confusing the present and the past) (Niederehe & Fruge, 1984). The Behavior Problem Upset Index summed the cross-product of the frequency of occurrence of 28 behaviors (1 = never to 5 = every day) with a 4-point scale rating the amount of upset created by each problem (0 = none to 3 = a lot). The scale range was 0 to 271, with a mean of 65.07 (SD = 18.2).

Task distress reflects the amount of effort or difficulty caregivers experience in performing caregiving-related tasks. The amount of distress, effort, or difficulty was assessed on a 5-point scale (1 = little or none to 5 = a great deal) for 12 tasks (personal care, assistance with mobility, emotional support, monitoring symptoms, managing finances, other household tasks, and planning or coordinating services). Scores were summed, with a potential range of 12 to 60. The mean level of direct care distress was 19.0 (SD = 8.6). Internal consistency reliability was .89 (Cronbach's alpha).

Resources were measured by social support (the number of helpers a caregiver had) and by a personality trait (i.e., caregiver mastery). Social supports was operationalized by asking caregivers to list all the persons who helped them in providing care for their care-receiver. The mean value for male caregivers was 6.7 (SD = 3.9) out of a range from 0 to 20.

Caregiver mastery expresses a general feeling of competence in caregiving (Lawton, Kleban, Moss, Rovine, & Glicksman, 1989). Based on a 4-point Likert scale of 1 = strongly disagree and 4 = strongly agree, caregivers were asked about the degree of uncertainty they experienced in knowing how to care, if they felt reassured that their care-receiver was getting proper care, if they felt they should be doing more for their care-receiver, if they felt able to handle most problems, and if they had a sense of understanding about what was needed. The sample mean was 14.1 (SD = 2.0). Similar to Lawton et al. (1992), the reliability was moderate (Cronbach's alpha = .58).

Reflecting a lack of consensus in the caregiving literature about the appropriate methods for measuring caregiving outcomes, we chose three caregiving outcomes: caregiver depression as a general measure of distress, caregiver role strain as an indicator of specific caregiver distress, and caregiver satisfaction. The general measure of distress is the Center for Epidemiologic Studies Depression Scale (CES-D), a 20-item, self-report, scale with a range from 0 to 60 (Radloff, 1977). The mean level of CES-D among male caregivers was 12.4 (SD = 9.9). Inter-item reliability was high for this sample (Cronbach's alpha =.90).

The Caregiver Global Role Strain scale is a 3-item summary measure that asks about (a) caregivers' reactions to the confinement associated with caregiving, (b) the general difficulty they experienced in caregiving, and (c) the overall stress they experienced from caregiving obligations (Archbold, Stewart, Greenlick, & Harvath, 1990). The mean score was 15.5 (SD = 4.5) out of a range from 7 to 26, with a moderate inter-item reliability (Cronbach's alpha = .79). The general (CES-D) and caregiver specific measures of distressed mood were moderately correlated (r = .60), as would be expected between two measures of the same concept. Caregiver satisfaction was a 7-item summary scale of Likert scales responses to items such as enjoying being with an older person, feeling closer to them, taking care of them because caregiver wanted to, etc. (Lawton et al., 1989). The mean score was 21 (SD = 2.5; range 14–28) with Cronbach's alpha reliability of .81.

RESULTS

Table 5.1 presents the means of the study variables by race. A series of *t* tests indicated that significant race differences occurred only on income and depression. Thus, Hypothesis 1, which posits race differences in depression, global role strain, and satisfaction was only partially supported. African American male caregivers reported significantly lower levels of depression compared to their Caucasian counterparts.

To test Hypothesis 2, we performed separate hierarchical regressions on depression, role strain, and satisfaction. We entered race and income as the first block, stressors (i.e., caregiver health, task distress, PADL limitations, and behavior problems upsets), and resources (i.e., mastery and number of helpers) as the second block. Changes in the coefficient of race between the two models were assessed to determine the extent to which race effects could be explained by the other variables in the model.

Table 5.2 presents the results of the regression analyses. There is a significant race difference in depression and global role strain that remains even after the other variables are entered into the model. African American male caregivers are less likely to report higher levels of depression or global role strain than are Caucasian male caregivers. The coefficient for race changes only slightly when the stressor and resource variables are included in the model. There are no significant race differences in caregiver satisfaction.

TABLE 5.1   Description of Study Variables by Race

Variables	African American (n = 22)		Caucasian (n = 56)	
	M	SD	M	SD
Income*	11.73	2.47	13.52	2.34
Caregiver Health	2.55	1.01	2.88	0.92
Caregiver's Task Distress	18.09	11.44	19.34	7.34
Care-Receiver's ADL	5.14	2.36	3.84	2.84
Care-Receiver's Behavior Problems	62.60	20.14	66.05	17.42
Caregiver Mastery	13.95	1.86	14.18	2.09
Number of Helpers	5.31	4.36	7.07	3.58
Caregiver Depression*	7.04	9.02	14.48	9.44
Caregiver Role Strain	14.13	4.89	15.96	4.23
Caregiver Satisfaction	21.14	1.45	20.94	2.74

* $p < .05$. t-test of differences by race.

The predictors of each caregiver outcome vary. In addition to race, higher levels of caregiver depression among male caregivers are associated with poorer caregiver health, higher levels of task distress, and lower levels of caregiver mastery. Higher levels of global role strain are associated with higher levels of task distress, more behavior problems of the care-receiver, and lower levels of caregiver mastery, in addition to race. Higher levels of caregiver satisfaction are associated primarily with lower levels of care-receiver's behavior problems and higher levels of caregiver mastery. Although the model variables explain more variance in the two distress outcomes compared to caregiver satisfaction, the amount of variance explained is significant and large for all three outcomes. Thus, these results contribute to identified literature gaps by suggesting that race, caregiver health, task distress, sense of mastery, and the extent of behavior problems in the care-receiver are sources of heterogeneity among male caregivers that are worthy of future study.

FUTURE RESEARCH

The literature review and empirical case study suggest that much remains to be known about patterns of male caregiving. As noted above, most of

TABLE 5.2 Hierarchical OLS Regressions of Predictors on Caregiver Depression, Caregiver Role Strain and Caregiver Satisfaction ($n = 78$)

Variable	Caregiver Depression		Caregiver Role Strain		Caregiver Satisfaction	
	Unstandardized Beta	SE	Unstandardized Beta	SE	Unstandardized Beta	SE
Model 1						
Race (1 = Black)	-8.12**	2.49	-22.56*	1.16	.296	.66
Income	-.383	.45	-.412*	.21	.005	.12
Model 2						
Race (1 = Black)	-7.71**	1.98	-2.33**	.81	.002	.61
Income	-.009	.38	-.281	.15	.105	.12
Caregiver Health	-2.58**	.99	-.411	.41	.002	.30
Caregiver's Task Distress	.509**	.11	.237**	.04	.001	.03
Care-Receiver's ADL	.141	.31	.216	.13	.008	.10
Care-Receiver's Behavior Problems	.003	.05	.007**	.02	-.003**	.02
Caregiver Mastery	-.832*	.42	-.595**	.17	.489**	.13
Number of Helpers	.203	.24	.002	.10	-.139	.07
Adjusted R^2	.380		.566		.253	

* $p \leq .05$
** $p \leq .001$

the studies reviewed were atheoretical and were qualitative or descriptive in nature; as such, they did not test specific models of male caregiving. Many of the qualitative studies, however, did identify variables that could be examined further in the context of different theoretical frameworks, such as anticipatory grief models, elaborated stress process frameworks, or masculinity theories. In exploring models of male caregiving, attention should be directed toward understanding the differences that exist between subgroups of male caregivers (i.e., older men's resistance to using formal social services vs. younger men's use of such services or the differences that appear to exist between African American men vs. Caucasian men as noted in the empirical case study above). By focusing on specific models of male caregiving and on the heterogeneity within male caregivers as a population, future studies would provide essential data to clinical practitioners in designing interventions to promote positive psychosocial adaptation in male caregivers.

With the exception of Kramer and Lambert (1999), the state of knowledge regarding male caregivers' psychosocial adjustment is limited to cross-sectional and qualitative descriptions. Thus, knowledge regarding male caregivers' adaptation over time is largely nonexistent. To answer questions regarding the timing of male caregivers' propensity toward negative psychosocial outcomes or the processes by which stressors and resources are causally linked to specific outcomes, longitudinal research designs are needed. Caregiving is clearly a process that shifts over time as the care-receiver's situation changes. More knowledge is needed about how male caregivers manage transitions in the caregiving experience and adapt to alternating periods of stability and change.

At the same time, the extent to which male caregiving experiences differ in quality from female caregivers in similar situations remains an unresolved issue. Our chapter and this book assume that male caregivers have different experiences from female caregivers and that gender differences in caregiving experiences are relevant and important for researchers, health professionals, and caregivers themselves. Men's caregiving roles are conditioned by the interplay of factors at many levels, ranging from the historical and social structural to the familial to social psychological to individual interactions between person and care situation. The role of gender as a social category at each level is unclear. We continue to know relatively little about the mechanisms by which social categories and socially constructed systems of thought and action occur and the extent to which they express continuity throughout the life course.

REFERENCES

Aneshensel, C. S., Pearlin, L. I., Mullan, J. T., Zarit, S. H., & Whitlatch, C. J. (1995). *Profiles in caregiving: The unexpected career.* San Diego, CA: Academic Press.

Applegate, J. S. (1997). Theorizing older men. In J. I. Kosberg, & L. W. Kaye (Eds.), *Elderly men: Special problems and professional challenges.* New York: Springer.

Applegate, J. S., & Kaye, L. W. (1993). Male elder caregivers. In C. L. Williams (Ed.), *Doing "women's work": Men in nontraditional occupations.* Newbury Park, CA: Sage.

Archbold, P. G., Stewart, B. J., Greenlick, M. R., & Harvath, T. (1990). Mutuality and preparedness as predictors of caregiver role strain. *Research in Nursing and Health, 13,* 375–384.

Archer, C. W., & MacLean, M. J. (1993). Husbands and sons as caregivers of chronically ill elderly women. *Journal of Gerontological Social Work, 21,* 5–23.

Barusch, A. S., & Spaid, W. A. (1989). Gender differences in caregiving: Why do wives report greater burden? *The Gerontologist, 29,* 667–676.

Biegel, D., Sales, E., & Schulz, R. (Eds.). (1991). *Theoretical perspectives on caregiving: Family caregiving in chronic illness.* Newbury Park, CA: Sage.

Blood, G. W., Simpson, K. C., Dineen, M., Kauffman, S. M., & Raimondi, S. C. (1994). Spouses of individuals with laryngeal cancer: Caregiver strain and burden. *Journal of Community Disorders, 27,* 19–35.

Cafferata, G. L., & Stone, R. (1989). The caregiving role: Dimensions of burden and benefits. *Comprehensive Gerontology: Section A, Clinical and Laboratory, 3,* 57–64.

Chatters, L. M., Taylor, R. J., & Jackson, J. S. (1986). Aged Blacks' choices for an informal helper network. *Journal of Gerontology, 41,* 94–100.

Coe, M., & Neufeld, A. (1999). Male caregivers' use of formal support. *Western Journal of Nursing Research, 21,* 568–588.

Collins, C., & Jones, R. (1997). Emotional distress and morbidity in dementia carers: A matched comparison of husbands and wives. *International Journal of Geriatric Psychiatry, 12,* 1168–1173.

Coward, R. T., & Dwyer, J. W. (1990). The association of gender, sibling network composition, and patterns of parent care by adult children. *Research on Aging, 12,* 158–181.

Dwyer, J. W., & Coward, R. T. (1991). A multivariate comparison of the involvement of adult sons versus daughters in the care of impaired parents. *Journal of Gerontology, Social Sciences, 40,* S259–S269.

Eisler, R. M. (1995). The relationship between masculine gender role stress and men's health risk: The validation of a construct. In R. F. Levant & W. S. Pollack (Eds.), *A new psychology of men* (pp. 207–228). New York: Basic Books.

Fitting, M., Rabins, P., Lucas, M. J., & Eastham, J. (1986). Caregivers for dementia patients: A comparison of husbands and wives. *The Gerontologist, 26,* 248–252.

Folkman, S., Chesney, M. A., & Christopher-Richards, A. (1994). Stress and coping in caregiving partners of men with AIDS. *Psychiatric Clinics of North America, 17,* 35–53.

Ford, G. R., Goode, K. T., Barrett, J. J., Harrell, L. E., & Haley, W. E. (1997). Gender roles and caregiving stress: An examination of subjective appraisals of specific primary stressor in Alzheimer's caregivers. *Aging and Mental Health, 1,* 158–165.

Fuller-Jonap, F., & Haley, W. E. (1995). Mental and physical health of male caregivers of a spouse with Alzheimer's Disease. *Journal of Aging and Health, 7,* 99–118.

Gallagher, D., Rose, J., Rivera, P., Lovett, S., & Thompson, L. W. (1989). Prevalence of depression in family caregivers. *The Gerontologist, 29,* 449–456.

Harris, P. B. (1993). The misunderstood caregiver? A qualitative study of the male caregiver of Alzheimer's disease victims. *The Gerontologist, 33,* 551–556.

Harris, P. B. (1995). Differences among husbands caring for their wives with Alzheimer's disease: Qualitative findings and counseling implications. *Journal of Clinical Geropsychology, 1,* 97–106.

Harris, P. B. (1998). Listening to caregiving sons: Misunderstood realities. *The Gerontologist, 38,* 342–352.

Hinrichsen, G. A. (1991). Adjustment to caregivers to depressed older adults. *Psychology and Aging, 6,* 631–639.

Hinrichsen, G. A., & Ramirez, M. (1992). Black and White dementia caregivers: A comparison of their adaptation, adjustment, and service utilization. *The Gerontologist, 32,* 375–381.

Hirsch, C. (1996). Understanding the influence of gender role identity on the assumption of family caregiving roles by men. *Journal of Aging and Human Development, 42,* 103–121.

Horowitz, A. (1985). Sons and daughters as caregivers to older parents: Differences in role performance and consequences. *The Gerontologist, 25,* 612–617.

Horowitz, A. (1992). Methodological issues in the study of gender within family caregiving relationships. In J. W. Dwyer & R. T. Coward (Eds.), *Gender, families, and elder care* (pp.132–150). Newbury Park, CA: Sage.

Ikels, C. (1983). The process of caretaker selection. *Research on Aging, 5,* 491–509.

Jutras, S., & Veilleux, F. (1991). Gender roles and care giving to the elderly: An empirical study. *Sex Roles, 25,* 1–18.

Kaye, L. W., & Applegate, J. S. (1990a). *Men as caregivers to the elderly:*

Understanding and aiding unrecognized family support. Lexington, MA: Lexington Books.

Kaye, L. W., & Applegate, J. S. (1990b). Men as elder caregivers: A response to changing families. *American Journal of Orthopsychiatry, 60,* 86–95.

Kaye, L. W., & Applegate, J. S. (1994). Older men and family caregiving orientation. In E. Thompson (Ed.), *Older men's lives.* Thousand Oaks, CA: Sage.

Kaye, L. W., & Applegate, J. S. (1995). Men's style of nurturing elders. In D. Sabo & D. F. Gordon (Eds.). *Men's health and illness: Gender, power, and the body.* Thousand Oaks, CA: Sage.

Kramer, B. J. (1997). Differential predictors of strain and gain among husbands caring for wives with dementia. *The Gerontologist, 37,* 239–249.

Kramer, B. J., & Kipnis, S. (1995). Eldercare and work role conflict: Toward an understanding of gender differences in caregiver burden. *The Gerontologist, 35,* 340–348.

Kramer, B. J., & Lambert, J. D. (1999). Caregiving as a lifecourse transition among older husbands: A prospective study. *The Gerontologist, 39,* 658–667.

Lawton, M. P., Kleban, M. H., Moss, M., Rovine, M., & Glicksman, A. (1989). Measuring caregiver appraisal. *Journal of Gerontology: Psychological Sciences, 44,* P61–P71.

Lawton, M. P., Rajagopal, D., Brody, E., & Kleban, M. (1992). The dynamics of caregiving for a demented elder among Black and White families. *Journal of Gerontology: Social Sciences, 47,* S156–S164.

Lutzky, S. M., & Knight, B. G. (1994). Explaining gender differences in caregiver distress: The roles of emotional attentiveness and coping styles. *Psychology and Aging, 9,* 513–519.

Marks, N. F. (1998). Does it hurt to care? Caregiving, work-family conflict, and midlife well-being. *Journal of Marriage and the Family, 60,* 951–966.

Mathew, L. J., Mattocks, K., & Slatt, L. M. (1990). Exploring the roles of men: Caring for demented relatives. *Journal of Gerontological Nursing, 16,* 19–25.

Matthews, S. H., & Heidorn, J. (1998). Meeting filial responsibilities in brothers-only sibling groups. *Journal of Gerontology: Social Sciences, 53B,* S278–S286.

Mays, G. D., & Lund, C. H. (1999). Male caregivers of mentally ill. *Perspectives in Psychiatric Care, 35,* 19–28.

Miller, B. (1989). Adult children's perceptions of caregiver stress and satisfaction. *The Journal of Applied Gerontology, 8,* 275–293.

Miller, B. (1991). Elderly married couples, gender, and caregiver strain. *Advances in Medical Sociology, 2,* 245–266.

Miller, B., & Cafasso, L. (1992). Gender differences in caregiving: Fact or artifact? *The Gerontologist, 32,* 498–507.

Miller, B., Campbell, R. T., Farran, C. T., Kaufman, J. E., & Davis, L. (1995). Race, control, mastery and caregiver distress. *Journal of Gerontology: Social Sciences, 50B,* S374–S382.

Miller, B., & Kaufman, J. E. (1996). Beyond gender stereotypes: Spouse caregivers of persons with dementia. *Journal of Aging Studies, 10,* 189–204.

Mintzer, J. E., & Macera, C. A. (1992). Prevalence of depressive symptoms among White and African American caregivers of demented patients. *American Journal of Psychiatry, 149,* 575–576.

Montgomery, R. J. V., & Kamo, Y. (1989). Parent care by sons and daughters. In J. A. Mancini. (Ed.), *Aging parents and adult children.* Lexington, MA: Lexington Books.

Motenko, A. K. (1988). Respite care and pride in caregiving: The experience of six older men caring for their wives. In S. Reinharz & G. D. Rowles (Eds.), *Qualitative gerontology.* New York: Springer.

Mui, A. C. (1995). Caring for frail elderly parents: A comparison of adult sons and daughters. *The Gerontologist, 35,* 86–93.

Niederehe, G., & Fruge, E. D. (1984). Dementia and family dynamics: Clinical research issues. *Journal of Geriatric Psychiatry, 17,* 21–56.

Parson, K. (1997). The male experience of caregiving for a family member with Alzheimer's disease. *Qualitative Health Research, 7,* 391–407.

Picot, S. J. F., Youngblut, J., & Zeller, R. (1997). Development and testing of a measure of perceived caregiver rewards in adults. *Journal of Nursing Measurement, 5,* 33–52.

Pruchno, R. A., & Potashnik, S. L. (1989). Caregiving spouses: Physical and mental health in perspective. *Journal of the American Geriatric Society, 37,* 697–705.

Pruchno, R., & Resch, N. (1989). Husbands and wives as caregivers: Antecedents of depression and burden. *The Gerontologist, 29,* 159–165.

Radloff, L. S. (1977). The CESD scale: A self report depression scale for research in the general population. *Applied Psychological Measurement, 1,* 385–401.

Scanlon, J. M., Vitaliano, P. P., Ochs, H., Savage, M. V., & Borson, S. (1998). CD4 and CD8 counts are associated with interactions of gender and psychosocial stress. *Psychosomatic Medicine, 60,* 644–653.

Schulz, R., O'Brien, A. T., Bookwala, M. S., & Fleissner, K. (1995). Psychiatric and physical morbidity effects of dementia caregiving: Prevalence, correlates, and causes. *The Gerontologist, 30,* 228–235.

Silverstein, M., & Waite, L. J. (1993). Are Blacks more likely than Whites to receive and provide social support in middle and old age? Yes, no, and maybe so. *Journal of Gerontology: Social Sciences, 48,* S212–S222.

Siriopoulos, G., Browne, Y., & Wright, K. (1999). Caregivers of wives with Alzheimer's disease: Husband's perspectives. *American Journal of Alzheimer's Disease, 14,* 79–87.

Smerglia, V., Deimling, G. T., & Barresi, C. M. (1988). Black/White family comparisons in helping and decision making networks of impaired elderly. *Family Relations, 37*, 305–309.

Starrels, M. E., Ingersoll-Dayton, B., Dowler, D. W., & Neal, M. B. (1997). The stress of caring for a parent: Effects of the elder's impairment on an employed adult child. *Journal of Marriage and the Family, 59*, 860–872.

Stoller, E. (1990). Males as helpers: The role of sons, relatives, and friends. *The Gerontologist, 35*, 771–791.

Stommel, M., Given, B. A., Given, C. W., Kalaian, H. A., Schulz, R., & McCorkel, R. (1993). Gender bias in the measurement properties of the Center for Epidemiologic Studies Depression Scale (CES-D). *Psychiatry Research, 49*, 239–250.

Taylor, R. J. (1988). Aging and supportive relationships among Black Americans. In J. Jackson (Ed.), *The Black American elderly.* New York: Springer.

Vinick, B. H. (1984). Elderly men as caretakers of wives. *Journal of Geriatric Psychiatry, 17*, 61–68.

Vitaliano, P. P., Russo, J., & Niaura, R. (1995). Plasma lipids and their relationships with psychosocial factors in older adults. *Journal of Gerontology: Psychological Sciences, 50B*, P18–P24.

Walker, A. J. (1992). Conceptual perspectives on gender and family caregiving. In J. W. Dwyer & R. T. Coward (Eds.), *Gender, families, and elder care.* Newbury Park, CA: Sage.

Williamson, G. M., & Schulz, R. (1990). Relationship orientation, quality of prior relationship, and distress among caregivers of Alzheimer's patients. *Psychology and Aging, 5*, 502–509.

Young, R. F., & Kahana, E. (1989). Specifying caregiver outcomes: Gender and relationship aspects of caregiving strain. *The Gerontologist, 29*, 660–666.

Zarit, S. H., Todd, P. A., & Zarit, J. M. (1986). Subjective burden of husbands and wives as caregivers: A longitudinal study. *The Gerontologist, 26*, 260–266.

Physiological Challenges Associated With Caregiving Among Men[1]

6

Karen A. Adler
Thomas L. Patterson
Igor Grant

INTRODUCTION

Although it is generally accepted that caregiving is a potent chronic stressor that can lead to significant psychological distress (e.g., Dura, Stukenberg, & Kiecolt-Glaser, 1990; Redinbaugh, MacCullum, & Kiecolt-Glaser, 1995; Vitaliano, Scanlan, Krenz, Schwartz, & Marcovina, 1996), a smaller but growing body of evidence suggests that caregiving also has important ramifications for physical health and well-being (Grant, 1999; Vitaliano, 1997). Several cross-sectional studies have shown that when compared to non-caregiving controls, caregivers report lower levels of perceived health (Schulz, O'Brien, Bookwala, & Fleissner, 1995), a greater number of physical symptoms (Cohen & Eisdorfer, 1988; Deimling, Bass, Townsend, & Noelker, 1989; Haley, Levine, Brown, Berry, & Hughes, 1987; Moritz, Kasl, & Berkman, 1989; Sainsbury & Grad de Alarcon, 1970; Satariano, Minkler, & Langhauser, 1984; Stone, Cafferata, & Sangle, 1987), and more chronic illnesses (Pruchno & Potashnik, 1989). In addition, it has been demonstrated that caregivers mount poorer immune responses to viral challenges (Glaser & Kiecolt-Glaser, 1997) and evidence slower rates of wound healing (Kiecolt-Glaser, Marucha, Malarkey, Mercado, & Glaser, 1995) than do age-matched controls.

Further evidence of the health hazards involved with caregiving comes from longitudinal studies. A survival analysis conducted with spousal caregivers of persons with Alzheimer's disease (AD) revealed that, as

This work was supported by National Institute on Aging of the National Institutes of Health Grant 9 RO1AG 15301 to I.G.

compared to age-matched controls, there was a trend (p < .08) for care-givers to experience a greater risk for developing a serious illness over a three-year period (Shaw et al., 1997). In a second, related study, caregivers were found to be at elevated risk for developing mild hypertension over a six-year interval (Shaw et al., 1999). Furthermore, a recent prospective study (Schulz & Beach, 1999) found that the relative risk for all-cause mortality among older spousal caregivers experiencing caregiver strain was 63% higher than that which was seen in non-caregiving controls.

Most studies in this area have not specifically examined the effect of caregiver gender on the physiological effects of providing care. However, the handful of studies that have addressed these issues appear to indicate that, in general, caregiving men are experiencing a greater level of physiological disturbance than caregiving women (Irwin et al., 1997; Mills et al., 1997; Moritz, Kasl, & Ostfeld, 1992; Scanlan, Vitaliano, Ochs, Savage, & Borson, 1998; Vitaliano, Russo, & Niaura, 1995). These findings run counter to those mentioned previously on the psychological well-being of caregiving men and women and underscore the importance of examining the effects of caregiving in multiple outcome domains before making any conclusive statements about which types of caregivers may be at elevated risk for experiencing decrements in health or well-being.

Although the majority of caregivers have traditionally been women, growing numbers of men (spouses, partners, sons, brothers) are now assuming the caregiving role (Hoffman & Mitchell, 1998). The implications of such a shift must be examined not only in terms of its social and psychological impact but also in terms of the consequences to the physical health of the caregiver. Furthermore, physical health needs to be assessed not only through the use of self-report instruments that could be subject to response bias but also through the measurement of objective physiological responses such as blood pressure and immune functioning.

Admittedly, there is a limited amount of evidence indicating that men who are caregivers may exhibit particularly pronounced physiological responses to the stressors involved with providing care. However, there is considerable evidence suggesting that men as a whole may be more physiologically reactive to psychosocial stressors when compared with women. A tendency toward a pronounced response to stress may serve to place men at particular risk for developing a stress-related physical illness in response to providing care for a chronically ill loved one.

DISEASE MORBIDITY AND MORTALITY

One reason that it is possible to speculate that caregiving would have particularly detrimental health consequences for men comes from the available statistics and research on the sex differential in the prevalence of several fatal diseases as well as in all-cause mortality rates. Even though women experience more illnesses, men have shorter life expectancies (Ory & Warner, 1990; Verbrugge 1985, 1989; Wingard, 1984). It appears that although women experience a greater number of acute and nonfatal chronic conditions, men have a higher prevalence for fatal diseases such as coronary heart disease and chronic obstructive pulmonary diseases (Verbrugge, 1989). In addition, the all-cause mortality rates for males are higher than those for females at every age group from infancy to 85 and older (see Wingard). Researchers have attempted to account for these differences by examining various social and lifestyle factors that differ as a function of gender and could contribute to women's excess morbidity on the one hand, and men's excess mortality, on the other. Some of these factors include those of lifestyle (exercise, smoking, drinking); roles, stress, and socioeconomic status; as well as health attitudes, psychological factors (mastery, self-esteem), structural-enabling factors (number of committed hours, having insurance or a regular physician); and, finally, health reporting behaviors.

When all of these factors were statistically equated across genders, however, instead of causing gender differences in morbidity and mortality to shrink or disappear, they actually widened (Verbrugge, 1989). If men and women were equal on all risk factors for illness and death, not only would men have higher mortality rates, but they would also have higher morbidity rates than women, as indexed by the number of illnesses, doctor's visits, prescription medication use, and days spent in bed reported. Verbrugge proposes that psychosocial factors can account for women's current excesses in morbidity, but biological factors apparently underlie men's higher mortality rates. She concludes that when psychosocial factors are adjusted for and equated between groups, men not only die at a younger age but also experience more illness than women, indicating an underlying vulnerability that cannot be accounted for by differences in access to care, lifestyle, psychological variables, or reporting behavior.

It is interesting to note that the gender difference in mortality rates has increased dramatically from 1920 to the present, a time frame that coincides with the shift in leading causes of death away from childbirth-related injury and infectious disease to diseases more strongly associated with stress, lifestyle factors, and health behaviors (diet, exercise, smoking). If these two trends are at all related, one could speculate that men may be particularly susceptible to acquiring fatal illnesses associated with stress and lifestyle factors, a hypothesis with serious implications for the male caregiver under chronic stress.

Another factor that may serve to place male spousal caregivers at elevated risk has to do with the protective effect of marriage upon health. It has been shown that the death rate from many illnesses, including heart disease and many forms of cancer, are consistently lower for married individuals than for those who are either single or divorced. Furthermore, the health benefits conferred by marriage have been shown to be considerably greater for married men than for married women (Berkson, 1962), implying that marriage may be a particularly salient factor for men's health. It has been suggested that the consequences of the alteration of the marital relationship that occurs in spousal caregivers, particularly those of persons with dementia, may prove to be especially difficult for men and may serve as an added risk for decrements in health (Vitaliano, 1997).

The remainder of the chapter will review research exploring the possibility that men may be particularly vulnerable to the physiological consequences of caregiving. The authors will also attempt to elucidate the mechanisms that may underie this effect. First, we will present a review of studies directly examining the effects of caregiving on men's physical and physiological well-being. Second, we will review the related research investigating physiological responses to acute stressors in men as a whole. We include the latter review because (a) the available literature specifically examining the relationship between gender and physiological correlates of caregiving is quite limited and (b) the findings from this broader but related field of study may have direct implications for men facing the chronic stress of caregiving. Finally, we will summarize and synthesize the findings presented and provide recommendations for future research.

PHYSIOLOGICAL CORRELATES OF STRESS AND CAREGIVING IN MEN

In 1997, Irwin and colleagues conducted a study examining the neurohormonal and immune functioning of a group of 100 spousal caregivers of persons with Alzheimer's disease as well as 33 age and gender-matched controls. Although the authors did not find significant group differences between caregivers and controls on natural killer cell activity (an index of the robustness of the immune response) or plasma neurohormones such as cortisol and epinephrine, it was found that both older age and male gender predicted elevated basal levels of adrenocorticotrophic hormone (ACTH) (Irwin et al., 1997). ACTH is a peptide hormone released by the pituitary gland under stressful circumstances. It in turn stimulates the adrenal cortex to secrete cortisol, which is the major stress hormone in humans. Thus, it appears that in this study, caregiving and control men were experiencing greater levels of stress (as measured by physiological indicators) than were caregiving or control women.

Various parameters of cardiovascular functioning have also been examined in men who are caregivers. Moritz et al. (1992) studied a group of 318 men and women providing in-home care for their spouse with a cognitive impairment. The authors examined the relationship between the level of cognitive impairment of the care recipient and the blood pressure and health status of the spousal caregiver. It was found that the level of cognitive impairment in wives predicted elevated systolic blood pressure and perceived declines in health status in their caregiving husbands. However, cognitive impairment in husbands that were being cared for was not associated with either systolic blood pressure or perceived declines in health status in the wives who were providing care. This study appears to indicate that men who are caregivers may be particularly responsive to parameters of the caregiving situation (e.g., level of cognitive impairment) in terms of both their cardiovascular functioning and physical well-being.

Further evidence of cardiovascular risk in caregiving men comes from a study linking psychosocial factors to plasma lipid levels in a group of men and women caring for a spouse with Alzheimer's disease as well as a control of group of age and gender-matched men and women whose spouses did not require care. For the group as a whole, it was found that both expressed and controlled anger, as well as anger held in (Type A behavior), avoidance coping, and being a caregiver predicted a less favorable lipid profile. It was also shown that male caregivers had higher triglyceride (TG) levels and lower levels of high-density lipoproteins (HDLC) when compared to male controls, whereas female caregivers did not differ as a group from female controls in terms of plasma lipid concentrations (Vitaliano et al., 1995). A favorable lipid profile includes low levels of total cholesterol, low-density lipoproteins, and triglycerides, with concomitantly high levels of high-density lipoproteins, or "good" cholesterol. The pattern exhibited by men who are caregivers is clearly in the opposite direction, indicating possible risk for atherosclerosis or other cardiac complications.

Psychosocial stress and immune function has also been studied in a group of men and women Alzheimer caregivers as well as a group of men and women age-matched controls (Scanlan et al., 1998). Data collection was conducted at a baseline visit and then repeated at a follow-up time point. The authors found that male caregivers had lower absolute counts of CD4 (helper) cells when compared to male controls; however, no such difference was evident for the women. In addition, at the first time point the ratio of CD4 (helper) cells to CD8 (suppressor) cells (CD4/CD8 ratio) was correlated to daily hassles for men but not for women. The authors concluded that, in the study, the majority of psychoimmunological relationships were dependent on male gender, indicating that men may be more vulnerable to the physiological consequences of caregiving stress.

The effects of chronic stress and life events on lymphocyte β-receptor sensitivity was examined in another group of older spousal caregivers of persons with Alzheimer's disease (Mills et al., 1997). It was determined that 30% of the variance in β-receptor sensitivity on the lymphocyte cells of the immune system could be accounted for by the combination of a high life stress rating, increased age, lower norepinephrine levels, and male gender, once again suggesting that male caregivers may be particularly vulnerable to immune alterations as a result of the chronic stress associated with caregiving.

Overall, studies examining caregiver gender as a predictor of various physiological correlates of neuroendocrine functioning, cardiovascular disease, and changes in immune functioning have found that men who are caregivers appear to have elevations in parameters that have traditionally been associated with increased risk for disease as well as decrements in parameters associated with good health. This suggests that the notion that men are protected from the adverse health effects of caregiving when compared to women does not generalize to physical health. Although there have been studies that have indicated that caregiving women report a greater number of physical symptoms or rate their health to be poorer than caregiving men (e.g., Pruchno & Potashnik, 1989; Rose-Rego, Strauss, & Smyth, 1998), these studies typically assessed physical health via self-report measures. It is possible that these measures were subject to response bias that may have been gender-related in origin. For example, it is known that depressed individuals have a tendency to experience some level of memory distortion, wherein negative events are recalled more readily than positive events. If the women caregivers in the sample had higher levels of depression than the men (which was often the case), they may have recalled their physical ailments and illnesses at a disproportionate rate, thus obscuring the true relationship between caregiver gender and physical health.

Regardless of the accuracy of gender differences in health as assessed by self-report measures, the studies reviewed above shed light on the possibility that men may be experiencing deleterious physiological alterations in response to caregiving, irrespective of the subjective level of stress that they are experiencing. In order to further assess the hypothesis that men may be particularly physiologically responsive to stress, below we review literature on gender differences in the response to acute psychosocial stressors. However, before presenting this literature, we will first provide readers with a brief overview of the human stress response.

THE HUMAN STRESS RESPONSE

The body's physiological response to stress can best be conceptualized as a broad-based neural and hormonal effort to quickly mobilize the resources necessary to survive an immediately threatening situation, while minimizing the effort spent on the slower, anabolic processes associated with long-term well-being. For example, when the stress response is activated, fats and sugars are released into the bloodstream, while digestion and the building of new muscle mass is halted (Selye, 1956). Obviously, this system works best for brief, discrete stressors that primarily require a physical response to the stressful stimuli, such as fighting with a rival or fleeing for one's life. It is less appropriate for mental challenges such as taking a difficult examination, and it is particularly unsuited for long-term psychosocial stressors such as caring for a sick relative. However, since the inception of stress research (Selye) it has been noted that the body's way of responding to markedly different stressors tends to be strikingly similar.

When a stressor is perceived in either the internal or external environment, two distinct but related neuroendocrine pathways are activated. In the first of these pathways, the hypothalamic-pituitary-adrenal (HPA) axis, the hypothalamus releases a hormone known as corticotrophin-releasing factor (CRF) into the portal circulation, which stimulates the corticotroph cells of the pituitary gland to release stores of ACTH. ACTH travels through the bloodstream until it arrives at the adrenal gland, at which point it triggers cells in the adrenal cortex to release cortisol, a glucocorticoid steroid hormone, and the major mediator of the stress response in humans. Cortisol then goes on to induce a number of important metabolic and physiologic changes, including increasing the levels of blood glucose, amino acids, and serum free fatty acids, while inhibiting the formation of glycogen and the synthesis of new proteins. In addition, cortisol interacts with receptors on immune cells, causing transient immune activation followed by immune suppression. Aldosterone, a mineralocorticoid hormone often released together with cortisol, acts to increase both sodium retention and potassium excretion, causing plasma volume to expand and systemic blood pressure to rise.

The second branch of the stress response, the sympatho-adrenal-medullary (SAM) axis, involves the sympathetic branch of the autonomic nervous system (ANS) that, along with the parasympathetic branch, helps to regulate essential involuntary processes such as heart rate, body temperature, respiration, and digestion. The sympathetic and parasympathetic components of the ANS tend to serve as two opposing arms of the same regulatory system, so that, for example, sympathetic activation causes the heart to contract harder and beat faster, while the parasympathetic vagus nerve fires in order to slow the heart down.

In general, the sympathetic nervous system is associated with catabolic, energy-expending endeavors such as running a race, while parasympathetic influence is most prominent during normal, daily functioning when the body is essentially at rest. When the sympathetic nervous system is activated by the presence of a stressor, the autonomic sympathetic ganglia are stimulated and release norepinephrine, which triggers the adrenal medulla to secrete epinephrine (adrenaline) into the peripheral circulation. Known collectively as catecholamines, norepinephrine and epinephrine act to mediate many of the same processes described above in relation to cortisol, including increasing blood glucose levels and suppressing insulin secretion. However, they also possess certain actions distinct from those of cortisol. Most prominently, catecholamines acting at α adrenergic receptors on blood vessels cause vasoconstriction, so that the diameter of the blood vessel is decreased and blood pressure is therefore increased. Epinephrine and norepinephrine also act at myocardial β-receptors to increase the rate and strength of heart muscle contractions, again raising blood pressure due to resultant increases in contractility, stroke volume, and cardiac output.

It is evident why such alterations are adaptive in the short term. If you are participating in a 100-meter dash, you would want your respiration rate and blood pressure to increase so that the maximum amount of oxygen can reach the muscles of your arms and legs. In addition, the higher levels of glucose and free fatty acids traveling through your bloodstream indicate that quick sources of energy are available to help power those muscles. However, if these changes persisted much past the end of the race, it is equally easy to see how they would quickly become maladaptive and deleterious.

Long-term stressors, such as providing care for a loved one with a chronic illness, can lead to chronic arousal and constant activation of the HPA and SAM axes, which can, in theory, provoke or exacerbate cardiovascular illness (increased cardiac output, total peripheral resistance, sodium, and serum lipids), immune dysfunction (e.g., suppression of natural killer cell activity), and diabetes (elevated serum glucose, insulin suppression).

It is possible that for men placed in the caregiving role a confluence of factors may create particular risk for developing a potentially fatal stress-related illness as a product of caregiving. Figure 6.1 provides a general model linking characteristics of the caregiver; to stressors, mediators, and physiologic outcomes. We will now turn to the literature on gender, health, and the physiological response to stress in an attempt to assess the validity of this statement and to identify the putative mechanisms underlying any detected gender differential in the stress response.

THE HYPOTHALAMIC-PITUITARY-ADRENAL AXIS

There have been a number of investigations aimed at determining whether gender differences in HPA activation exist at the level of the hypothalamus,

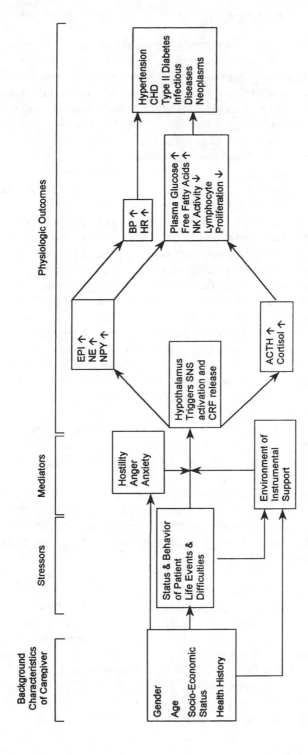

FIGURE 6.1 General model linking perceived stress to physiological response (adapted from Grant, 1999). ACTH = adrenocorti-cotropic hormone; BP = blood pressure; CNS = central nervous system; CRF = corticotrophin releasing factor; EPI = epinephrine; HR = heart rate; CHD = coronary heart disease; NK = natural killer cells; NPY = Neuropeptide Y.

pituitary, or adrenal gland. In a study designed to assess sex differences in both pituitary and adrenal responses to stimulation, Gallucci et al. (1993) administered a standardized bolus injection of ovine-corticotropic-releasing hormone (o-CRH) to a group of men and women and examined their subsequent total plasma ACTH and cortisol responses over a 120-minute time period. Although there were no differences in resting levels of ACTH, the authors found that men had a significantly lower peak ACTH response to o-CRH and greater total (total area under the concentration-time curve) and net (area under the concentration-time curve corrected for baseline) ACTH levels over the course of the sampling period. By contrast, cortisol levels did not differ significantly as a function of gender, both at rest and in response to challenge, despite the smaller amount of ACTH produced by the male participants. There were no differences in men and women in either peak or total cortisol responses over time, although men's net cortisol response was marginally lower than women's (p < .07), mostly owing to the fact that women's plasma cortisol levels remained significantly more elevated than men's at the 90- and 120-minute sampling points. These findings imply that sex differences in the pituitary and adrenal responses to a purely pharmacological challenge do not exist or are relatively minor. Furthermore, where differences do occur, the direction of the detected differences indicates that men's HPA axes may be less responsive than women's.

In a series of studies that included psychosocial tasks as well as pharmacological and physical challenges, however, it appears that men may actually be more reactive to acute psychosocial stress. Kirschbaum, Wust, and Hellhammer (1992) measured salivary-free cortisol at rest and in response to a variety of stressors, including public speaking, mental arithmetic in front of an audience, anticipation of making a speech, a bolus injection of human-CRF, and bicycle ergometry until exhaustion. The study participants consisted of postpubertal adolescent and young adult males and females at random places in their menstrual cycle. A very interesting pattern of results emerged from these studies. Although there were no gender differences in baseline measures of cortisol or in peak cortisol responses to h-CRH or bicycle ergometry, men had significantly higher peak cortisol levels in response to all three psychosocial challenges. Both men and women experienced significant elevations from baseline during public speaking and mental arithmetic; however, men experienced a 3- to 3.5-fold elevation, while the elevation for women was between 1.5 and 2.5 that of baseline levels, a difference that was significant at the .05 level. It is important to reiterate that men and women were equivalent on resting levels of cortisol for all psychological challenges, so differential ceiling or floor effects need not be considered. Furthermore, in response to the challenge that involved preparing to deliver a speech but then being told that one did not actually have to deliver it, men's cortisol levels rose substantially, while women's levels actually dropped from baseline.

When the results of the two studies are taken together, it appears that although there is not a pronounced *sex* difference in the biological sensitivity of the HPA axis to pharmacological and physical challenges, there is a notable *gender* difference in the level of cortisol produced in response to psychosocial stressors. There are several potential explanations for why such a gender difference may exist. It may be that men cognitively appraised the psychosocial tasks to be more challenging than women did and thus experienced a greater level of stress in response. However, this hypothesis is unlikely because a majority of studies have found that men report lower levels of subjective distress in response to acute laboratory stressors than women (Baum & Grunberg, 1991). Of course, it is possible that men are consistently underreporting their level of distress, potentially masking the magnitude of their true responses. Alternatively, men may not be fully aware of their subjective level of task-induced distress, and this process of repression may actually lead to heightened physiological responsivity in and of itself (Niaura, Herbert, McMahon, & Sommerville, 1992).

It is fairly well established that estrogen can alter the sensitivity of the HPA axis (Kirschbaum et al., 1996; Manin & Delost, 1984; Norman, Smith, Pappas, & Hall, 1992). Therefore, it is possible that the effects described earlier with younger study participants may not be identical to what occurs with older adults who have experienced a decline in reproductive hormone levels. Studies assessing gender effects on the HPA responsivity of older adults have been somewhat inconclusive and possibly inconsistent to that seen with younger samples. Seeman, Singer, and Charpentier (1995) have hypothesized that although HPA responses tend to be greater in young men than in young women, at older ages women's HPA responses exceed that of men's. The authors suggest that such a shift could partially explain the increase in women's levels of risk for diabetes, heart disease, and hypertension after menopause. Some evidence supporting this age-shift has been gained from studies examining gender differences in the response to pharmacological challenges (Greenspan, Rowe, Maitland, McAloon-Dyke, & Elahi, 1993; Heuser et al., 1994).

Seeman et al. (1995) tested the validity of the hypothesis using a more naturalistic stressor. They exposed older (70–79 years) men and women drivers to a driving simulation challenge and measured the resultant levels of plasma ACTH and cortisol. The results of the study confirmed their hypothesis insofar as when the data were analyzed in terms of the likelihood to be above the median for both ACTH and cortisol, there were significantly more female high-responders. However, traditional analysis of variance (ANOVA) techniques revealed no significant gender differences in response to the challenge. Also, given the advanced age of the participants, it is not unreasonable to question if the men in the sample may have had more years of driving experience and would therefore be somewhat more familiar or comfortable with the experimental task. In addition, a similar study examining HPA reactivity in older men and women (mean age 67.6) demonstrated that older men had greater ACTH and salivary cortisol responses to psychosocial stress in a pattern that was almost identical to that seen in younger adults (Kudielka et al., 1998). Because of the limited number of studies that have been conducted, it is difficult to ascertain to what degree gender differences in the HPA response of younger adults generalizes to an older population. It is important for future research into gender and HPA response to include older participants, not only to gain a better understanding of the underlying mechanisms of the response but also to better assess the physiological risks that older men providing care for their spouses are likely to face.

SYMPATHETIC ACTIVATION AND CARDIOVASCULAR REACTIVITY

Exaggerated sympathetic activation in response to stress is thought to be linked to the development of essential hypertension (Fredrikson & Matthews, 1990), which is, in turn, a leading risk factor for coronary heart disease (CHD) (Kannel, Gordon, & Schwartz, 1971), a condition that afflicts more men than women. It has been hypothesized that men may exhibit heightened endocrine and cardiovascular responses to stressors, and this tendency may account for a portion of the variance in the gender difference in CHD prevalence (Stoney, Davis, & Matthews, 1987). In a meta-analytic review, Stoney et al. (1987) concluded that men had consistently greater blood pressure (BP) and urinary catecholamine increases during acute stress, while women tend to be higher in terms of heart rate (HR). Men's excesses in BP reactivity in particular have been confirmed by most (Allen, Stoney, Owens, & Matthews, 1993; Lai & Linden, 1992; Lash, Gillespie, Eisler, & Southard, 1991; Lawler, Harralson, Amstead, & Schmied, 1993; Matthews & Stoney, 1988; McAdoo, Weinberger, Miller, Fineberg, & Grim, 1990; Stoney, Matthews, McDonald, & Johnson, 1988; Treiber et al., 1993) but not all subsequent studies (e.g., Jones et al., 1996).

In addition, it appears that gender moderates the explanatory power of certain risk factors to predict the cardiovascular response to stress. For example, it was shown prospectively that among boys, but not girls, larger systolic blood pressure (SBP) and diastolic blood pressure (DBP) responses to challenge were predictive of higher resting blood pressure levels at subsequent time points (Matthews, Woodall, & Allen, 1993). Similarly, men with a positive family history for hypertension were found to exhibit higher levels of systolic blood pressure in response to stress than men with a negative family history. However, the SBP reactivity of women participants was unrelated to family history (Lawler, Lacy, Armstead, & Lawler, 1991). In a similar vein, a study investigating children's cardiovascular responses to challenging tasks and the angry behavior of adults found that while the sons of hypertensive parents responded to inter-adult anger with greater SBP reactivity than sons of normotensive parents, there was no clear pattern for daughters (Ballard, Cummings, & Larkin, 1993).

In terms of psychological risk factors and the cardiovascular response to challenge, Houston (1988) found that among men, having a Type A behavior pattern was associated with an exaggerated cardiovascular response to stress, whereas Type A did not predict increased responsivity in women. Burns and Katkin (1993) conducted a study in which participants were randomized to perform a stressful reaction time task under one of two conditions: harassment or social evaluation. Subjects' responses were measured in terms of SBP, DBP, and HR changes from a resting baseline. In addition, instruments were used to assess anger expression, hostility, and social-evaluative anxiety. Multiple regression analyses revealed that expressed anger was predictive of cardiovascular reactivity only for men in the harassment condition. Furthermore, hostile men who express anger were found to have the highest levels of cardiovascular reactivity across both situations, while for women, the traits assessed were unable to predict cardiovascular responses to either situation. In a similar study conducted by Lawler and colleagues (1993), it was found that in men, but not women, high expressed hostility was associated with greater diastolic reactivity to both the Stroop color-word conflict challenge and an anger recall interview.

Vogele, Jarvis, and Cheeseman (1997) found that for male college students, the combination of hypertension risk (as indexed by high-normal resting mean arterial pressure) and anger suppression resulted in the largest cardiovascular response to a variety of stressors (cold pressor, mental arithmetic, mirror-tracing). For female college students, however, anger-in scores had no relationship to reactivity, although hypertension risk was able to predict subsequent levels of SBP and DBP reactivity. It is important to note that the groups were equivalent in age, body mass index (BMI), and responses to the psychological questionnaires. In other words, men and women responded to the tasks with equal levels of anger, frustration, and anxiety and exhibited equal levels of trait anger, so the gender differential in the predictive power of anger suppression cannot be attributed to a gender difference in the prevalence of the trait.

It is not only anger and hostility that appear to be differentially linked to cardiovascular reactivity as a function of gender, but negative emotions as well. A prospective study assessing cardiovascular morbidity found that anxiety levels at baseline predicted hypertension 18–20 years later for middle-aged men, but not women (Markovitz, Matthews, Kannel, Cobb, & D'Agostino, 1993).

The observed gender difference in cardiovascular reactivity has been attributed to a number of factors, including differing levels of aggression, hostility, and anger between men and women as well as the protective effects of ovarian hormones, particularly estrogen (e.g., Vogele et al., 1997). Owens, Stoney, and Matthews (1993) conducted a study examining the effect of ovarian hormones on cardiovascular reactivity. Age-matched groups of men, premenopausal women, and postmenopausal women not engaging in hormone replacement therapy were given a series of stressful mental challenges during which time their BP, HR, plasma catecholamines, serum lipids, and lipoproteins were measured. Following this, each participant was fitted with an ambulatory blood pressure monitor that they wore for two consecutive workdays. Postmenopausal women evidenced significantly higher SBP and DBP reactivity when compared with both age-matched men and premenopausal women. Furthermore, postmenopausal women and men showed greater mean ambulatory DBP than premenopausal women. Although this study was cross-sectional in nature, it provides preliminary support that at least a component of the difference in men and women's levels of sympathetic activation in response to stress is mediated by ovarian hormones.

Another indication that estrogen may promote a dampening of the SNS comes from a study involving stress and heart period variability (HPV) (Rossy & Thayer, 1998). HPV refers to the cyclic variations in the length of consecutive regular rate (RR) intervals that occur as a function of different internal physiological rhythms and has been used for the past 30 years to assess the autonomic modulation of the heart. Essentially, the differences in RR interval lengths form a wave pattern that can be decomposed into a series of sine waves of different frequencies through the use of a Fourier transformation. Each frequency component represents the contribution of a different physiological process to the overall level of HPV. For example, high-frequency (HF) power reflects parasympathetic modulation of the heart while low frequency (LF) power reflects a mix of sympathetic and parasympathetic (vagal) influences (Stein & Kleiger, 1999).

In a study examining HPV at rest and then in the context of three different experimental stress tasks designed to differentially activate the sympathetic and vagal branches of the ANS, it was found that at rest and across all three tasks, women evidenced more vagal control of the heart (greater percent HF power), while men evidenced a predominance of sympathetic control of heart rate (greater percent LF power) (Rossy & Thayer, 1998). The authors noted that the pattern of men exhibiting elevated LF power combined with reduced HF power has previously been associated with numerous cardiopathologies (Guzzetti et al., 1991; Langewitz, Ruddel, & Schachinger, 1994; Liao et al., 1996; Tusji et al., 1994, 1996), and posits a pathway by which men find themselves at particular risk for cardiovascular disease morbidity and mortality. The women participating in this study were all premenopausal, and the authors suggest that estrogen is most likely responsible for the gender differences in autonomic control of the heart they observed. This is supported by previous research that indicates that estrogen provides vagal cardiac control in women (Du, Riemersma, & Dart, 1995).

Generally speaking, the hypothesis that estrogen affords protection against the development of atherosclerosis has received wide support. It has been known epidemiologically for quite some time that, relative to men, women are protected from coronary heart disease and coronary artery atherosclerosis during the reproductive years particularly. The increased incidence of coronary artery disease in older women has traditionally been attributed to the reduction in female reproductive hormones, particularly estrogen. However, it should be mentioned that the results of the Heart and Estrogen/progestin Replacement Study (HERS), a randomized controlled trial of the efficacy of hormone replacement therapy in reducing the risk for coronary heart disease events in postmenopausal women with established coronary disease, failed to detect significant differences in risk between placebo and treatment groups (Hulley et al., 1998).

Nevertheless, animal models of coronary heart disease as well as basic research on the mechanisms of action have provided consistent evidence in support of the role of estrogen in protecting against atherosclerotic damage. Extensive research on both animals and humans has revealed much about the mechanisms by which estrogen may confer protection. First, and most notably, estrogen affects serum lipid composition, such that LDL and lipoprotein A levels are lowered while HDL (or "good" cholesterol) and apolipoprotein A-1 are increased. Second, estrogen is a potent oxidant that appears to prevent LDL from being oxidized to a form that is common and pathogenic in atherosclerosis. Oxidized LDL can no longer be recognized by its normal receptor and is instead recognized by the macrophage receptor whose actions are not regulated by the cholesterol content of the cell. This, in turn, allows massive amounts of cholesterol to be taken up into macrophages, which become known as foam cells owing to their appearance once they have been loaded with cholesterol. It is these foam cells that comprise the fatty streak that becomes the site for the later development of fibrofatty lesion and the fibrous plaque which mark clinically significant atherosclerotic disease (Nathan & Chaudhuri, 1997).

Although the effects of estrogens on lipids are substantial, they only account for 25–50% of the observed overall reduction in cardiovascular risk (Nasr & Breckwoldt, 1998). Other important mechanisms include decreasing factors that promote vascular smooth muscle proliferation, such as insulin and plasminogen activator inhibitor (PAI-1), as well as those that affect blood viscosity and fibrinolysis, such as serum fibrinogen and factor VII. In addition, estrogen decreases the expression of certain adhesion molecules that are associated with the inflammatory atherosclerotic process. Estrogen also enhances vasodilation and inhibits vasoconstriction by a number of actions, including by increasing nitric oxide release and by inhibiting voltage-gated calcium channels. Nitric oxide also prevents the migration of vascular smooth muscle cells, which is one of the crucial steps in the development of the atherosclerotic lesion.

Estrogen also protects the integrity of the vascular endothelial cells by promoting healing and angiogenesis and inhibiting tumor necrosis factor, which is responsible for inducing apoptosis in damaged cells. A number of other activities of estrogen have been identified as playing a role in protecting against atherosclerosis, including inhibiting adrenergic responses, downregulating platelet and monocyte reactivity, decreasing serum renin, increasing serum relaxin, and lowering overall systemic blood pressure (Nasr & Breckwoldt, 1998; Nathan & Chaudhuri, 1997).

When the discussion on the mechanisms of action of estrogen is linked with the earlier review of gender differences in sympathetic activation and cardiovascular reactivity, it becomes apparent how estrogen may be responsible for some of the gender effects we presented. For example, the tendency for men to experience greater increases in systolic and diastolic blood pressure in response to a challenge can be better understood by factoring in the effects of estrogen. Imagine that a group of young adult men and women are exposed to an identical stressor that is perceived and appraised in an identical manner by all group members. One would still expect the men to experience more steep increases in blood pressure. The men experience an increase in blood pressure that stems from sympathetic activation roughly equivalent to the perceived magnitude of the stressor. However, even though the women of the group perceive the stressor to be of the same magnitude as the men did, their higher levels of estrogen are more effectively downregulating their adrenergic responses, causing the epinephrine and norepinephrine released by their sympathetic nervous systems to be less effective in causing their blood vessels to narrow and their hearts to beat harder and faster. At the same time, estrogen is promoting nitric oxide release, which causes their blood vessels to widen in diameter, further lessening the cardiovascular load.

The observed gender differences in the ability of psychological constructs such as anxiety and hostility to predict the magnitude of the cardiovascular response may be explained in a similar manner. If a group of young adult men and women are presented with an identical stressor that

they respond to with identical levels of anger, it is unlikely that the resulting increases in autonomic arousal and blood pressure will be identical.
For men, the experience of stress and anger will cause sympathetic nervous system activation, leading to increased catecholamines in circulation
that then bind to receptors which cause the heart to beat faster and with
more strength, leading more blood to be pumped into the circulation. The
catecholamines also bind to a second set of receptors that cause the blood
vessels to constrict in diameter. Now, the increased volume of blood must
flow through a narrower opening, creating a pressure increase that is
vaguely in proportion to the level of stress and anger which initiated the
response. For women, stress and anger will also lead to sympathetic activation. However, when the catecholamines bind to their receptors, less of
a response is generated. The signal telling the blood vessels to narrow is
attenuated by estrogen; first, because it leads adrenergic receptors to
downregulate (decrease in number or become less sensitive), and second,
because estrogen releases nitric oxide that is simultaneously instructing
blood vessels to widen. Therefore, the pathway linking stress and stress-
induced anger to autonomic arousal and a rise in blood pressure is direct
in men but is buffered by the actions of estrogen in women, leading the
overall association between anger and cardiovascular risk to be stronger
and more apparent in men.

These examples demonstrate that when all else is equal, it is predicted
that men will have stronger cardiovascular reactions to stress and that their
level of anxiety, anger, and hostility will be more directly associated with
their blood pressure. However, all else is not equal. Men tend to have
higher levels of hostility than women do (Matthews et al., 1992), confer-
ring additional gender-related risk beyond the sex-related risk of having a reproductive hormone profile that affords less protection than that
of women.

To summarize the role of gender in sympathetic arousal and cardiovascular responses to stress, men often exhibit heightened blood pressure
and catecholamine reactivity and tend to have higher rates of hypertension, atherosclerosis, and coronary heart disease than their female counterparts, particularly during the reproductive years. In addition, certain
risk factors such as family history of hypertension, anger suppression,
hostility, anxiety, and Type A behavior predict blood pressure responses
and subsequent hypertension more accurately for men than for women.
Estrogen has been shown to have many actions that appear to be cardio-
protective and may explain a sizable portion of the observed differences
in cardiovascular functioning between men and women. Despite these
effects, differential risk for death from coronary heart disease cannot be
entirely explained by reproductive hormones (Kannel, 1987; Stoney et al.,
1987). Psychological factors such as cognitive appraisal of stress and level

of anger as well as the proclivity for engaging in risk behaviors (e.g., smoking) must not be discounted. Only by examining the physiological consequences of psychosocial variables can we truly understand the mechanisms by which a complex construct such as gender can influence the body's response to stress.

SUMMARY AND CONCLUSIONS

In this chapter, we have reviewed several sets of findings that indicate that caregiving men may be at particular risk for developing a stress-related illness. Specifically, there is evidence to suggest that caregiving husbands experienced increases in blood pressure and declines in perceived health in response to worsening cognitive abilities in their wives, and men who are caregivers had lipid profiles that were significantly less favorable than those of non-caregiving men. Male caregivers also had higher levels of the stress hormone ACTH than did their female counterparts. The immune system of men caregivers may also be vulnerable. Male caregivers were found to have lowered CD4 counts when compared to male controls, and caregiving men were shown to have alterations in lymphocyte beta-receptor sensitivity.

Although it may be premature to state definitively that men are at increased risk of morbidity and mortality associated with caregiving, evidence suggests the need to pay particular attention to the physical well-being of men who are caregivers. Men have higher all-cause mortality rates than women and past research on gender differences in the response to stress appear to indicate that men tend to have greater increases in blood pressure and cortisol when faced with psychosocial challenges. Sociocultural factors may compound the risk associated with being male as well as the chronic stress associated with caregiving. Specifically, men are less likely than women to be socialized as caregivers; therefore, the nature of the role and the demands that it entails may be somewhat more difficult for a man to adjust to than for a woman, thus creating even greater strain for the male caregiver. Past research into explanatory factors for apparent gender differences in the psychological response to caregiving have identified factors such as differences in emotional awareness and coping style to account for why women caregivers report more distress (Lutzky & Knight, 1994). It is possible that the same factors that lead men to report less psychological distress from caregiving may actually be contributing to their greater levels of physiological distress. Future research should be aimed at directly assessing the interaction of gender and caregiving on physiological responses and physical health to determine if, in fact, male caregivers do suffer disproportionately and if so, why.

Furthermore, the gender of the caregiver should be included as a factor when designing interventions so that the particular needs of men and women caregivers can be assessed and adequately met.

REFERENCES

Allen, M. T., Stoney, C. M., Owens, J. F., & Matthews, K. A. (1993). Hemodynamic adjustments to laboratory stress: The influence of gender and personality. *Psychosomatic Medicine, 55*, 505–517.

Ballard, M. E., Cummings, E. M., & Larkin, K. (1993). Emotional and cardiovascular responses to adults' angry behavior and to challenging tasks in children of hypertensive and normotensive parents. *Child Development, 64*, 500–515.

Baum A., & Grunberg, N. E. (1991). Gender, stress, and health. *Health Psychology, 10*, 80–85.

Berkson, J. (1962). Mortality and marital status. Reflections on the derivation of etiology from statistics. *American Journal of Public Health, 52*, 1318–1324.

Burns, J. W., & Katkin, E. S. (1993). Psychological, situational, and gender predictors of cardiovascular reactivity to stress: A multivariate approach. *Journal of Behavioral Medicine, 16*, 445–465.

Cohen, D., & Eisdorfer, C. (1988). Depression in family members caring for a relative with Alzheimer's disease. *Journal of the American Geriatric Society, 36*, 885–889.

Collins, C. (1992). Carers: Gender and caring for the elderly. In T. Arie (Ed.), *Recent Advances in Psychogeriatrics 2*. London: Churchill Livingstone.

Deimling, G. T., Bass, D. M., Townsend, A. L., & Noelker, L. S. (1989). Care-related stress: A comparison of spouse and adult-child caregivers in shared and separate households. *Journal of Aging and Health, 1*, 67–82.

Du, X., Riemersma, R. A., & Dart, A. M. (1995). Cardiovascular protection by estrogen is partly mediated through modulation of autonomic nervous function. *Cardiovascular Research, 26*, 713–719.

Dura, J. R., Stukenberg, K. W., & Kiecolt-Glaser, J. K. (1990). Chronic stress and depressive disorders in older adults. *Journal of Abnormal Psychology, 99*, 284–290.

Fredrikson, M., & Matthews, K. A. (1990). Cardiovascular responses to behavioral stress and hypertension: A meta-analytic review. *Annals of Behavioral Medicine, 12*, 30–39.

Gallucci, W. T., Baum, A., Lane, L., Rabin, D. S., Chrousos, G. P., Gold, P. W., & Kling, M. A. (1993). Sex differences in the sensitivity of the hypothalamic-pituitary adrenal axis. *Health Psychology, 12*, 420–425.

Glaser, R., & Kiecolt-Glaser, J. K. (1997). Chronic stress modulates the virus-specific immune response to latent herpes simplex virus Type I. *Annals of Behavioral Medicine, 19,* 78–82.

Grant, I. (1999). Caregiving may be hazardous to your health. *Psychosomatic Medicine, 61,* 420–423.

Greenspan, S. L., Rowe, J. W., Maitland, L. A., McAloon-Dyke, M., & Elahi, D. (1993). The pituitary-adrenal glucocorticoid response is altered by gender and disease. *Journal of Gerontology, 48,* M72–M77.

Guzzetti, S., Dassi, S., Pecis, M., Casati, R., Masu, A. M., Longoni, P., Tinelli, M., Cerutti, S., Pagani, M., & Malliani, A. (1991). Altered pattern of circadian neural control of heart period in mild hypertension. *Journal of Hypertension, 9,* 831–838.

Haley, W. E., Levine, E. G., Brown, S., Berry, J. W., & Hughes, G. H. (1987). Psychological, social, and health consequences of caring for a relative with senile dementia. *Journal of the American Geriatric Society, 35,* 405–411.

Heuser, I. J., Gotthardt, U., Schweiger, U., Schmider J., Lammers, C. H., Dettling, M., & Holsboer, F. (1994). Age-associated changes of pituitary-adrenocortical hormone regulation in humans: importance of gender. *Neurobiology of Aging, 15,* 227–231.

Hoffman, R. L., & Mitchell, A. M. (1998). Caregiver burden: historical development. *Nursing Forum, 33,* 5–11.

Houston, B. K. (1988). Cardiovascular and neuroendocrine reactivity, global Type A, and components of Type A behavior. In B. K. Houston & C. R. Snyder (Eds.), *Type A behavior pattern: Research, theory, and intervention* (pp. 212–253). New York: Wiley.

Hulley, S., Grady, D., Bush, T., Furberg, C., Herrington, D., Riggs, B., & Vittinghoff, E. (1998). Randomized trial of estrogen plus progestin for secondary prevention of coronary heart disease in postmenopausal women. Heart and Estrogen/progestin Replacement Study (HERS) Research Group. *Journal of the American Medical Association, 280,* 605–613.

Irwin, M., Hauger, R., Patterson, T. L., Semple, S., Ziegler, M., & Grant, I. (1997). Alzheimer caregiver stress: Basal natural killer cell activity, pituitary-adrenal cortical function, and sympathetic tone. *Annals of Behavioral Medicine, 19,* 83–90.

Jones, P. P., Spraul, M., Matt, K. S., Seals, D. R., Skinner, J. S., & Ravussin, E. (1996). Gender does not influence sympathetic neural reactivity to stress in healthy humans. *American Journal of Physiology, 270,* H350–H357.

Kannel, W. B. (1987). Hypertension and other risk factors in coronary heart disease. *The American Heart Journal, 114,* 918–928.

Kannel, W. B., Gordon, T., & Schwartz, M. J. (1971). Systolic versus diastolic blood pressure and risk of coronary artery disease. *American Journal of Cardiology, 27,* 335–343.

Kiecolt-Glaser, J. K., Marucha, P. T., Malarkey, W. B., Mercado, A. M., & Glaser, R. (1995). Slowing of wound healing by psychological stress. *Lancet, 346,* 1194–1196.

Kirschbaum, C., Schommer, N., Federenko, I., Gaab, J., Neumann, O., Oellers, M., Rohleder, N., Untiedt, A., Hanker, J., Pirke, K. M., & Hellhammer, D. H. (1996). Short-term estradiol treatment enhances pituitary-adrenal axis and sympathetic responses to psychosocial stress in healthy young men. *The Journal of Clinical Endocrinology & Metabolism, 83,* 1756–1761.

Kirschbaum, C., Wust, S., & Hellhammer, D. (1992). Consistent sex differences in cortisol responses to psychological stress. *Psychosomatic Medicine, 54,* 648–657.

Kudielka, B. M., Hellhammer, J., Hellhammer, D. H., Wolf, O. T., Pirke, K. M., Varadi, E., Pilz, J., & Kirschbaum, C. (1998). Sex differences in endocrine and psychological responses to psychosocial stress in healthy elderly subjects and the impact of a 2-week dehydroepiandrosterone treatment. *Journal of Clinical Endocrinology and Metabolism, 83,* 1756–1761.

Lai, J. Y., & Linden, W. (1992). Gender, age, expression style, and opportunity for anger release determine cardiovascular reaction to and recovery from anger provocation. *Psychosomatic Medicine, 54,* 297–310.

Langewitz, W., Ruddel, H., & Schachinger, H. (1994). Reduced parasympathetic cardiac control in patients with hypertension at rest and under mental stress. *The American Heart Journal, 127,* 122–128.

Lash, S. J., Gillespie, B. L., Eisler, R. M., & Southard, D. M. (1991). Sex differences in cardiovascular reactivity: effects of the gender relevance of the stressor. *Health Psychology, 10,* 392–398.

Lawler, K. A., Harralson, T. L., Armstead, C. A., & Schmied, L. A. (1993). Gender and cardiovascular responses: What is the role of hostility? *Journal of Psychosomatic Research, 37,* 603–613.

Lawler, K. A., Lacy, J., Armstead, C. A., & Lawler, J. E. (1991). Family history of hypertension, gender, and cardiovascular responsivity during stress. *Journal of Behavioral Medicine, 14,* 169–186.

Liao, D., Cai, J., Rosamond, W. D., Barnes, R. W., Hutchinson, R. G., Whitsel, E. A., Rautaharju, P., & Heiss, G. (1997). Cardiac autonomic function and incident coronary heart disease: A population-based case-cohort study. *American Journal of Epidemiology, 145,* 696–706.

Lutzky, S. M., & Knight, B. G. (1994). Explaining gender differences in caregiver distress: The roles of emotional attentiveness and coping styles. *Psychology and Aging, 9,* 513–519.

Manin, M., & Delost, P. (1984). Dynamic measure of production rate of cortisol in the mature Guinea pig in response to the stress of anesthesia: Effect of estradiol. *Steroids, 43,* 101–110.

Markovitz, J. H., Matthews, K. A., Kannel, W. B., Cobb, J. L., & D'Agostino, R. B. (1993). Psychological predictors of hypertension in the Framingham Study: Is there tension in hypertension? *The Journal of the American Medical Association, 270*, 2439–2443.

Matthews, K. A., & Stoney, C. M. (1988). Influences of sex and age on cardiovascular responses during stress. *Psychophysiology, 50*, 46–56.

Matthews, K. A., Woodall, K. L., & Allen, M. T. (1993). Cardiovascular reactivity to stress predicts future blood pressure status. *Hypertension, 22*, 479–485.

Matthews, K. A., Woodall, K. L., Engebretson, T. O., McCann, B. S., Stoney, C. M., Manuck, S. B., & Saab, P. G. (1992). Influence of age, sex, and family on Type A and hostile attitudes and behaviors. *Health Psychology, 11*, 317–323.

McAdoo, W. G., Weinberger, M. H., Miller, J. Z., Fineberg, N. S., & Grim, C. E. (1990). Race and gender influence hemodynamic responses to psychological and physical stimuli. *Journal of Hypertension, 8*, 961–967.

Mills, P. J., Ziegler, M. G., Patterson, T. L., Dimsdale, J. E., Hauger, R., Irwin, M., & Grant, I. (1997). Plasma catecholamine and lymphocyte beta2-adrenergic receptor alterations in elderly Alzheimer caregivers under stress. *Psychosomatic Medicine, 59*, 251–256.

Moritz, D. J., Kasl, S. V., & Berkman, L. F. (1989). The health impact of living with a cognitively impaired elderly spouse: Depressive symptoms and social functioning. *Journal of Gerontology: Social Sciences, 44*, S17–S27.

Moritz, D. J., Kasl, S. V., & Ostfeld, A. M. (1992). The health impact of living with a cognitively impaired elderly spouse. *Journal of Aging and Health, 4*, 244–267.

Morris, R. G., Woods, R. T., Davies, K. S., & Morris, L. W. (1991). Gender differences in carers of dementia sufferers. *The British Journal of Psychiatry, 158*, 69–74.

Nasr, A., & Breckwoldt, M. (1998). Estrogen replacement therapy and cardiovascular protection: Lipid mechanisms are the tip of an iceberg. *Gynecological Endocrinology, 12*, 43–59.

Nathan, L., & Chaudhuri, G. (1997). Estrogens and atherosclerosis. *Annual Review of Pharmacology and Toxicology, 37*, 477–515.

Niaura, R., Herbert, P. N., McMahon, N., & Sommerville, L. (1992). Repressive coping and blood lipids in men and women. *Psychosomatic Medicine, 54*, 698–706.

Norman, R. L., Smith, C. J., Pappas, J. D., & Hall, J. (1992). Exposure to ovarian steroids elicits a female pattern of cortisol levels in castrated male macaques. *Steroids, 57*, 37–43.

Ory, M. G., & Warner, H. R. (1990). *Gender, health and longevity: Multidisciplinary perspectives.* New York: Springer.

Owens, J. F., Stoney, C. M., & Matthews, K. A. (1993). Menopausal status influences ambulatory blood pressure levels and blood pressure changes during mental stress. *Circulation, 88*, 2794–2802.

Pruchno, R. A., & Potashnik, S. L. (1989). Caregiving spouses: Physical and mental health in perspective. *Journal of the American Geriatric Society, 37*, 697–705.

Redinbaugh, E. M., MacCullum, R. C., & Kiecolt-Glaser, J. K. (1995). Recurrent syndromal depression in caregivers. *Psychology and Aging, 10*, 358–368.

Rose-Rego, S. K., Strauss, M. E., & Smyth, K. A. (1998). Differences in the perceived well-being of wives and husbands caring for persons with Alzheimer's disease. *The Gerontologist, 38*, 224–230.

Rossy, L. A., & Thayer, J. F. (1998). Fitness and gender-related differences in heart period variability. *Psychosomatic Medicine, 60*, 773–781.

Sainsbury, P., & Grad de Alarcon, J. (1970). The psychiatrist and the geriatric patient. The effects of community care on the family of the geriatric patient. *Journal of Geriatric Psychiatry, 4*, 23–41.

Satariano, W. A., Minkler, M. A., & Langhauser, C. (1984). The significance of an ill spouse for assessing health differences in an elderly population. *Journal of the American Geriatrics Society, 32*, 187–190.

Scanlan, J. M., Vitaliano, P. P., Ochs, H., Savage, M. V., & Borson, S. (1998). CD4 and CD8 counts are associated with interactions of gender and psychosocial stress. *Psychosomatic Med, 60*, 644–653.

Schulz, R., & Beach, S. R. (1999). Caregiving as a risk factor for mortality: The Caregiver Health Effects Study. *The Journal of the American Medical Association, 282*, 2215–2219.

Schulz, R., O'Brien, A. T., Bookwala, J., & Fleissner, K. (1995). Psychiatric and physical morbidity effects of dementia caregiving: Prevalence, correlates, and causes. *The Gerontologist, 35*, 771–791.

Seeman, T. E., Singer, B., & Charpentier, P. (1995). Gender differences in patterns of HPA axis response to challenge: Macarthur studies of successful aging. *Psychoneuroendocrinology, 20*, 711–725.

Selye, H. (1956). *The stress of life*. New York: McGraw-Hill.

Shaw, W. S., Patterson, T. L., Ziegler, M. G., Dimsdale, J. E., Semple, S. J., & Grant, I. (1999). Accelerated risk of hypertensive blood pressure recordings among Alzheimer caregivers. *Journal of Psychosomatic Research, 46*, 215–227.

Shaw, W. S., Patterson, T. L., Semple, S. J., Ho, S., Irwin, M. R., Hauger, R. L., & Grant, I. (1997). Longitudinal analysis of multiple indicators of health decline among spousal caregivers. *Annals of Behavioral Medicine, 19*, 101–109.

Stein, P. K., & Kleiger, R. E. (1999). Insights from the study of heart period variability. *Annual Review of Medicine, 50*, 249–261.

Stone, R., Cafferata, G. L., & Sangle, J. (1987). Caregivers of frail elderly: A national profile. *The Gerontologist, 27*, 616–626.

Stoney, C. M., Davis, M. C., & Matthews, K. A. (1987). Sex differences in physiological responses to stress and in coronary heart disease: A causal link? *Psychophysiology, 24*, 127–131.

Stoney, C. M., Matthews, K. A., McDonald, R. H., & Johnson, C. A. (1988). Sex differences in lipid, lipoprotein, cardiovascular, and neuroendocrine responses to acute stress. *Psychophysiology, 25*, 645–656.

Treiber, F. A., Davis, H., Musante, L., Raunikar, R. A., Strong, W. B., McCaffrey, F., Meeks, M. C., & Vandernoord, R. (1993). Ethnicity, gender, family history of myocardial infarction, and hemodynamic responses to laboratory stressors in children. *Health Psychology, 12*, 6–15.

Tusji, H., Larson, M. G., Venditti, F. J., Jr., Manders, E. S., Evans, J. C., Feldman, C. L., & Levy, D. (1996). Impact of reduced heart rate variability on risk for cardiac events. The Framingham Heart Study. *Circulation, 94*, 2850–2855.

Tusji, H., Venditti, F. J., Jr., Manders, E. S., Evans, J. C., Larson, M. G., Feldman, C. L., & Levy, D. (1994). Reduced heart rate variability and mortality risk in an elderly cohort. The Framingham Heart Study. *Circulation, 90*, 878–883.

Verbrugge, L. M. (1985). Gender and health: An update on hypotheses and evidence. *Journal of Health and Social Behavior, 26*, 156–182.

Verbrugge, L. M. (1989). The twain meet: Empirical explanations of sex differences in health and mortality. *Journal of Health and Social Behavior, 30*, 282–304.

Vitaliano, P. P. (1997). Physiological and physical concomitants to caregiving: Introduction to special issue. *Annals of Behavioral Medicine, 19*, 75–77.

Vitaliano, P. P., Russo, J., & Niaura, R. (1995). Plasma lipids and their relationships with psychosocial factors in older adults. *The Journals of Gerontology. Series B, Psychological Sciences and Social Sciences, 50*, P18–P24.

Vitaliano, P. P., Scanlan, J. M., Krenz, C., Schwartz, R. S., & Marcovina, S. M. (1996). Psychological distress, caregiving, and metabolic variables. *The Journals of Gerontology. Series B, Psychological Sciences and Social Sciences, 51*, P290–P299.

Vogele, C., Jarvis, A., & Cheeseman, K. (1997). Anger suppression, reactivity, and hypertension risk: Gender makes a difference. *Annals of Behavioral Medicine, 19*, 61–69.

Wingard, D. L. (1984). The sex differential in morbidity, mortality, and lifestyle. *Annual Review of Public Health, 5*, 433–458.

The Experiences and Relationships of Gay Male Caregivers Who Provide Care for Their Partners with AIDS

7

Carolyn Sidwell Sipes

INTRODUCTION

As the epidemic of Human Immunodeficiency Virus (HIV) disease continues to grow, the need for better understanding of the male caregiver of persons with HIV and Acquired Immunodeficiency Syndrome (AIDS) is crucial. Historically, the first 100,000 cases of HIV were reported over an eight-year period with a rapid increase in the second 100,000 cases seen in only two years. The task of providing care for persons or partners with AIDS (PWA) is enormous. Little is known about how gay male caregivers provide care for their partners, how caregiving impacts their lives, or how they manage on a daily basis. This knowledge can be crucial if the health care community is to support them and provide interventions that maximize the caregiver functioning and skills. The purpose of the study reported on in this chapter is to provide a better understanding of the caregiving relationship between gay male caregivers and their infected partners. These relationships were examined in the context of AIDS, an often fatal, chronic illness. AIDS remains most frequently seen in populations of young adult males, and may pose problems unlike those seen in other populations of caregivers. The study is significant because men as caregivers have been minimally studied, especially in the context of gender, age, homosexuality, and AIDS.

Biegel, Sales, and Schulz (1991) have suggested that the most appropriate definition of caregiving is the provision of assistance and support

151

by one family member to another as a normal part of the family interaction. The definition of family differs within the AIDS populations in that society does not view homosexual partnerships within the framework of traditional heterosexual marriages. Nonetheless, within either type of family relationship, having a terminal, chronic illness requires extraordinary care demands on the caregivers that go beyond the bounds of normal or usual care. The informal caregiver of a PWA is the individual who provides care for the person infected with AIDS; in the context of this study it was the gay male who provided care to his partner with AIDS. There are varied terms used to define the gay relationship including lover, spouse, partner, and less frequently, significant other. The person or partner with AIDS is the person who is infected with the HIV virus and is symptomatic for AIDS as defined by the Centers for Disease Control diagnostic criteria (CDC, 1992).

Problem Statement

Although HIV infection rates are decreasing in the gay community, men who had sex with men still accounted for 50% of newly diagnosed cases of AIDS through 1996 (CDC, 1997). This percentage increased to 55% when men who had sex with men and injected drugs were included. In California, 80% of the AIDS cases are gay men, but they receive less than 10% of the AIDS funding and support services (Sowell, 1995). These numbers cause a great deal of concern for those who provide care for PWA. Although half of those diagnosed with AIDS have died, the illness is becoming more chronic. As a result of increased knowledge and more effective management and treatment of the disease, there is now the possibility of the person being HIV-infected for as long as 10 years before developing AIDS (CDC, 1997; Durham & Lashley, 2000; Flaskerud & Ungvarski, 1992).

Social support from family, friends, nurses, and physicians for caregivers and PWA continues to be sporadic to nonexistent. This is thought to be due to the fear of contagion of the virus, and the social stigma surrounding homosexuality and intravenous drug use (Barrick, 1988; Matheny, Mehr, & Brown, 1997). In addition to providing care and coping with several health care system challenges, gay male caregivers face what has been referred to as the "triple negative." The triple negative is defined as the stigmatization of being gay, possibly being HIV positive themselves, and having to face the death of many friends who also have HIV and AIDS. Partners of PWA have expressed fear of watching their loved ones die, and typically those impacted by AIDS have experienced the loss of many gay friends.

AIDS is considered a nursing-intensive disease by formal caregivers. However, according to Durham and Lashley (2000), nursing care and treatment for PWA has shifted from long hospital stays to the provision of more care in the home. The shift was due to cost containment measures implemented or recommended by health care policy planners, insurers, and economists (Koch, 1994; Little, Long, & Kehoe, 1990). With this shift to home care, there is an increasing reliance on the informal caregiver to provide the care. These caregivers, along with their PWA, face a long course of illness with repeated exacerbation of many opportunistic infections, fatigue, weakness, pain, and HIV encephalopathy (dementia) (Pantaleo, Graziosi, & Fauci, 1993). Folkman, Chesney, and Christopher-Richards (1994) suggested that male caregivers of PWA may experience dysphoria when they lack the confidence to handle complex health care tasks and that many experience role conflict and feel challenged by the uncontrollable nature of the disease.

Although there is a plethora of literature related to issues of informal caregivers of other chronic illnesses, little is known about how gay male caregivers provide care for partners with AIDS, how such caregiving impacts their lives, or how they manage on a daily basis. Flaskerud and Ungvarski (1992) have discussed the fact that these caregivers face not only the challenges experienced by other informal caregivers but also face stressors unique to AIDS. These include such factors as the age of the PWA, the stigmatization of being gay, the disfigurement and debilitation of the disease, as well as the grief and bereavement from the loss of same-age friends. Because caregiver research involving PWA is in the early stages of development, more descriptive research is needed to gain a deeper understanding of the experiences of gay male caregivers. Increased knowledge about caregiver issues will sensitize formal caregivers, such as nurses and doctors, to caregiver and patient needs. Then models of care and, ultimately, appropriate therapeutic interventions can be developed.

Conceptual Framework

In an initial pilot investigation exploring the needs and experiences of male caregivers of PWA, a conceptual framework consisting of five primary domains emerged (Sipes & Farran, 1995). These included the male caregiver's perception of: (a) self, his role, needs, feelings, and behaviors; (b) his partner, including his needs, feelings, and behaviors; (c) formal health care providers; (d) the gay community, family, and friends; and, (e) the larger societal influences. This chapter will focus on the first two domains by presenting results from a grounded theory study that explored the relationships between gay male caregivers and their PWA in terms of the caregiver's role, needs, feelings, and behaviors, and the caregiver's perceptions of the infected partner's needs, feelings, and behaviors. As will be described below, the theoretical approach underlying this study was symbolic interactionism, appropriate for the study because the participants are actors in the world and defined their reality through the actions and interactions of others, the gay couple. Symbolic interactionism provides the basis for grounded theory assumptions (Strauss & Corbin, 1990).

METHODS

Research Design: Goal and Rationale of Method

For this study, several grounded theory methods provided the systematic process and procedures to guide data collection and analysis. The grounded theory approach was used to describe and expand the perceptions identified in the pilot study and their effect since the caregiving process began. Using the grounded theory approach was appropriate because the goal of grounded theory is to describe and elicit data about perceptions and social interactions (Strauss & Corbin). Strauss and Corbin (1990) described grounded theory as a transactional system, or as a method of analysis that allows for examinations of the interactive nature of events and answers the question, "Why is this . . . ." In this study, the described experiences of the participants (the male caregivers) and the context within which those experiences occurred, such as AIDS, were critical to answering the research questions. Additionally, they were critical to eliciting extensive descriptions and connections about the caregiving experiences of gay male caregivers of PWA.

According to Strauss and Corbin (1990), the grounded theory process involves linking sequences of actions or interactions and responses to a specific phenomenon in terms of the changing conditions and then identifying the consequences. The grounded theory analysis procedures that facilitate the development of thick descriptions and that were attended to in this study include: (a) sample selection; (b) identification of subcategories in terms of events, actions, and interactions that explain major categories; (c) identification of major emerging categories through the coding process; (d) use of theoretical sampling as categories emerge; (e) identification and explanation of how the major categories and subcategories are grounded or linked back to the literature and identification of linkages between categories and subcategories; and (f) the direct linking of categories to the phenomenon by evaluating the outcomes. These procedures were created by Glaser and Strauss (1967) and expanded upon by Strauss and Corbin (1990, 1994).

Theoretical Framework: Symbolic Interactionism

Symbolic interactionism, as an approach to the study of human group life and conduct, suggests that the investigator will understand and determine how individuals take and derive meaning from gestures and words from people as they interact with one another or define "What is this process . . . ." (Baker, Wuest, & Stern, 1992; Blumer, 1969; Denzin, 1987; Denzin & Lincoln, 1994). The theoretical assumptions, concepts, and content for this study were derived from the process of symbolic interactionism, which is the theoretical underpinning of grounded theory.

According to Blumer (1969), symbolic interactionism consists of three premises: (a) that human beings act toward things based on the meanings things have for them; (b) that meaning derives from the process of social interactions; and (c) that meanings evolve through interpretations. The end result of symbolic interactionism is the formation of propositions about relationships or shared meanings among categories of data, from which theories are derived or are woven into "theoretical schemes" (Blumer, p. 48). Next, the process of grounded theory enables prediction and explanation of the meanings and behaviors. Using grounded theory method moves symbolic interactionism further to make the connections among the categories of data. This is accomplished through the process described below of coding, categorizing, theoretical sampling (the hallmark of grounded theory), and finally deriving theory (Miles & Huberman, 1994). For the purposes of this study, only coding and categorizing to derive themes was done, as this was primarily a descriptive study. The role of this investigator, as a symbolic interactionism researcher, was to provide the lens or interpretation for the caregivers' stories.

Sampling Procedures

According to Strauss and Corbin (1990), sampling in grounded theory is about gathering data about what people "do or don't do" (p. 177). Theoretical sampling is a hallmark of grounded theory and involves taking emerging codes, categories, or concepts and asking specific questions about them in subsequent interviews with different, comparative groups (Glaser & Strauss, 1967; Hutchinson, 1986; Wilson & Hutchinson, 1996). In this study, pilot interviews provided beginning description and the set of interview questions were derived from the findings of that study. However, theoretical sampling to develop theory was not done, because the purpose was not to develop theory but to provide a thick description of the caregiving relationships between two people.

A purposive, convenience sample of 28 participants were recruited in Chicago ($n = 9$) and Denver ($n = 19$). Initial sampling efforts were aimed at collecting data and beginning to identify and analyze categories associated with the caregiving experiences. Gay men, currently caring for a partner diagnosed as HIV positive and self-identified as the caregivers, were recruited for this study through AIDS service agencies in Chicago and Denver as well as other sources. In Chicago, participants were recruited through a counselor at a large AIDS service provider in the gay community. They were also recruited through the investigator's networking process in the gay community, through an AIDS physician's office, and through snowball sampling techniques, with one participant personally recruiting another or identifying others appropriate for the study. Snowball sampling is a strategy that benefits theory building as does intensity sampling or looking for information-rich exemplar cases (Miles & Huberman, 1994). In addition, advertisements were placed in the local gay newspapers and stores frequented by the gay community ($n = 9$). In Denver, participants were recruited through an AIDS clinic by nurses and counselors, through the metropolitan AIDS service agency, and through snowball sampling ($n = 19$).

Using the principle of saturation of categories (a hallmark of grounded theory), participants were recruited until no new or relevant data emerged necessitating additional categories (Glaser, 1978; Glaser & Strauss, 1967; Strauss & Corbin, 1990, 1994). In this study, the majority of the information was obtained from the first 18 participants, but to assure saturation, 10 additional participants were interviewed in an attempt to obtain additional data from those with divergent population characteristics. This included deliberately searching for extreme or deviant cases or confirming or nonconfirmatory cases, which serves to increase confidence in the conclusions (Miles & Huberman, 1994). For example, an African American male with an older White partner, in the relationship for only two years, was an example of one such case that was deliberately sought out. Overall, the sample varied in terms of duration of relationship, living arrangements, ethnicity, age, and caregiver HIV status, which permitted richer data and more diverse categories. When sampling was discontinued, the categories were diverse; the relationships between the categories were established as new, short-term caregivers were validating similar stories as the more experienced caregivers; and no new data seemed to be emerging, regardless of the category.

Sample Characteristics

Characteristics of the male caregivers and their partners are described below and summarized in Table 7.1.

Age.   Although the primary focus of this study was on caregivers for partners with HIV disease and AIDS, it is also important to understand

TABLE 7.1   Caregiver Characteristics

Caregiver Characteristics	M (years)	SD (years)
Caregiver's age: 25–56 years	40.8	8.4
Partner's age: 24–63 years	40.3	7.7
Year partner diagnosed: 1984 (oldest) 1994 (youngest)	7.3	2.2
Length of relationship:		
Short term: 1–9 years (n = 19)	3.7	1.9
Long term: 10–18½ years (n = 9)	13.6	3.5

Aspects of the Caregiving Relationship	n	%
Relationship with partner viewed as:		
Marriage	12	43
Friend/lover/significant other	16	57
Relationship:		
Monogamous	23	82
Open	5	18
Partner HIV+ before you entered the relationship?		
Yes	19	68
No/did not know/did not tell	9	32
Participant HIV+ status:		
Positive	17	61
Negative	11	39
Family relationships:		
Good	10	36
Fair	6	21
Nonexistent/divorced	12	43
Relationships with your partner's family:		
Good/supportive	13	47
Fair/accepting	9	32
Estranged/No contact	6	21

the partner or care-receiver's background. A total of 28 men participated in this research study. The caregivers' ages ranged from 25 to 56 years ($M = 40.8$; $SD = 8.4$). The partners or care-receivers ages ranged from 24 to 63 years of age ($M = 40.3$; SD = 7.7).

Year of diagnosis.   Many of the couples decided to be tested as they entered into the relationship because they wanted to be aware of their HIV status as they took on a new partner. The partners had been diagnosed as being HIV positive ranging from 1984 to the most recent in 1994; the majority (n = 17) were diagnosed in 1990 and after; the average number of years since diagnosis was 7.3 (SD = 2.2). According to the caregivers, 19 (68%) of the partners knew they were infected and HIV positive prior to entering into the current relationship, and did not consider being HIV positive a barrier to making a commitment to the relationship and new partner. In other cases it was not clear when the partners made their diagnosis known to the caregiver. Also, 17 (61%) of the caregivers identified themselves as being HIV positive at the time they began the process of caregiving for their partners.

Duration of relationship.   Length of time in the relationship between caregivers and PWA ranged from 1 to 18½ years (M = 7.7); the majority, 68% (n = 19), had been in short-term relationships from 1 to 9 years, and 32% (n = 9) had been in long-term relationships that ranged from 10 to 18½ years.

Relationships with partner and family defined.   The relationships were first defined in terms of the couple and then with their families, because these relationships did not exist without outside influences. Twelve of the 28 couples (43%) viewed their relationships with their partners as a marriage; one stated that he was in the process of getting a divorce. Five (18%) of the participants defined the relationships with their partners as open, meaning that they continued to have more than one sexual partner even though they were in a committed relationship.

As the men shared their stories, they frequently included things that were happening with their families. Four (14%) of the caregivers had their teenage children from their heterosexual marriages living with them. Relationships with families were less than satisfactory for the majority of the caregivers. Six of 28 (21%) of the caregivers rated their family relationships as "fair" to "do not discuss them." Further, 12 of 28 (43%) of the partners defined their relationships with their families as strained, "nonexistent" or even "divorced," meaning that they had no contact with them.

Data Collection

Interview procedures.   In-depth, face-to-face intensive interviews were conducted with the participants at time and site of their convenience. Most of the interviews were scheduled and conducted after work in the evenings, before or after their doctor's appointments, at the AIDS services agencies, or during lunch hours. This was done to limit problems with stigma, anxiety, and stress related to the situation and to maintain confidentiality and privacy. Prior to each interview, the potential participant was called and screened for willingness to participate, and given an overview of the questions, questioning format, and audiotaping procedure. It was explained that the interviews would take at least 1 hour; most averaged 1½–2 hours.

As recommended by May (1991), anticipating issues and biases that may be encountered during the interview process is key to "getting the story." This investigator provided consistency and used language similar to that used in the gay culture in the interviews, such as reference to the relationship as lovers and acknowledging the marriage, if applicable. In order to have comparable data across all interviews, similar questions were asked of all participants using the questions as guidelines. In previous work, some participants refused to be interviewed, even when referred by a friend; others canceled previously scheduled appointments; and still others failed to appear for scheduled interviews. Therefore, based on this past experience, flexibility with regard to the interview setting and timing, content, and structure of the interviews became an important detail of conducting the interviews. Since the study focus was on a vulnerable and difficult-to-access population, it was also recognized from past pilot work that potential participants might employ self-protective behaviors and provide other challenges to obtaining data.

For some participants, establishing trust was difficult. They initially asked for credentials such as what my previous background work had been in the area of AIDS. One caregiver initially assured me that he was only a friend of an infected person and was adamant that he was heterosexual. Approximately 30 minutes into the interview he started crying as he told me that he was really gay, deeply in love with this person, and that he was indeed the caregiver. He had exhibited the self-protective behaviors also found in the previous study by this investigator (Sipes & Farran, 1995). At this point every effort was made to assure quality for the data by reviewing any areas where there may have been questions. This demonstrated to this investigator the importance of establishing a trusting relationship with research participants. In addition, participants were allowed to control the interview process as much as possible by not interrupting an important train of thought and they were asked to expand on what they determined were important points.

A semistructured interview guide was used that allowed for open listening, but still provided a format of similar questions for all participants related to their relationships with their partners. The major question was "Can you tell me about your relationship with your partner?" A total of 13 questions were developed from past personal experience working with caregivers and PWA, which additionally drew upon past interviews conducted by the investigator in pilot work, the AIDS and caregiving literature, questions used in caregiver research by Farran, Keane-Hagerty, Salloway,

Kupferer, and Wilken (1991), and use of qualitative methodology identified by Morse (1992). Asking the same questions of all participants and gathering similar data allowed for comparisons among participants and provided greater assurance of validity.

At the beginning of the interview the participants completed the demographic and consent forms, then were given a copy of the interview questions to follow if they wished. However, none of them used the interview guide; as soon as they began telling their stories, they became totally engrossed in sharing their experiences. Some were almost in a trance-like state; others cried and seemed relieved to share their experiences. Hutchinson, Wilson, and Wilson (1994) have emphasized that intense interviews provide an opportunity to describe experiences and through this, validate a person's self-worth and provide catharsis or a sense of relief that comes from having an accepting listener.

Audiotaping of interviews during data collection is a recommended procedure to ensure auditability of the data to establish credibility and was done in this study to eliminate any issue of bias that might be introduced through researcher control of data collection. Advantages of audiotaping the interviews prevented interference and distractions from the investigator when taking notes, ensured a more natural one-on-one interaction, and assured that everything being stated was accurately captured. Only one informant did not want to be audiotaped but agreed to write out all responses. These answers were reviewed in the face-to-face interview situation and copious notes and memos were taken. As mentioned earlier, many of the participants were unaware of the taping as they were very engrossed and eager to tell their stories.

Data Analysis

Data processing.   The grounded theory method of data analysis was used for data reduction and interpretation. However, only the first two levels of description including defining codes (subcategories, categories) and themes were identified in this study. After assigning each participant a study number, the audiotapes were transcribed verbatim by the interviewer into a Microsoft Access Relational Database Management System, which has sorting and association capabilities. Each tape was transcribed verbatim and coded at the completion of the each interview. The transcripts were reviewed for accuracy by reading the transcripts while replaying the tapes, and each line of the transcript was numbered for easy tracking.

Substantive or open coding.   The basic coding process is based on generic content analysis. Glaser (1978) defined coding on two levels, substantive and theoretical. Substantive or open codes are concepts of empirical substance in the area of research and theoretical codes conceptualize how substantive codes relate to one another. Substantive coding opens or "fractures" the data; theoretical codes link them back together. As the first step of analysis the data were fractured in a line-by-line analysis, closely examined, and compared for similarities and differences with other data and initially, across six interviews (Strauss & Corbin, 1990, 1994). During initial coding, a code book was developed that contained labeling of a code (fears, anger, uncertainty) rationale for decisions, memos, definitions for codes, and other data exemplifying the category code. Next, the code labels were used to code further transcripts by assigning the codes to line-by-line units of information. For example, in this study, after preliminary data reduction, 2,166 unique lines of data were coded from 28 transcripts using the line-by-line, open coding process. Initially, the caregivers spoke of the physical things they had to do to take care of their partners, such as "I had to bathe and dress him," others spoke in terms of "providing emotional support and love." These were originally coded as "physical caregiving and emotional caregiving." Finally, 103 codes were developed. With further refinement and data reduction, such as combining codes like "affect" and "allowing" into other appropriate categories, the codes were reduced to 61.

Strauss (1987) stressed the importance of open coding, looking at the minutia. If this were not accomplished, critical elements such as contexts, strategies, interactions, conditions, or consequences would be lost. Using the computer application, Access, the codes were used to retrieve and cluster data in a variety of ways using a process called "drill down." Using Access and the unique application design, all of the data could be retrieved by specific code, category, or theme. It can be tracked back to raw data or exact quotes of participants and can be linked in any of a variety of ways such as, code to code, theme to theme, and theme to category to code.

Theoretical/axial thematic coding.   The second step in analysis involved theoretical/thematic or axial coding. Axial coding, defined by Strauss and Corbin (1990), puts the data back together in new ways making the connections between categories and subcategories. Categories are broadly defined as classifications of concepts or code groupings that have some commonality and are combined under a single abstract concept. For example, *fears* as a concept or category had subcategories such as fear of disease, dying, impact of disease, caregiver involvement, and finding out. Combining data, using the open codes, created more abstract groups of information about the caregiving relationships and was done to reduce the number of indicators. After additional transcripts were analyzed, it was noted that the two concepts of physical and emotional caregiving were consistently identified by the caregivers and were provisionally labeled as the category, "care types." From this point on, all of the codes that were indicators of the care types category were compared and labeled as such and became part of the definition of that category, if they "fit." Three outside reviewers and the investigator discussed and mutually agreed upon, after several revisions, the initial substantive–open codes from the first six transcripts. Having outside reviewers strengthened and added credibility for the study This is the beginning of comprehension and synthesis of the data as defined by Morse (1994).

The first six transcripts were recoded using Level I coding, and with further reduction, resulted in 63 codes; an additional three transcripts were coded verifying the 63 codes and added to the codebook. The code-book was again reviewed by the outside reviewers and some categories were collapsed into others with similar meanings (e.g., *defense* was combined with *denial*). The ongoing process of identifying properties and dimensions with additional transcripts confirmed the relationships between categories and subcategories (Strauss & Corbin, 1990). Coding and data analysis were considered complete only when all of the critical categories were defined and relationships and themes had been described. At the second level emerging themes and categories were also reviewed by three outside reviewers. This provided assurance that the categories and themes were recognizable and represented an accurate description of the experiences of the study participants. The themes, subthemes, and categories generated from the data are presented in Table 7.2.

RESULTS

This group of gay men described their relationships in terms of how caregiving influenced them from the perspective of a caregiver. These relationships were viewed as different from usual gay male relationships because it was in the context of AIDS and caregiving. They described the relationships in terms of the caregiving process, emotions, feelings, and behaviors related to how they dealt with these while in the context of dealing with HIV and AIDS. Four major themes and subthemes that emerged from the stories can be found in Table 7.2. The themes are significant because these were the major concepts consistently found in the stories and experiences of what it was like to be a gay male caregiver who cared for a partner with AIDS. The stories were told both by men who had been in the relationship only a short time and by those who had been long-term caregivers. It was significant that the short-term, less experienced caregivers frequently validated the stories and experiences of the more experienced, long-term caregivers.

TABLE 7.2 Themes, Subthemes, and Categories

Themes	Subthemes and Categories

Dealing with the Caregiving Relationships	Key components affecting the relationship
	1. Committing to the relationship
	2. Accepting in the relationship
	3. Accommodating and adapting to the relationship
	4. Giving up control
	5. Recognizing the effect of society on the relationship
	  a. Stigma and discrimination
	  b. Isolation
	  c. Distrusting society
	  d. Support

Dealing with the Caregiving Process	1. Context of providing care
	2. Characteristics of the caregiving process
	  a. Involvement in caregiving
	  b. Commitment to caregiving
	  c. Care tasks/responsibilities/requirements
	  d. Outcomes of caregiving
	3. Key components of the caregiving process
	  a. Knowing
	  b. Identifying/anticipating needs
	  c. Being there
	  d. Maintaining hope
	  e. Maintaining reciprocal communication
	  f. Recognizing the effect of society on the caregiving process

(continued)

TABLE 7.2 Themes, Subthemes, and Categories (*Continued*)

Themes	Subthemes and Categories

Dealing with Emotions and Feelings	1. Grieving
	   a. Anticipatory grieving
	   b. Experiencing losses
	   c. Regrets
	2. Emotional responses to grief
	   a. Fears
	   b. Anger
	   c. Powerlessness

Dealing with Behaviors	1. Reclusive/secretive behaviors
	   a. Keeping secret with regard to HIV status
	2. Distancing behaviors
	   a. Distancing by caregiver
	   b. Distancing by family and friends
	   c. Shelving
	   d. Denial
	   e. Avoiding
	3. Coming to terms
	   a. Caregiver influence over quality of life
	   b. Partner control over dying
	   c. Resigning to end of life
	   d. Dependency
	   e. Growing and transforming
	   f. Dying

Furthermore, the caregivers described caregiving as a series of phases that were differentiated from one phase to the next and which were typically triggered by some critical event; these phases have been integrated into the four major themes. The phases integrated into the themes were identified by two caregivers who described the caregiving process as "a journey down the path." Growing and transforming, as one of the final and most poignant subthemes, took place as the caregivers spoke of the difficulties caring for someone who was dying. They described their feelings and explained how their experiences transformed their lives forever, providing them with an "incredible deep, growing experience." As their partners were dying, the long-term caregivers discussed the meaning of the experience, how it had transformed their lives, and the final attitudes and emotions they had shared with their partner. For the caregivers who were infected themselves, it was viewing their own mortality.

DEALING WITH THE CAREGIVING RELATIONSHIPS

The first essential theme that emerged in the data is Dealing with the Caregiving Relationships. The subtheme and categories that best supported the major theme were identified by the caregivers as key components that affected the caregiving relationships. The caregivers who had been in long-term relationships of more than 10 years provided retrospective, in-depth descriptions of how their relationships changed over the course of the disease and defined key components that were responsible for and affected the changes. Those who had been in shorter term relationships of 3 to 4 years shared similar but less in-depth stories due to lack of experience and time in the relationship. Caregivers described key components they felt were necessary to make the changing relationship work; the unique relationship that now included caregiving as a major factor. The key components required in the dynamic caregiving relationship included the following: making a commitment to the relationship; accepting the relational part of both the partner and caregiver; accommodating and adapting; giving up control by both the caregiver and care receiver; and dealing with societal influences (i.e., stigma and discrimination, isolation, distrust for society, and familial or community supports). The age of the caregiver is included in parentheses at the end of each substantial quote, which defines the context of the quote.

Committing to the Relationship

The first key component that affected the caregiving relationships and described by the caregivers was commitment. It was defined as being obligated to their partners for a long-term relationship and the expectation that they would grow old together. One 53-year-old caregiver stated that he wanted to impress upon people that the commitment side of gay life is just like that of heterosexual life. Because a primary concern for gay couples was to have a long-term relationship, many of the couples had made the commitment to spend the rest of their lives with each other, often before they knew they were HIV positive. As the caregivers discovered that their partners were HIV positive, all of the couples in this study stayed together because of the commitment they had made to each other:

> you just do these things as part of life, when you commit to somebody . . .
> you do what it takes, it's just a matter of your commitment, deepening; our
> commitment to each other . . . the commitment, marriage, things like that
> absolutely mean something . . . it's not something you easily make.

Some new caregivers hesitated and questioned making a long-term commitment if they learned of the diagnosis just as they were entering into the relationship:

> you don't know if you want to stay with it or not when you find out the
> diagnosis, it would just be easier to leave; I'm afraid of getting involved
> with somebody who might die on me, that there would be a loss I don't
> want to experience; I will do this now but never again. (ages 29, 30, and 36)

Finding out about the diagnosis while trying to make a commitment was devastating and ultimately changed the unexpected caregivers and their partners' long-range plans.

Accepting in the Relationship

The second key component was learning to accept the reality of what was happening in their lives. The long-term caregivers identified dimensions of acceptance, such as acceptance of the illness and help, and how they varied over the course of the disease. The caregivers stated that part of the responsibility for making the relationship work also included that their partners be accepting of the illness and help. At first, new caregivers of 3 to 4 years had great difficulty accepting that the disease existed, as did their partners, especially when symptoms of disease were not evident. From the caregivers' perspectives, they felt they had to accept the fact that their partners might try to exert control over them by always wanting and needing the caregiver there. From the partners' perspectives, acceptance meant that they did not try to do things they were incapable of any more. Acceptance also included not ignoring the diagnosis. As one caregiver of 6 years shared, his infected partner had tried to convince him that he did not have AIDS "because I don't have any of the infections."

As the disease progressed, caregivers identified that they had to learn to accept the reality of the disease, that part of becoming an experienced caregiver was to acknowledge and accept the fact that they could not be self-sufficient, and that they had to be more open and ask for help to care for their partners. In the longer-term relationships, there was acceptance and recognition that the partner was dying because physical decline was obvious. From this they learned how to prioritize what was important in life such as "it's letting go of life noise, and not getting upset by things that are just 'noise.'"

Accommodating and adapting to the relationship. After the caregivers learned to accept the diagnoses and the limitations imposed by the disease, the next step was learning to accommodate and adapt. Another key component to making the relationship work was accommodating and adapting to the various situations as they changed with disease progression. Accommodating and adapting meant learning to live with AIDS, accommodating to partners' abilities, and changes in their sex lives. Although learning to deal with the disease was described as devastating, the couples learned to change and adapt from the free and spontaneous lifestyles they had once enjoyed prior to illness, to a more regimented life due to treatment and medication schedules.

The long-term caregivers discussed the changes in their sex lives as the disease progressed, causing both physical and psychological changes that led to a loss of intimacy and affection. This influenced and dramatically changed the relationship from what it once had been because they now had to plan around partners' needs and demands rather than be spontaneous. As the caregivers became more experienced, they felt they could function better and address their partners' physical needs as they gained an increased understanding of psychological and emotional components required to adapt to the changes in the relationship.

Giving Up Control in the Relationship

Giving up control meant that caregivers stayed in the supporting role rather than trying to control or dominate the relationship. They allowed their partners to make decisions and do things, such as driving, dressing, and bathing on their own as much as possible to maintain their independence and a sense of normalcy. With more experience, caregivers recognized that relinquishing control and allowing the partners to maintain control over their lives for as long as possible was very important to maintaining the relationship, "to let him do that because it's one of the last things he has control over" (caregiver ages 36, 37, 39, 42, 49, 49, 53, 56).

Experienced caregivers learned to be extremely sensitive to ways they offered physical and emotional help for their partners as the partners gradually relinquished control for important functions in their lives such as driving a car. And finally, part of giving up control but not letting the disease be in control for both the caregiver and care receiver was to maintain a positive attitude and find ways to vent frustrations through support groups. Other ways of not letting the disease take control were to maintain medication schedules or doctors' appointments and to deal with new symptoms as they came up and not ignore them.

Recognizing the Effect of Society on the Relationship

Because the relationship did not exist in a vacuum and was affected by outside factors, it is important to identify and discuss how the external environment affected it. Being able to recognize that stigma and discrimination from outside influences, such as society, surrounded and affected the relationship and, in part, led to isolation and issues of trust or distrust for the couples. In a more positive sense, the couples recognized the importance of outside support in the relationship, which included that from families.

From a broader view of the society and the medical profession, a few caregivers felt that the medical profession did not accept AIDS, although the majority of the caregivers did not identify specific issues with the medical society. The overall sentiment was expressed as, "I would like to see us live in a society that is more accepting of others, no matter what their lifestyle is or what color they are or what religion they are, who they choose to have sex with, or if they're sick . . . that they would just be more accepting."

Stigma and discrimination. To discriminate against someone involves separating out, not treating the same, or setting them apart from others and involves more action. Stigma and discrimination were predominant factors throughout gay males' lives; therefore, these factors cannot be ignored because they had tremendous influence on the caregiving relationships and were experienced in a variety of forms, including behaviors of parents, the community, other gays, and in the work environment. A 50-year-old caregiver of 4 years shared his experience from the community, that:

> not only is it AIDS, it could be cancer too, there was stigma associated with other illness, such as cancer or heart attacks or people with any illness, but that the stigma may not be as intense as with AIDS. And you hope when they do stare that they're feeling some compassion and not some kind of negative feeling.

They often sought protection by hiding from the stigma in the community such as not telling others they were gay or HIV positive. At other times they did not hide, but it resulted in a lack of support from other gay friends and families.

Isolation.   Isolation is the verbal or physical voluntary or involuntary refusal to interact with caregivers and partners. Some of the couples with both long- and short-term caregiving relationships felt isolated and alone because of outside circumstances; others made a conscious choice to be isolated and alone. Dimensions of isolation were isolation by the person with AIDS, caregiver isolation and familial isolation.

Distrusting society.   Another key subcomponent that affected the relationship with regard to securing support and help with care was the issue of trust versus distrust for what others were trying to do. This included the medical community, family, and friends. For some caregivers, past experiences had led to feelings of distrust for the medical community whose variety of medical interventions and treatments always seemed to fail despite promises made. With distrust for the medical community, caregivers discussed how they went through periods where they were suspect, critical, and nontrusting with the treatments and care offered for the disease. As one 56-year-old, long-term caregiver of 18 years shared:

> I will trust my own intuitions and my own medical knowledge more . . . you have an intuitive knowledge of what is right and what is wrong . . . I wouldn't let doctors in the emergency room or the clinic tell me what should or shouldn't be, I don't trust that they will do a good job, I have learned to be very aggressive to get what he needs.

Distrust occurred because of the ways gay men had previously been treated by the community, family, and friends. Long-term caregivers, whose family and friends wanted to help but were inexperienced, were concerned because they felt they could not trust them to provide the appropriate care.

Support.   There were three dimensions of support discussed by the caregivers: two negative views that support was there but inappropriate, or that it was not there at all; the third view was positive and included support from work, family, and friends who offered help. Other support issues centered on dealing with partners' families and their nonsupportive homophobia. When they would come to visit, the caregivers wanted their families to be supportive of them as a couple, but often found they supported the partner but not the caregiver. The caregivers also shared positive stories about receiving support from fellow workers, friends, and family, which was provided in a variety of ways.

DEALING WITH THE CAREGIVING PROCESS

The second major theme, Dealing with the Caregiving Process, was defined by the caregivers as having to deal with a multitude of complex factors that complicated and compounded the caregiving relationship, and ultimately affected the caregiving process. Dealing with the Caregiving Process was couched in the context of providing care for a partner with AIDS; the characteristics of that process are presented in terms of involvement and commitment to caregiving; the care tasks, responsibilities and requirements; and the outcomes of caregiving as identified by the caregivers. These all were influenced by the length of time in the relationship, which was ultimately the length of time spent as a caregiver and by the key components of the caregiving process such as knowing, identifying and anticipating needs, being there, maintaining hope, and reciprocal communication. It did not depend on the overall age of the couple. Caregivers also described how societal influences affect the caregiving process. For example, one caregiver was older, 54 years, but in the relationship only 3 years, whereas another caregiver was 39 years old and in the relationship for 10 years.

Context of Providing Care

Understanding the context or circumstances and environment that surrounded care provision provided insight into the caregiving process. The majority of the caregivers reported that they had not thought about having to assume the role of a caregiver for their partner when they entered into the relationship because they assumed they would enjoy a normal gay lifestyle. It was explained as:

> in the gay world so much is based on the physical . . . hard bodies, looking young, looking great . . . that gay relationships start out 80% physical and 20% cerebral, but they are not as deep and loving at first, they're superficial and not lasting if they stay this way.

After caregivers assumed the caregiving role, they discussed how they were offended with attitudes and assumptions made by others that men are not capable of caring. For example, "I still sometimes get very upset when fathers are maligned; fathers—men are capable of giving care, sometimes it's just a matter of learning how to boil water without burning it." They frequently felt that they were viewed in terms of certain role models. As one 49 year-old caregiver of 15 years expressed it:

> I have always been gay, but I was married at one time because I was trying to prove that I wasn't gay; the whole point of this is that I get very upset

when fathers are made fun of in this society, we don't have any more "father-knows-best" fathers who were obviously very capable of being caregivers and providing.

Frequently, after the longer-term caregivers assumed the role and responsibility for caregiving, they felt they were not given the credit they deserved and were overly criticized, such as:

> men aren't taught to be caregivers in their early years, and in our society's case, we're taught to be providers, we're taught to be strong and macho. And then when the need comes, we're really all thumbs, father doesn't know how to do anything, our society tends to make fun of that . . . we need to give our male members of our society a little more credit than they're given, we need to give ourselves more support, we need to know that it's OK to be all thumbs once in a while. And the rest of our society needs to know that's OK because they're not perfect either. (age 56)

Thus, there were many complex issues and attitudes such as dealing with physical changes and having to assume an unexpected role that influenced the caregiving for these men.

Characteristics of the Caregiving Process

Specific characteristics of providing care include: involvement in caregiving, commitment to caregiving, definition of care tasks, responsibilities and requirements, and outcomes of caregiving. These defined and characterized the caregiving processes for this particular group of AIDS caregivers because these views were frequently identified in their stories as being critical to making the process work.

Involvement in caregiving.   Becoming involved in providing care was the first step in the caregiving process. Involvement was described by the caregivers in terms of their level of interest, concern, participation, which included various roles that were assumed as they were gradually drawn in as caregivers for their partners. Levels of participation evolved from the superficial, with minimal involvement, to being very involved in care as the partner became more debilitated with the progression of the disease.

Commitment to caregiving.   Commitment to caregiving was different from committing to the relationship because it meant committing to something such as caregiving for a partner who was dying. This was not considered normal in these relationships because these men were in the age group where they were considered to be in the prime of life and without illness, unlike older populations. Commitment levels, whether superficial or deep, frequently were based on the amount of love the caregivers felt and expressed for their partners and the care they provided in turn. As the caregiving process began, few actual caregiving functions were needed. At this point, the focus was more on what was going to happen in the future to both partners in the relationship, their lives, and what would be required as the caregiver role was assumed. At this phase, the commitment was more superficial but later deepened, because the caregivers became more involved and empathetic as their partners became sicker.

One described it as "caring for" as "at first I was providing 'anti-care,' not understanding what was going on and not necessarily being cooperative or supportive." Others described their commitment as "caring about" and said "it's how much we care about each other." Caregivers assured their partners of their love, making sure they were aware of their feelings; that was a critical element in the caregiving process.

Responsibility was recognized and often described as a dimension of commitment. For example, "there are different phases of responsibility and there is responsibility that, no, I did not give this disease to him but there are still responsibilities if there is going to be a partnership here." Another key dimension of commitment identified by the long-term caregivers was that "if you don't have a sense of caring for the other person, there's no point in doing it."

Later, as illness progressed, caregiving work took on other aspects because the caregiving process required greater involvement. At the end of caregiving, with increased empathy and understanding for the partner with AIDS, caregivers' involvement intensified as they assumed more responsibility for their partners' lives. This was partially due to denial of what was coming and partially due to the realization that the end was near. At the end of caregiving, caregivers talked more about the meaning of the experience, the transformation that had occurred, and the need to be truly committed to providing care. The caregivers spoke less about specific tasks that had been required. Several long-term caregivers spoke of not being a caregiver again, or that they would have to strongly evaluate making such a commitment in the future.

Care tasks, responsibilities, and requirements. Care tasks were the duties the caregivers felt their partners expected and needed from them during the caregiving process. These care tasks were described in terms of the changes and demands that occurred during the caregiving process identified earlier. They were categorized by caregivers as being psychological-emotional, financial, and physical. Care tasks included dealing with the physical changes that increased caregiving work. A 49-year-old, long-term caregiver of 10 years commented:

> I asked what he was scared of, is it death? He said no, it's the mutilation, the disfiguration; he told me there are times he looks at himself while brushing his teeth and he thinks he looks hideous. I told him he is still beautiful in the eyes of Jesus and mine too.

As one new caregiver settled into the caregiving process, he shared that, while he had not been aware that he had the ability to care for someone, he had become comfortable with it. Other caregivers expressed feelings of inadequacy in their abilities. Another caregiver commented that "he made me very aware of the fact that I don't know what it's like to go through this; 'I'm not walking in his shoes,' even though I'm sick too. I try to relate to that when I take care of him."

Outcomes of caregiving. Four of the long-term caregivers shared that it would not have been as a deep and meaningful experience if they had not been as committed to their partners. They also shared various reasons why they would not be caregivers again, that "you need to be aware that you have limitations as a caregiver and you [must] learn to recognize these." Only 2 of the 28 caregivers talked about the burden of caregiving near the end stages of AIDS. This was at the point where they became more involved with the physical tasks of caregiving as they assumed more responsibilities. Not viewing caregiving as a burden allowed them to commit more to caregiving. Two other short-term caregivers of 2 to 3 years stated that, "burden, there's no burden, not yet; I'm not sure about in the future, but not true burden yet." And "I don't feel there is a burden at all; it is a task of love. I am not afraid to deal with him, or touch him, and am not afraid to take care of him."

Key Components of the Caregiving Process

As the caregivers previously described key components that affected the caregiving relationship and characteristics of the caregiving process, they also identified key components that influenced the caregiving process. Caregivers described key components of the caregiving process they felt were basic to providing good care and that needed to be consistent and present in all caregiving functions. The key components that characterized the dynamic caregiving process included: Knowing, or being aware; the ability to identify and anticipate needs; Being there; maintaining hope; and maintaining reciprocal communication. Recognizing the effects of society such as families' good intentions and how they affected the caregiving process were also described.

Knowing. Caregivers defined 'Knowing' as requiring intuition, being informed and knowledgeable about conditions, the disease, and treatments.

It also included understanding, empathy, and being perceptive. The first key component of caregiving was being perceptive to the partner's needs such as, "not asking him what he wants, but just knowing what he needs, knowing, just knowing, not having to always be bugging him about what he wants." And further, "knowing how much to give, both from his need and from how much I feel I can give at any one time is very important and something I had to learn."

Knowing and being more perceptive and empathetic to needs and feelings was a hard lesson to learn for some caregivers and was key to providing good care. Conversely, there was a sense of not knowing "especially the powerlessness, you never know what's going to happen, what disease will come up next" from those who were caregivers for 8 to 10 years as they watched the disease progress.

Identifying and anticipating needs. Another component in the caregiving process included identifying and anticipating needs for both the caregiver and partner. It also required gradual transition to assume more care and responsibility. It was important that caregivers identified emotional needs of their partners such as the need to maintain control, independence, and dignity as the caregivers became more involved with the caregiving process. When identifying needs of the caregivers, long-term caregivers shared how important it was to think of themselves and give credit, to not feel guilty about doing the right thing, as they assumed more of the care for their partners.

Caregivers wanted reassurance; "in order to continue, I need to know that there is still hope, that this isn't just a futile effort." Caregivers identified their own needs in terms of the need to be encouraged and reassured they were doing the right thing for their partners.

Being there. Being there, providing both physical and emotional support, was perceived by the caregivers as an important part of the caregiving process for partners. Partners wanted assurances that the caregiver would be there and available in case there was a need, thus providing a sense of support, understanding, peace, and security. Being there, providing physical and, more often, emotional support, was expressed as "it's not just true with AIDS, it's true with other illnesses as well; if you don't have the support, you don't survive."

Other components of the caregiving process included discussions of maintaining hope and reciprocal communications between partner and caregiver. In addition, it included recognizing the effect of society on the caregiving process.

DEALING WITH EMOTIONS AND FEELINGS

The third major theme, Dealing with Emotions and Feelings, required that the caregivers identified emotions and feelings, then that they discussed openly in order to deal with them appropriately. The emotions and feelings found to be common in many of the stories were dimensions of grieving such as anticipatory grieving, experiencing losses and regrets, and the emotional responses to grief such as the fears, anger, and powerlessness.

Grieving

The concept of grieving had many dimensions for these caregivers. They described it in terms of grief or sorrow over a loss, or in the case of anticipatory grieving, an anticipated or expected loss. Regrets were also described as a dimension of grief.

Anticipatory grieving. The concept of anticipatory grieving changed over the course of the interviews. Anticipatory grieving was frequently discussed by the long-term caregivers who had watched as their partners deteriorated over the years and now realized that they were near death:

> there's the sadness of watching them watching you; it's so sad for me watching him . . . I can see it in his eyes, hear it in his voice, you know these things. (age 49)

Currently, with new AIDS treatments, couples previously had learned to prepare for death and were in the process of anticipatory grieving. But now, with the new medications and treatments, the partners who are on the new treatments show no signs of HIV and appear healthy. For example, one 45-year-old caregiver of 10 years shared:

> there is dealing with living and all of a sudden you're dealing with . . . I don't know how to live with him living because he's been dying for years . . . everything was planned and was developing. My whole existence was of him dying and about 6 months ago it was like I didn't know how to live because our life was not based on him living. Now he's living because he's on these new meds, he was so sick for so long and now he's healthier than I can remember and he's not dying, so I don't know what to do, what to plan for, life or death.

Experiencing losses. Experiencing losses were expressed in terms of: (a) loss associated with the disease, (b) loss of friends, (c) loss of intimacy, and (d) loss of other freedoms such as independence and ability to do things. The loss associated with the disease were those related to loss of a lifestyle and the uncertainty surrounding the multiple crises. Other types of loss included gay friends and came from two perspectives—loss by death and loss by disassociation. Loss by dissociation, as gay friends pulled away with the realization of what may happen to them, was expressed as "there's a great deal of loss by contact and of support from our gay friends. I've found more support from my heterosexual friends than my gay friends. Because he is a threat of what might happen to them and they don't want to acknowledge that. So we don't get emotional support from our gay friends."

The loss of intimacy in the relationship did not occur until the disease was well advanced and physical changes were very evident in their partners. Another dimension of grieving and experiencing losses was expressed as the loss of independence and abilities. Caregivers spoke of loss of other freedoms such as being able to make plans for the future. A long-term caregiver shared that the loss of freedom in terms "the freedom to do things like take a shower, shave, eat, all of the things of life that we don't even think about."

Finally, another long-term caregiver shared that he had not done any grieving during his partner's death process until near the end and used other things as excuses, such as hiding behind caregiving tasks, keeping himself too busy to confront what was happening. He had not grieved the individual losses until the very end when it became cumulative and overwhelming.

Regrets. Regrets, as a third subcategory of grieving, were expressed by all the caregivers and varied along the disease continuum. Initially, regrets stemmed from not using safe sex to finding out both partner and caregivers were HIV positive; as the disease progressed regrets were at giving up freedoms previously discussed. There were regrets related to the loss of the relationship to self and partner both physically and emotionally; loss of own abilities due to disease; feeling alone; rejection by family; and regrets for those things they had not been able to accomplish. The long-term caregivers regretted that they soon would be alone. "I'm finally coming to the point where I realize that my life will continue but as one person, and very alone."

Emotional Responses to Grief

Of the primary emotional responses identified by the caregivers, the multiple dimensions of fears and anger were most dependent on the length of time in the relationship and where the partner was in terms of the stage of disease. Many of the caregivers described similar experiences of how fears and anger changed with disease progression. At the beginning of the caregiving relationship, fears were of finding out the diagnosis and at the end, fears and anger were focused on losing a partner and of death. Anger also varied across the course of disease. At first anger was due to finding out the diagnosis, then projected on the influence of past experiences on the relationship. Finally, caregivers spoke of their anger at the disease and losing a partner. The third primary emotional response was of a sense of powerlessness.

DEALING WITH BEHAVIORS

The three themes described previously have cumulative and interrelated influences on both the caregiver and the care-receiver behaviors. For example, stigma and discrimination, involvement and commitment, fears and anger all have a profound effect on behaviors and the ease with which these can be dealt with. Dealing with Behaviors, as the fourth major theme, emerged from the caregivers descriptions of the caregiving relationships for their partners with AIDS. Caregivers and partners alike exhibited reclusive and secretive behaviors (e.g., keeping secret and not disclosing HIV status), which influenced behaviors in other aspects of their lives. Caregivers described behaviors they dealt with such as distancing and other types of denial, shelving, and avoiding by both the caregivers, their partners, and family or friends.

Further, caregivers talked about such things as coming to terms with the disease and their view of the caregiving relationship. This view was given from the perspective of things the caregiver had to do or deal with such as influencing quality of life, dealing with the increased dependency of their partner, and coping with the end of life. Additionally, the caregiver viewed his own mortality and the growth and transformation that had taken place for the caregiver.

Reclusive and secretive behaviors. Reclusive and secretive behaviors were viewed as protective mechanisms, which included withdrawal and not telling the truth about the diagnosis. Another dimension of reclusive and secretive behaviors included "keeping secret" with regard to disclosure of HIV status to others. Reclusive behaviors for the partners and caregivers were mostly protective and identified by both. For the partners, some made a conscious choice to be alone and were very selective about the people they included in their closed circle. For caregivers, withdrawal or not, dealing with issues was a type of reclusive behavior and is different from distancing described later. Secretive behaviors were described as, "we told them cancer, we don't tell people AIDS and we found that we've had more acceptance that way than if we'd ever told the truth."

Keeping secrets.   Keeping secrets with regard to HIV status was described by the caregivers as multidimensional. The dimensions were being open and honest about being infected, understanding what it means to be infected, and the implications of revealing HIV status which also meant exposing their gay lifestyle, particularly to their immediate family.

Twenty-seven out of 28 (96%) of the caregivers were in denial or tried to keep secret their diagnosis of HIV and the possibility that they and their partners were infected.

Distancing Behaviors

Distancing behaviors were defined as pulling away or continuing to participate in activities and interactions, but not at a high level. It included behaviors such as gradually decreasing involvement for the caregiver, care-receiver, and by family and friends. For example, one caregiver stated that, "the sicker he becomes, the more his friends don't come around." Another type of distancing behavior identified by these caregivers was the concept of shelving.

Shelving.   Shelving was used by caregivers to put aside things that they choose not to deal with immediately and then "pull off the shelf a little at a time" when they could deal with them. Caregivers "shelved" as life changes compounded and multiplied such as "putting" life on hold or putting aside future worry, compromises, not making plans, and even shelving related to acknowledging the diagnosis of HIV. Putting life on hold means:

> you live their life plus your own. Two lives at one time and you have to put yours on hold because they come first . . . it's just something you just have to set aside and just say this is it, you gotta deal with it, deal with the current, with what's going on now. There's a lot of future worry, so I try to just focus on being in the present and put that aside for now. (age 35)

The long-term caregivers spoke about compromises they made for not dealing with it now, as part of shelving in the caregiving relationship, that "the closeness, the intimacy part is very important . . . the physical part, you put on a shelf . . . our love for each other has become secondary, put aside."

Caregivers shelved feelings in order to cope. And finally, shelving, as a degree of distancing, was discussed by one new 42-year-old caregiver as, "I don't really view myself as an HIV positive person, I just feel myself as me, who happens to be HIV positive and who is going through this traumatic experience." This last notion can be dangerous if there is a potential to infect others in a sexual relationship since he does not view himself as being HIV positive.

Denial.   Denial, as not accepting or admitting things, was described in a variety of different ways; for some it was related to the notion of "what you don't know won't hurt you." For the caregivers, some tried to deny that the partner was dying but were frequently confronted with it. A 49-year-old caregiver of 10 years expressed it as:

> It's just easier to pretend that he's not sick . . . no one is ever prepared for death . . . I don't want to look at him and see how sick he is because you are just reminded that this is really happening and this is really coming . . . until it happens you always have this idea that it's out there somewhere else but not here.

There was an attitude of ignoring used as a denial mechanism, that if you do not know about AIDS, then you will not get it. Denial continued to be a big part of trying to maintain normalcy in the relationship; there was global denial by many that the disease exists. From a 50-year-old caregiver of 8 years:

> I don't want to know anything about AIDS, because if you know, you have to accept the realities of it and I don't want to think that people die from this, I don't want to know about the disease or these drugs . . . because what you don't know won't hurt you . . . I stayed away from it because I didn't want the reality, it was somebody's else's reality, not ours and I thought that if we didn't bring it into our house, that it wouldn't contaminate him . . . We just didn't discuss it.

Frequently, when HIV was discussed, the caregivers still did not understand or ignored what it meant to be HIV positive. This type of denial was best expressed by a 40-year-old caregiver of 6 years:

> I knew he was positive when I met him . . . he told me, but I didn't really understand what that meant because I don't know anyone with AIDS or anyone who had died from it or what the definition of AIDS was . . . the fact that he was asymptomatic, and something about T-cells, and he made the comment that "I don't have AIDS because I don't have any of the infections" . . . he looked so young and healthy . . . it was stupidity on our part . . . there's a lot of that out there [lack of understanding], and even gay people who are supposed to be better educated on this subject but it doesn't get through. It's partly a denial and partly it's real hard for them to understand what's going on, that test for HIV is not well explained. Or there's so much anxiety they can't hear what's going on.

For partners, denial manifested in interesting ways, such as trying to escape the reality of the disease, to their newly diagnosed partners not seeking medical care, or to not making plans for the future. There also were many forms of denial from the families such as, "they can't seem to break away from their lives to come to see him and maybe that's denial on their part, but they don't realize how serious this is."

Coming to Terms

Coming to terms was a category that included concepts exhibited at the end of life. These included controlling quality of life, resignation at the end of life, and increased dependency. Finally, the caregivers who had gone through this experience or journey talked about the growth and transformation they had experienced and the dying behaviors.

Caregiver influence over quality of life. Couples were coming to terms and dealing with overall quality-of-life issues while still trying to maintain some quality of life for themselves and their dying partners. Caregivers talked about aspects of control over quality of life and whether they could deal with it.

Partners' control over dying. Caregivers spoke in terms of how the disease had controlled their lives, and how they felt rewarded as they tried to assist their partners to maintain some sense of control over dying. This control was best expressed by a 49-year-old caregiver of 10 years, "it's rewarding to allow him to control his own death and make the [funeral] arrangements, when to stop taking meds . . . that he wants to die at home, not a hospital or hospice, deciding when enough is enough." And that "death is very personal."

Resigning to the end of life. Ultimately, caregivers came to terms with final resignation when they finally realized that their partner was dying. In resignation, a 39-year-old caregiver of 10 years shared that:

> AIDS is not God's punishment or revenge, it is just God's way for him to leave, if it wasn't AIDS it would be something else . . . feeling this or saying it helps me when I think of him dying . . . I think about how much happier he will be in a much better place than this, free of pain, free of all of this, if he can't be healthy here, there's a better place . . . I'm tired of this whole thing and why is he hanging on. I just tell him that you have to allow yourself to let go, I can't deal with him suffering anymore.

Growing and transforming. The experience of caregiving provided many positive things such as growth and transformation of a person. As one caregiver shared, "this is a tremendous gift, even though it is tremendously sad that you have to go through the experience to receive the gift." The disease also intensified experiences and fostered emotional and spiritual growth for several caregivers. One 36-year-old caregiver of 14 years expressed the transformation as "... unless you go through this walk with somebody, you don't realize what they have to give up between the time they get sick and the time they die."

As caregivers began to prepare for the end, they shared "be sure that you say everything you ever want to say to them before they die, everything good, bad, or indifferent, because once they're gone you can't say it, then you feel guilty." The long-term caregivers acknowledged that this was a valuable experience best explained by this 42-year-old caregiver of 17 years:

> this experience is preparing me for much more good . . . I wouldn't trade this experience for anything, I'd want the same people, the same friends, the same relationship over again. Because each person has taught me so much individually, about emotions, life, and living life and without that from those same people, I wouldn't be the person I am . . . there is loss and gain through this experience. Our relationship over the last several years has actually gotten better because it has evolved so much and now I know it won't continue, there's anger about AIDS, I can't deny that.

Dying. The long-term caregivers spoke of dying behaviors. Defined as those exhibited by partners at the end of life or the final things that needed to be accomplished at the end, it included as not making their partners feel guilty, giving them permission to die, or spending extra time with them. A 48-year-old caregiver of 5 years stated that, "I'm a hospice chaplain so I've had experience. Lot's of people hang on for other people, not for themselves. People hang on for other reasons, that's why it's so important that we make sure everybody tells them it's OK for them to go. I'm going to miss him but I have to give him permission." Caregivers wanted time alone at the end. "One of my friends who has lost someone said that as he's dying you will want to spend time with him, just tell everybody to leave and spend time with him you need that." And acceptance at the end such as, "I can deal with losing the sick C., but I can't accept losing the well one, it's so overwhelmingly sad; people with this die at such a young age." And finally, "with this illness, it's all over for him and I think he'll be fine where he's going, it will be better there."

DISCUSSION

This study sought to describe the relationships of gay male caregivers who provide care for their partners with AIDS. Four major themes emerged from the data that provide a rich and complex picture of how these caregivers dealt with their partners' illness and how it influenced their relationships. Within the theory and framework of caregiving as a process, caregivers described how the experience influenced and transformed their lives. The caregiving themes occurred within the caregiving process and were used to describe subthemes and categories including caregiver involvement and relationships, attitudes, emotions and feelings, and behaviors as they were identified by the caregivers. Findings suggest the value of implementing a caregiving model that more fully defines and explains phases of caregiving in order to help focus needs where appropriate, provide guidelines, and help caregivers anticipate the course of disease. The purpose of this section is to present a discussion of the results of this study through an overview of study and themes, to compare findings with previous research, and to discuss implications of the study for best supporting the male caregiver to PWA.

As noted elsewhere in this text, caregiving researchers typically have not studied men as caregivers. Several investigators have reported that men are underrepresented relative to the total number of caregivers (Fitting, Rabins, Lucas, & Eastham, 1986; Horowitz, 1985; Pruchno & Resch, 1989; Schulz, Williamson, Morycz, & Biegel, 1992), that men are not generally involved in personal care tasks (Chang & White-Means, 1991; Horowitz, 1985), that primary caregivers are likely to be women over 55 years of age (Stone, Cafferata, & Sangle, 1987), and that "caregiving is women's work" (Rutman, 1996, p. 90). Findings from this study suggest that there are male caregivers who are highly committed and involved in caregiving functions, that men caring for PWA are likely to be young to middle-aged gay males, that their experience is often complex and challenging, and that they have significant needs which might be addressed by health and social service providers. Men in this study were offended that they were not viewed as "capable of giving care" or were not given credit for nurturing and caring attributes because neither they nor society have been taught to value caregiving skills. In this study, the majority of the men had no previous experience as caregivers. Overall, as some complained later, they had no "guidelines" for care but desperately needed some guidance. Some had little knowledge of the implications of having HIV or AIDS; thus, when they agreed to do "whatever was needed," they had no idea what that meant. Many did not know that the caregiving commitment would extend beyond several months and that the caregiving could consume years of their lives. They did not know and were not educated about what was involved, what it meant to be a caregiver, what the tasks might be, or what AIDS as a disease meant physically or emotionally. They did not know and frequently were not told where or how to seek help.

Dealing with Relationships

Most caregivers viewed their relationships as life-long commitments similar to traditional, heterosexual marriages and many referred to their partners as spouses. Caregivers and their partners were similar in age. Most of the men entered into the relationship with the assumption that it would be a relationship that paralleled the traditional relationships of marriage. When the majority of the men committed to the relationship, they typically decided to be tested for HIV. Therefore, most of the men were not aware of their HIV status until after they were in the committed relationship. When they discovered that their partners were HIV positive, they made the decision to stay in the relationship because of the commitment they had made. It was from this point that the caregiving process began to evolve, as they became "accidental caregivers." The men shared how they had never intended to become caregivers, with the exception of one couple, and described how the process evolved over the years as their partners became sicker with AIDS.

More than 40% of the male caregivers considered their relationship as a marriage, whereas Brody, Kleban, Johnsen, Hoffman, and Schoonover (1987) and Brody and Schoonover (1986) reported that 70% of the Alzheimer's caregivers were married. All of the male caregivers in this study were employed, as were most of the partners, until they were unable to continue work due to physical decline. This is in contrast to Horowitz's (1985) study where only one-third of the informal, family caregivers were employed. Pruchno and Resch (1989) reported that for those who had poor financial circumstances, the caregiving process was more complicated due to the limited resources. That was not the case in this study, which may be related to the fact that most of the partners had some form of health care insurance from employment. One could conclude that having insurance and other types of financial support were key to assisting the caregiving process.

Dealing with the Caregiving Process

Men in this study assumed all tasks of caregiving, including bathing, feeding, and other nurturing tasks, especially at the later phases of caregiving as their partners became more debilitated. It is important to recognize this as it was raised as an issue by the gay male caregivers who felt they had been ignored as the primary person who provided care. This finding was contrary to the stereotype that males take a hands-off approach to personal care and are uninvolved in domestic tasks. Men described an intuitive and sensitive approach to caring for their partners, an approach that involved being empathetic to needs and feelings. Findings suggested that many of these caregivers could benefit from validation of their experience from service providers, by receiving encouragement and reassurance that they are doing the right thing for their partners.

Dealing with Emotions and Feelings

Male caregivers of PWA in this study reported many similar feelings of other primary caregivers, such as fears, anger, and denial; however, they did not seem to focus on stress, burden, or strain. Only two talked about the burden of caregiving near the end stages of AIDS. There appeared to be several emotional responses that may be unique to this population. For example, expressed fears were related to lack of knowledge about HIV disease, fear related to uncertainty for the future related to the disease course, and fears about rejection and contagion. Fears were described by two caregivers who thought they could transmit HIV by touching food in a grocery store. There was fear of rejection by family and friends and discrimination with housing and receiving proper medical care. Other AIDS researchers described more fear and stigma from the perspective of contagion and transmission through blood and body fluids for professional health care workers when caring for PWA (Altman, 1988; Brennan, 1988). The other types of fears the caregivers discussed were similar to previous research such as their partner dying, maintaining quality of life, and being left alone.

"Uncertainty," a recognized response among other caregiving populations, was described as a subcategory of fears. The male caregivers in this study spoke of their fears of uncertainty, of what was going to happen, continuously and throughout the phases of caregiving that occurred over the years, including the uncertainty associated with dying. These caregivers did not adapt to the issues of uncertainty that were related to HIV disease progression and loss of their partner and relationships. This is different from the study by Zarit, Todd, and Zarit (1986). In that study, it was reported that caregivers appeared to adapt to the illness and initial differences in morale between male and female caregivers diminished over time, suggesting that family caregivers do adapt to caregiving demands over time. And in other qualitative studies conducted by King and Mishel (1986), and in contrast to the study by Stetz (1987), it was found that the longer caregivers and care-receivers lived with continual uncertainty, the more positively they evaluated the uncertainty. Previous research suggested that the continual appraisal and reappraisal of uncertainty may evolve over time, but this was not reported by male caregivers in the current study.

Anger and frustration related to the partner finding out and being confronted with his HIV status; being infected and feeling powerless were not dissimilar to patients with other diseases. And at the end phase of caregiving, anger was expressed toward the disease because of realization that the partner was dying. In past research, a variety of similar behaviors and emotions were identified for caregivers of Alzheimer's patients, including anger and uncertainty (Gwyther & George, 1986; Mishel, 1990; Oberst & Scott, 1988; Rabins, Fitting, Eastham, & Fettig, 1990).

Trust versus nontrust and skepticism of the medical community because of bad experiences was noted in this study as well as the preliminary study by this investigator (Sipes & Farran, 1995). In this study, however, there was a noticeable difference in attitudes. The caregivers at any phase of the study were not as negative regarding professional care issues as they previously had been. One caregiver did mention that today society seems to be more tolerant and educated about HIV disease. However, it is not known if the increased tolerance was due to the geographic location or other factors such as time, although all data between the two locations was collected within one year.

Dealing with Behaviors

In previous research, denial was frequently identified as a key issue when dealing with many diseases. In this study, denial may be similar to other research in that partners denied they were infected with HIV, as did families and friends. The outcomes of denial were evident when they did not seek information about the disease, how it is transmitted, or when they assumed the attitude that, if they did not know about HIV, they did not have to accept the reality of the disease. Denial was described as actively not seeking medical care or hiding behind the tasks of caregiving so that they did not have to think about what was happening. Finally, denial was not making plans for the future—or from families and friends—denial was staying away, similar to other chronic diseases.

Other behaviors identified and described in this study have not been well defined in the literature but are integrated into discussions with many other behaviors. The specific concepts of reclusive and secretive behaviors as well as distancing and dying behaviors of those with other chronic illnesses were beyond the focus of this study, although they were identified by these caregivers as behaviors seen in their partners. Shelving, a dimension of denial, did emerge as a coping behavior described by the caregivers and would be interesting to compare to other literature. The caregivers in this study were emphatic about the fact they were not in denial and described the shelving as a mechanism whereby they could deal with issues a little at a time.

Physical Morbidity

Although physical morbidity was not a factor in this study, it is important to acknowledge since it was used as a key indicator of physiologic stress determinations by other caregiving investigators. The issue of evaluating physical morbidity would have posed an almost impossible task for the group of gay male caregivers in this study due to the fact that over 61% of them were HIV positive or had AIDS. Although most of the information was volunteered freely, there were several cases where this investigator was first told one thing and then another about HIV status. Therefore, clear information about HIV status, critical to establishing physiologic health status, should be considered suspect unless documented. There were studies of other caregivers that relied on monitoring immune status to determine levels of stress such as Snyder and Keefe (1985) who reported that approximately 70% of the caregivers they evaluated reported a negative change in their physical health status because of the caregiving role. In summary, it would be very difficult to conduct similar studies with subjects who already have compromised to nonexistent immune systems.

Implications for practice.   Two key implications for practice come from this study. First, in order for clinicians to be more effective providers to this population of caregivers, they must value the gay relationships and put aside any personal issues that may exist with regard to dealing with gay populations. Second, men must be viewed and valued as capable of giving care and as having nurturing and caring attributes. Gay men are intuitive and sensitive to partners' needs, and clinicians need to validate this by offering reassurances and support for the care they provide. Finally, to be more effective practitioners, we need to establish a trusting environment and provide them with the tools necessary to be more proficient such as guidelines for care and setting realistic expectations for all aspects of care.

REFERENCES

Altman, D. (1988). Legitimation through disaster: AIDS and the gay movement. In E. Fee & D. Fox (Eds.), *AIDS: The burdens of history* (pp. 301–315). Berkeley, CA: University of California Press.

Baker, C., Wuest, J., & Stern, P. (1992). Method slurring: The grounded theory/phenomenology example. *Journal of Advanced Nursing, 17,* 1355–1360.

Barrick, B. (1988). The willingness of nursing personnel to care for patients with acquired immune deficiency syndrome. *Journal of Professional Nursing, 4,* 366–372.

Biegel, D., Sales, E., & Schulz, R. (1991). *Family caregiving in chronic illness.* Newbury Park, CA: Sage.

Blumer, H. (1969). *Symbolic interactionism: Perspective and method.* Englewood Cliffs, NJ: Prentice Hall.

Brennan, L. (1988). The battle against AIDS: A report from the nursing front. *Nursing, 18*(4), 60–64.

Brody, E., Kleban, M., Johnsen, P., Hoffman, C., & Schoonover, C. (1987). Work status and parent care: A comparison of four groups of women. *The Gerontologist, 27,* 201–208.

Brody E., & Schoonover, C. (1986). Patterns of parent-care when adult daughters work and when they do not. *The Gerontologist, 26,* 372–381.

Centers for Disease Control (1992). 1993 revised classification system for HIV infection and expanded surveillance case definition for AIDS among adolescents and adults. *Morbidity & Mortality Weekly Review, 41:* No. RR-17, pp. 1–19.

Centers for Disease Control (1997). Update: Trends in AIDS incidence, deaths, and prevalence—United States, 1996. *Morbidity & Mortality Weekly Review, 46,* 165–173.

Chang, C., & White-Means, S. (1991). The men who care: An analysis of male primary caregivers who care for frail elderly at home. *The Journal of Applied Gerontology, 10,* 343–358.

Denzin, N. (1987). *Sociological methods: A source book.* (2nd ed.). New York: McGraw-Hill.

Denzin, N., & Lincoln, Y. (Eds.). (1994). *Handbook of qualitative research.* Thousand Oaks, CA: Sage.

Durham, J., & Lashley, F. (Eds.). (2000). *The person with HIV/AIDS: Nursing perspectives.* New York: Springer.

Farran, C., Keane-Hagerty, E., Salloway, S., Kupferer, S., & Wilken, C. (1991). Finding meaning: An alternative paradigm for Alzheimer's disease family caregivers. *The Gerontologist, 31,* 483–489.

Fitting, M., Rabins, P., Lucas, M., & Eastham, J. (1986). Caregivers of dementia patients: A comparison of husbands and wives. *The Gerontologist, 26,* 248–252.

Flaskerud, J., & Ungvarski, P. (1992). *HIV/AIDS: A guide to nursing care* (2nd ed.). Philadelphia: W. B. Saunders.

Folkman, S., Chesney, M. A., & Christopher-Richards, A. (1994). Stress and coping in caregiving partners of men with AIDS. *Psychiatric Clinics of North America, 17,* 35–55.

Glaser, B. (1978). *Theoretical sensitivity: Advances in methodology of grounded theory.* Mill Valley, CA: Sociology Press.

Glaser, B., & Strauss, A. (1967). *The discovery of grounded theory: Strategies for qualitative research.* New York: Aldine DeGruyter.

Gwyther, L., & George, L. (1986). Caregivers for dementia patients: Complex determinants of well-being and burden. *The Gerontologist, 26,* 245–247.

Horowitz, A. (1985). Sons and daughters as caregivers to older parents: Differences in role performance and consequences. *The Gerontologist, 25,* 612–617.

Hutchinson, S. (1986). Grounded theory. The method. In P. Munhall & C.

Oiler (Eds.), *Nursing research: A qualitative perspective* (pp. 111–130). Norwalk, CT: Appleton-Century-Crofts.

Hutchinson, S., Wilson, M., & Wilson, H. (1994). Benefits of participation in research interviews. *IMAGE: Journal of Nursing Scholarship, 26,* 161–164.

King, B., & Mishel, M. (1986). *Uncertainty appraisal and management in chronic illness.* Paper presented at the Nineteenth Communicating Nursing Research conference, Western Society for Research in Nursing, Portland, Oregon.

Koch, T. (1994). Establishing rigor in qualitative research: The decision trail. *Journal of Advanced Nursing, 19,* 976–986.

Kvale, S. (1988). The 1000-page question. *Phenomenology and Pedagogy, 6*(2), 90–106.

Lincoln, Y., & Guba, E. (1985). *Naturalistic inquiry.* Newbury Park, CA: Sage.

Little, J., Long, A., & Kehoe, B. (1990). AIDS home health, attendant and hospice care pilot project. *Physician Association in AIDS Care (PAAC) Notes, 2*(1), 32–57.

Marshall, C., & Rossman, G. (1995). *Doing qualitative research.* (2nd ed.). Newbury Park, CA: Sage.

Matheny, S., Mehr, M., & Brown, G. (1997). Caregivers and HIV infection: Services and issues. *Primary Care, 24,* 677–690.

May, K. (1991). Interview techniques in qualitative research: Concerns and challenges. In J. Morse (Ed.), *Qualitative nursing research: A contemporary dialogue* (rev. ed.) (pp. 188–201). Newbury Park, CA: Sage.

Miles, M., & Huberman, A. (1994). *An expanded sourcebook: Qualitative data analysis* (2nd ed.). Thousand Oaks, CA: Sage.

Mishel, M. (1990). Reconceptualization of the uncertainty in illness theory. *Image: Journal of Nursing Scholarship, 22,* 256–262.

Morse, J. (Ed.). (1992). *Critical issues in qualitative research methods.* Thousand Oaks, CA: Sage.

Noelker, L., & Wallace, R. (1985). The organization of family care for impaired elderly. *Journal of Family Issues, 6,* 23–44.

Oberst, M., & Scott, D. (1988). Post discharge distress in surgically treated cancer patients and their spouses. *Research in Nursing and Health, 11,* 223–233.

Omery, A. (1983). Phenomenology: A method for nursing research. *Advances in Nursing Science, 5*(2), 49–63.

Pantaleo, G., Graziosi C., & Fauci, A. S. (1993). New concepts in the immunopathogenesis of human immunodeficiency virus (HIV) infection. *The New England Journal of Medicine, 328,* 327–335.

Pruchno, R., & Resch, N. (1989). Aberrant behaviors and Alzheimer's disease: Mental health effects on spouse caregivers. *Journal of Gerontology: Social Science, 44*(5) S177–S182.

Rabins, P., Fitting, M., Eastham, J., & Fettig, J. (1990). The emotional impact of caring for the chronically ill. *Psychosomatics, 31*, 331–336.

Rutman, D. (1996). Caregiving as women's work: Women's experiences of powerfulness and powerlessness as caregivers. *Qualitative Health Research, 6*, 90–111.

Schulz, R., Williamson, G., Morycz, R., & Biegel, D. (1992). A longitudinal study of the costs and benefits of providing care to Alzheimer's patients. In S. Oskamp & S. Spacapan (Eds.), *The Social Psychology of Helping*. Newbury Park, CA: Sage.

Sipes, C., & Farran, C. (1995). *Experiences of gay male caregivers who provide care for their partners with AIDS*. Unpublished manuscript, Rush University College of Nursing, Chicago, Illinois.

Snyder, B., & Keefe, K. (1985). The unmet needs of family caregivers for frail and disabled adults. *Social Work in Health Care, 10*(3), 1–14.

Sowell, R. (1995). The view from here: Gay men should not be forgotten. *Journal of Association of Nurses in AIDS Care, 6*(1), 15–16.

Stetz, K. (1987). Caregiving demands during advanced cancer: The spouses needs. *Cancer Nursing, 10*, 260–268.

Stone, R., Cafferata, G., & Sangle, J. (1987). Caregivers of the frail elderly: A national profile. *The Gerontologist, 27*, 616–626.

Strauss, A. (1987). *Qualitative analysis for social scientists*. Cambridge, UK: Cambridge University Press.

Strauss, A., & Corbin, J. (1990). *Basics of qualitative research: Grounded theory procedures and techniques*. Newbury Park, CA: Sage.

Strauss, A., & Corbin, J. (1994). Grounded theory methodology: An overview. In N. Denzin & Y. Lincoln (Eds.), *Handbook of qualitative research* (pp. 273–285). Newbury Park, CA: Sage.

Wilson, H., & Hutchinson, S. (1996). Methodologic mistakes in grounded theory. *Nursing Research, 45*, 122–124.

Zarit, S., Todd, P., & Zarit, J. (1986). Subjective burdens of husbands and wives as caregivers: A longitudinal study. *The Gerontologist, 26*, 260–267.

AIDS Caregiving Stress Among HIV-Infected Men[1]

8

Richard G. Wight

INTRODUCTION

This chapter summarizes findings from a longitudinal study of 376 gay-identified men who cared for a partner or friend living with HIV or AIDS. The focus is on sources of stress among caregivers whose risk of adverse effects may be especially pronounced—men who are themselves infected with HIV (HIV+). Comparable HIV negative (HIV–) caregivers are also examined, permitting the identification of factors that are specific to HIV+ caregivers. The gay male community has been especially involved in informal AIDS caregiving because, to date, they account for the largest proportion of reported AIDS cases in the United States (Centers for Disease Control and Prevention [CDCP], 2000). Gay men may care for partners and friends because of relationship commitments and because ties to "traditional" extended family networks have often been severed (Mullan, 1998; Wardlaw, 1994), engendering an unprecedented juxtaposition of families of choice and families of origin.

Gay men who care for a friend or partner with AIDS are subject to unique sources of caregiving stress because they enter into the caregiving role at a relatively early stage in the life course (LeBlanc & Wight, 2000), are subject to AIDS stigma, which stems from homophobia and fear of contagion (Herek & Glunt, 1988), and must deal with unpredictable illness trajectories on the part of the care recipient (Folkman, Chesney, Cooke, Boccellari, & Collette, 1994; Pearlin, Mullen, Aneshensel, Wardlaw, & Harrington, 1994; Wardlaw, 1994). Their mental health also may be

[1] This research was supported by a grant from the National Institute of Mental Health (R01 MH 44600, Leonard I. Pearlin, Principal Investigator).

affected by varying degrees of homophobia, or negative reactions to their homosexuality, which may be external or internal in origin (Cass, 1996; Gonsiorek, 1995; Herek, 1995; Rothblum, 1994), or multiple experiences of AIDS-related deaths within their social networks (Gluhoski, Fishman, & Perry, 1997; Martin, Dean, Garcia, & Hall, 1989; Vedhara & Nott, 1996). For caregivers who are themselves infected with HIV, the stress experience may be magnified by its precursive nature (Wight, 2000). HIV infected men provide care knowing the roles may well have been reversed, or with some certainty that they too will require care in the future.

The distinction between HIV and AIDS is important because it defines the individual's illness trajectory. There may be little or no initial sympto-matology in the immediate aftermath of infection with HIV. A person may feel healthy and live with HIV infection for many years, and is not diag-nosed with AIDS unless they are HIV+ *and* meet the clinical criteria as designated by the CDCP. Caregiving assistance is usually required only after a person has been infected with HIV for an extended period of time. Most persons with AIDS experience a variety of opportunistic health prob-lems that range from fairly mild (oral candidiasis) to quite debilitating (toxoplasmosis of the brain) or disfiguring (Kaposi's sarcoma). There are more than twenty clinical conditions that are included in AIDS surveillance case definitions (LACDHS, 2000), each with varying degrees of severity and complication. Persons with AIDS constantly struggle to maintain their health, and the ups and downs in their health create chronic stress that affects the degree to which they can function (Folkman, 1993; Griffin, Rabkin, Remien, & Williams, 1998).

As a result of the heterogeneity of the HIV experience, the functional status of persons living with HIV (PLH) is quite varied. For example, PLH may be employed at times or they may be home bound; they may need assistance with activities of daily living (ADL), or they may be able to func-tion independently all of the time. The types of assistance they may require occur along a continuum of care (Benjamin, 1989), in which intense care provision is necessitated at some points in time but not at others. In the past, most PLH have eventually needed assistance with virtually all aspects of daily living as their health deteriorated (Raveis & Siegel, 1991; Weitz, 1989). This scenario has changed more recently with the intro-duction of highly active anti-retroviral therapy (HAART), but the case fatality rate for AIDS remains about 60% (CDCP, 2000). Whereas AIDS is a terminal illness, persons with HIV do not fit into traditional models of death and dying (see, e.g., Kubler-Ross, 1969). Their illness trajectories are not clearly or uniformly defined and their functional abilities are vari-able and fluctuating.

Thus, young age, stigma, homophobia, unpredictable illness trajecto-ries, multiple experiences of AIDS-related bereavements, and HIV status may negatively affect the caregiver's mental health in addition to and in conjunction with other care-related stressors. In other words, these caregivers are exposed to stressors that impinge on the lives of caregivers in general and also encounter stressors that are unique to gay caregivers to PLH. In this chapter, the effects of both general sources of caregiving stress and these unique sources of stress are documented among HIV+ caregivers, in comparison to HIV− caregivers.

CONCEPTUAL FRAMEWORK

This study was based on the concept of stress proliferation as described by Pearlin and associates (1990, 1997). The stress proliferation model evolved out of investigations of the stress process in general, and as it specifically pertains to caregivers to persons with Alzheimer's disease and AIDS (Aneshensel, 1992; Aneshensel et al., 1995; Pearlin, 1989; Pearlin et al., 1990, 1997). The main premise of stress proliferation is that some stressful life experiences generate more stress, setting in motion a series of events and circumstances that compound the original source of stress and lead to psychological distress (Pearlin et al., 1997). Primary stressors are the original source of stress, in this instance care-related activities, and secondary stressors grow out of the dislocations that accompany these activities. Secondary stressors are no less pervasive than primary stressors but are secondary in the sense that they are consequences of the original stressor. Thus, stressors tend to beget other stressors, which, in turn, affect emotional well-being (Pearlin et al., 1990, 1997).

Primary stressors associated with AIDS caregiving are located in the actual activities of caregiving: the need for assistance by the PLH because of declining functional status (see Figure 8.1). These stressors may be objective (e.g., assistance provided with personal care), or subjective (e.g., feelings of burden or overload that flow from these activities) in nature (Pearlin et al., 1990, 1997). Secondary stressors associated with AIDS caregiving are located in other realms of the caregiver's life. For example, the demand for care may tax the caregiver's monetary resources, leading to financial worry, especially if the caregiver or PLH is unemployed. Primary and secondary stressors are preceded conceptually by background and contextual characteristics of the caregiver and PLH. Social statuses and resources, such as age and income, may affect the stress proliferation process by influencing exposure to stress or access to coping resources. Especially important for this study are background characteristics such as gay acceptance and AIDS-related stigma that uniquely influence the stress process for HIV+ gay caregivers. The proliferation of stress may be mediated by factors that are internal (coping) or external (social support) in origin

BACKGROUND
CHARACTERISTICS

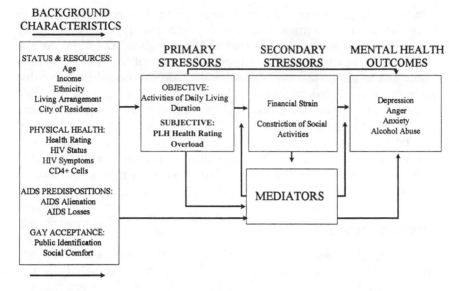

FIGURE 8.1   Conceptual Framework.

(Pearlin et al., 1990). Stress mediators are not assessed for the present analysis, but it is important to note that these mediators may facilitate caregivers in the fulfillment of their roles by intervening in the stress-distress relationship (Turner & Catania, 1997).

For this chapter, sources of stress proliferation were traced over time among HIV+ caregivers, in comparison to HIV– caregivers. These analyses established the effects of background characteristics on primary and secondary stressors, the effects of primary stressors on secondary stressors, and subsequent effects of all sources of stress on caregiver mental health.

METHODS

Field Procedures

Data were from personal interviews conducted with primary caregivers to PLH in two sites: San Francisco and Los Angeles. Data were collected at three points in time, at six month intervals, from 1991 to 1993. Structured interviews were conducted by lay persons trained specifically for this research. Study participants were typically interviewed in their homes, interviews lasted approximately two hours, and each caregiver was paid $25 upon completion. Caregivers were reinterviewed at each time point regardless of changes in assistance requirements or the PLH's death.

Study participants were primary caregivers providing ongoing practical assistance with activities of daily living to a friend, partner, or family member. Physical activity on the part of the caregiver was required; the exclusive provision of emotional support was not sufficient to qualify for the study. A total of 642 caregivers self-selected into the study. Forty-five percent were recruited in Los Angeles and 55% were recruited in San Francisco. Participants were obtained through a variety of recruitment channels. Most responded to mass media announcements in newspapers, radio, or television (32%), or were referred through community-based AIDS organizations (32%). The remaining caregivers were recruited through doctor's offices, clinics, health fairs, gay pride festivals, and other miscellaneous sources (36%).

Analytic Subsample

For this chapter, analyses were limited to caregiving men who were gay-identified, not blood relatives of the PLH, and caring for a male PLH (i.e., a significant partner or friend). Caregivers were asked, "Do you identify yourself as gay/lesbian, bisexual, or heterosexual?" Only those who selected the "gay" response (n_1 = 376; HIV+ = 153; HIV– = 223) were included in this analysis. This operationalization of "gay caregivers" excludes those who identify as bisexual to maintain sample homogeneity on this important characteristic. Note that HIV+ caregivers are themselves PLH, but are primarily the donors rather than the recipients of care. Thus, in these analyses, the phrase PLH generally refers to the care-receiver. The sample size decreased at each data collection point due to attrition and caregiver death (n_2 = 340, n_3 = 307). Attrition effects are discussed below. Although caregiving activities ceased when the care-receiver died, bereaved caregivers were nevertheless reinterviewed. At the second interview, 214 men continued to provide care (95 HIV+, 119 HIV–) and 126 were bereaved (40 HIV+, 86 HIV–). At the third interview, 143 men continued to provide care (62 HIV+, 81 HIV–), and 164 were bereaved (56 HIV+, 108 HIV–).

As shown in Table 8.1 under the heading "Statuses and Resources," the average caregiver in this subsample was middle aged, with some college education, and low-middle income. HIV+ caregivers were significantly younger, less educated, and had significantly lower incomes than the HIV–. Over half were co-residing significant partners, with HIV+ caregivers significantly more likely than HIV– caregivers to share this living arrangement with the PLH. Ethnic minorities were represented in one-third of the caregiver-PLH dyads, and this type of ethnic representation was significantly more likely to occur among HIV+ caregivers. Over one-third of all caregivers were unemployed, with the HIV+ significantly more likely than the HIV– to be out of work.

TABLE 8.1 Sample Characteristics at Baseline (Means/Proportions)

Baseline Characteristics	Total (N = 376) M (SD)		HIV+ (N = 153) M (SD)		HIV– (N = 223) M (SD)	
Statuses & Resources						
CG age (years)	38.90	(8.60)	37.24	(6.66)	40.03	(9.56)***
CG education (years)	14.98	(2.14)	14.50	(2.23)	15.30	(2.01)***
CG income (thousands of dollars)	27.65	(20.29)	20.88	(16.26)	32.30	(21.47)***
CG and/or PLH minority (/non-Hispanic White)	.33		.42		.28**	
CG and PLH co-residing partners (/no)	.54		.61		.49*	
CG unemployed	.36		.47		.29***	
CG lives in Los Angeles (/San Francisco)	.43		.39		.46	
Physical Health						
CG poor health rating (1–5)	2.31	(.96)	2.81	(.93)	1.97	(.82)***
HIV+ symptomatic[a]			.65			
CD4+ count[a,b]			422.40	(270.76)		
AIDS Predispositions						
AIDS alienation (1–4)	3.02	(.41)	3.01	(.42)	3.02	(.42)
Number of close friends who died from AIDS	6.84	(9.58)	9.05	(11.67)	5.33	(7.49)***
Gay Acceptance						
Comfort with other gay people (1–4)	2.75	(.59)	2.77	(.59)	2.73	(.59)
Degree of "outness" (1–4)	3.38	(.63)	3.51	(.56)	3.30	(.66)**
Primary Stressors						
ADL assistance (1–4)	1.90	(.53)	1.91	(.51)	1.89	(.55)
Years CG has been helping PLH	1.78	(1.66)	1.73	(1.60)	1.81	(1.69)
Role overload (1–4)	2.78	(.70)	2.76	(.67)	2.80	(.73)
PLH poor health rating (1–5)	3.73	(.87)	3.71	(.86)	3.75	(.88)
Secondary Stressors						
Financial worry (1–4)	2.50	(.85)	2.66	(.81)	2.40	(.87)**
Constriction of social life (1–4)	2.33	(.77)	2.33	(.72)	2.34	(.80)
Mental Health Outcomes						
Depression (1–4)	1.99	(.67)	2.09	(.68)	1.92	(.65)*
Anger (1–4)	1.72	(.58)	1.73	(.59)	1.71	(.57)
Anxiety (1–4)	2.11	(.84)	2.18	(.81)	2.07	(.85)
Heavy alcohol use (/no)	.27		.32		.24	

Note. CG = Caregiver; PLH = Person Living with HIV.

[a] HIV+ only.

[b] Truncated at 1,000; less than 6 months since last test.

* $p < .05$. ** $p < .01$. *** $p < .001$; HIV+ differ from HIV–.

Measures

Physical health.   The caregiver's health rating ranged from poor (5) to excellent (1). As shown in Table 8.1, the average score was 2.31 (SD = .96), corresponding to a health rating of "very good," and HIV+ caregivers were in significantly poorer health than the HIV−. Caregivers who reported being infected with HIV were subsequently asked about HIV-related symptoms and illnesses. Nearly two-thirds of HIV+ caregivers had experienced HIV-related symptoms. HIV infected caregivers were also asked if they had CD4+ counts completed, and if so, the result. CD4+ cell counts, also called "helper-cells" or "T-helper cells" or "T-cells," are well-accepted indicators of the impact of HIV disease on the immune system (Perkins et al., 1995). CD4+ counts are considered low if they drop below 500, and, as of 1993, those with counts lower than 200 are formally diagnosed with AIDS (CDC, 2000). CD4+ counts were included as measures of caregiver health only if they were obtained less than six months prior to the interview. The mean number of CD4+ cells was less than 500 among those who had recently been tested, indicative of compromised immune function.

AIDS-related dispositions.   An 8-item scale measured feelings of AIDS alienation-stigma with response categories of strongly disagree (1) to strongly agree (4). Its mean score was equivalent to a response of "agree" among both the HIV+ and the HIV−. Caregivers were also asked how many of their close friends died from AIDS, which averaged 6.84 (SD = 9.58), a huge loss to any individual's social network, and the HIV+ had lost significantly more close friends to AIDS than the HIV−.

Gay acceptance.   Gay public identification, or "outness," was measured through a 3-item scale that ascertained the proportion of the caregiver's friends, family members, and acquaintances or neighbors who knew about his homosexuality (α = .70). The average score indicated that most members of the caregiver's social network were aware that he was gay and that the HIV+ were significantly more "out" than the HIV−. Social comfort with other gay people was measured with a 4-item scale (α = .74) and its mean score indicated fairly high comfort levels among both the HIV+ and HIV−. Gay acceptance and "outness" were only assessed at baseline, and, therefore, changes in these variables over time cannot be ascertained.

Objective primary stressors.   Global need for assistance with activities of daily life (ADL) was measured by combining three dimensions: Personal ADL (α = .88; Katz & Lyerly, 1963) (eating, dressing, and toileting); Instrumental ADL (α = .81; Lawton, Lipton, & Kleban, 1969) (housework, laundry, and transportation); and Affairs Management (α = .78; Pearlin et al., 1990). Its mean score was indicative of an average response of "helps with some of it in the past few weeks" (α = .88). As shown in Table 8.1, caregivers had been at these tasks for an average of 1.78 years (SD = 1.66), although some had been providing care for over a decade (range = .03 to 12 years). Objective primary stressors did not differ significantly between HIV+ and HIV– caregivers.

Subjective primary stressors.   Role overload was measured with a 4-item scale (α = .82; Pearlin et al., 1990) that assessed agreement with items such as "you have more things to do than you can handle" and "you don't have enough time just for yourself." The mean score indicated overall agreement. The caregiver's perception of the PLH's health was a primary stressor because it established the demand for care and the mean score was equivalent to a response of "poor." HIV+ and HIV– caregivers reported similar levels of subjective primary stress.

Secondary stressors.   Financial worry was a 5-item scale that asked how concerned respondents were about money (α = .78; Pearlin and Radabaugh, 1985). As shown in Table 8.1, the mean score showed that caregivers were moderately concerned about finances, and the HIV+ were significantly more concerned than the HIV–. Constriction of social life was a 6-item scale that reflected the extent to which caregivers had to give up social and leisure activities (e.g., vacations, exercise, and hobbies; α = .84), and its mean score indicated that, on average, both HIV+ and HIV– caregivers had to give up a few activities.

Mental health outcomes.   Depression, anxiety, and anger were each assessed by modified subscales of the Hopkins Symptom Checklist (HSCL) (Derogatis, Lipman, Rickels, Uhlenhuth, & Covi, 1974). The mean score for depression (6 items, α = .82) indicated that the average caregiver experienced symptoms of depression during one or two days in the previous week, with the HIV+ experiencing significantly greater levels than the HIV–. The mean score for anger (4 items, α = .74) indicated a response equivalent to experiencing anger during "1 or 2 days" in the past week. The mean score for anxiety (4 items, α = .84), indicated that, like depression and anger, the average caregiver experienced anxiety during one or two days in the previous week.

Findings from epidemiologic surveys suggest that men may be more prone to abuse alcohol in response to social stressors than to feel depressed (Aneshensel, Rutter, & Lachenbruch, 1991; Kessler et al., 1994). Therefore, a composite alcohol abuse variable was created from measures of typical frequency and number of alcoholic drinks consumed. Analyses summarized here utilized a dichotomous measure of alcohol abuse, coded 1 for heavy use and 0 for abstains, light, or moderate use. As shown in Table 8.1, well over one-quarter of the caregivers in this sample were heavy alcohol users, and the HIV+ did not significantly differ from the HIV–.

Data Analysis

Data were examined through multivariate regression analyses (ordinary least squares regression for continuous outcomes, logistic regression for alcohol abuse). Independent correlates of primary stressors, secondary stressors, and mental health outcomes were assessed by regressing the outcomes on variables that preceded them in the conceptual framework (see Figure 8.1). Stepwise selection was used to obtain a parsimonious set of independent variables. For longitudinal analyses, baseline values of the dependent variable were controlled so that the coefficients for independent variables were effects on change in the dependent variable between two time points. In addition, baseline values for independent variables were forced into any regression models where change scores were significant. When a change score is included as a predictor of a subsequent outcome, baseline scores represent the amount of the score that is stable between two time points, and the change score represents variation between the two time points. Change was computed as Time 2 minus Time 1, or Time 3 minus Time 1.

Regression analyses were stratified by HIV infection status because the variance-covariance matrices for HIV+ and HIV– caregivers could not be pooled (Time 1 $\chi^2 = 288.75$, $df = 171$, $p < .0001$; Time 2 $\chi^2 = 510.88$, $df = 351$, $p < .0001$; Time 3 $\chi^2 = 429.07$, $df = 351$, $p < .01$). Longitudinal models were first assessed for those who continued to provide care at follow-up (i.e., nonbereaved, referred to as "continuing care"). Subsequent analyses combined the continuing care and bereaved groups, but because these analyses included both the bereaved and nonbereaved, care-related variables were removed and bereavement status was controlled. Comparisons between HIV+ and HIV– caregivers were made by replicating significant regression models for the HIV infected group among the HIV– and highlighting dissimilarities. Analyses were conducted among multiple subsamples because some aspects of stress proliferation were relevant to only some caregivers.

Effects of Attrition Over Time

Attrition was of concern because the men most at risk for care-related stress were those in the poorest health, which may have made them unavailable for reinterview. To assess the impact of attrition, subsequent participation status was used in a logistic regression with prior risk factors (Time 1 or Time 2) used as independent variables to determine whether loss was systematic. The logistic regression model was not statistically significant for either Time 2 or Time 3, indicating a low probability of systematic loss.

RESULTS

Independent effects of statuses and resources, physical health, AIDS predispositions, and gay acceptance on primary stressors, secondary stressors, and mental health as well as primary and secondary stressors on mental health are summarized below. The effects of the variables, as they emerged in multivariate regressions, are described in the order in which they appear in the conceptual model (see Figure 8.1). For each variable, significant effects (< .05) found among HIV+ caregivers are described first, and congruence or divergence in findings with HIV– caregivers are then noted. As discussed earlier, multivariate regressions were conducted separately at each wave of data collection for HIV+ and HIV– caregivers. In addition, regressions were further stratified at Times 2 and 3 for: (a) the continuing care, and (b) the continuing care combined with the bereaved. The former allows for the identification of longitudinal effects of contemporaneous caregiving activities, and the latter allows for assessments of stress that may extend beyond the cessation of caregiving. These summaries necessarily omit statistical detail and are intended to provide a general overview of the potential origins of stress among these caregiving men.

Statuses and Resources

Caregiver age. Caregiver age was negatively associated with anger at Time 1 and increasing anger at Time 3 among the HIV+ continuing care. A similar effect was found for the HIV–, indicating that younger caregivers were more likely to experience anger and increasing anger than older caregivers, regardless of their HIV status.

Caregiver education. Caregiver education was negatively associated with anxiety at Time 2 among the HIV+ continuing care, and among the total HIV+ subsample at Time 3. Additionally, education was negatively associated with heavy alcohol use at Time 3 among only the HIV+ continuing care. Education was not associated with anxiety or alcohol use among the HIV– at the multivariate level. These results indicate that education may have played a minimal role in containing the mental impact of AIDS-related caregiving and that this role was largely exerted through other components of the stress proliferation process.

Caregiver income.   Caregiver income was negatively associated with financial worry at Times 2 and 3 among the total HIV+ subsample (i.e., the continuing care combined with the bereaved) and among the HIV–. At Time
2, increasing income was associated with increasing anxiety and increasing anger among the HIV+ continuing care. These findings may have been
due to the effects of added role demands associated with the source of the
increasing income. HIV– caregivers also experienced increasing anxiety
with increasing income at Time 2, but their anger levels did not also
increase. Thus, the effects of income on caregiver mental health are complex and not simply a matter of income serving as a resource.

Minority status.   Minority status of the caregiver, the PLH, or both individuals influenced only depression at Time 1 among the HIV+. Minority
status was negatively associated with depression, indicating that depression was lower among caregivers who were ethnic minority members or
who cared for a minority PLH, than in caregiving dyads where both individuals were non-Hispanic White. This association held true for HIV–
caregivers as well. The contribution of minority status to depression was
fairly strong, but the finding could be spurious. AIDS caregivers who
were ethnic minorities or cared for ethnic minority PLHs could have been
less prone to depression than their counterparts. Minority status was not
associated with depression longitudinally, or with any other mental health
outcomes, so this finding was most likely not robust.

Co-residence as significant partners.   Co-residence with the PLH as his significant partner consistently emerged as an independent correlate of
stress proliferation among HIV+ caregivers who were not bereaved. This
living arrangement was positively associated with ADL assistance at
Times 2 and 3, negatively associated with the PLH's poor health at Time
1, negatively associated with role overload at Time 2, positively associated
with social constriction at Time 1, and negatively associated with heavy
alcohol use at Time 1.

In contrast to HIV+ caregivers, co-residence with the PLH as his significant partner was not associated with ADL assistance, the PLH's poor
health, or role overload among HIV– caregivers. In addition, the association between this living arrangement and heavy alcohol use among the
HIV– was positive, a finding opposite to that for the HIV+. Thus, HIV+
caregivers who lived with the PLH as his significant partner were less
likely to be heavy drinkers than HIV+ caregivers who did not share this
living arrangement, whereas HIV– caregivers who lived with the PLH as
his significant partner were more likely to be heavy drinkers than HIV–
caregivers who did not share this living arrangement.

Caregiver unemployment.   Caregiver unemployment did not influence the stress proliferation process directly and was only occasionally an independent correlate of caregiver mental health among HIV+ caregivers. Unemployment was associated with baseline depression and with increasing depression at Time 3 among the total HIV+ subsample (i.e., continuing care and bereaved). Unemployment was also associated with baseline anger among the continuing care. Unemployment did not similarly affect mental health among the HIV–. These sporadic effects indicated no uniform influence of unemployment on caregiver stress and mental health.

City of residence.   Living in Los Angeles versus living in San Francisco had no independent effects on stress proliferation or caregiver mental health at the multivariate level.

Physical Health

Poor caregiver health.   Poor or deteriorating caregiver health influenced primary stressors, secondary stressors, and mental health outcomes among HIV+ caregivers. The strongest impact of poor health on primary stressors occurred with role overload at Time 1. The strongest impact of poor health on secondary stressors occurred with financial worry at Time 2. The strongest impacts of poor health on mental health occurred with depression, anxiety, and anger at Time 3. Thus, the magnitude of the effects of poor health appeared to be a function of both time and the expansion of caregiver stressors. That is, the strength of the effects of poor health followed the sequence of stress proliferation. Poor health strongly influenced perceptions of burden early in the caregiving trajectory. Several months later, consistently poor or deteriorating health influenced feelings of financial worry. Still later, consistently poor or deteriorating health was strongly associated with emotional distress.

In sharp contrast, poor and deteriorating physical health did not similarly influence the stress process among HIV– caregivers. HIV– caregivers may have felt anxious if they were in poor or declining physical health, but poor health did not influence their feelings of burden, financial worry, social constriction, depression, or anger as it did among the HIV+. These findings demonstrate the unique compounding effects of poor health and increasing burden on caregiver mental health among HIV+ caregivers. Both sources of stress were independently associated with emotional distress, and poor health indirectly influenced caregiver mental health through covariation with role overload.

CD4+ counts.   Perceptions of poor health influenced stress proliferation and mental health more extensively than self-reported CD4+ counts among

HIV+ caregivers. High CD4+ counts were associated with high levels of ADL assistance at Time 2, suggesting that healthier caregivers were able to provide higher levels of assistance than those who were less healthy (i.e., had low CD4+ counts). Anxiety and anger were a function of persistently low and decreasing CD4+ counts, but only when the analytic sample size was increased by inclusion of bereaved caregivers. That is, there was no independent contribution of CD4+ counts to anxiety or anger among only those caregivers who continued care at Times 2 and 3. The directions of the associations between CD4+ counts and ADL assistance (positive) and emotional distress (negative) were logical. Regression coefficients for the effects of CD4+ counts were fairly small, however. Therefore, self-reported CD4+ counts were useful to the extent that they demonstrated mental health consequences of declining immune system function, but they did not appear to meaningfully add to the study of caregiving stress.

HIV symptomatology. Perceptions of poor health also influenced stress proliferation and mental health more extensively than HIV symptomatology. HIV symptomatology did not independently influence primary stressors or secondary stressors but was positively associated with increasing anger at Time 3. Additionally, HIV+ symptomatic caregivers were more likely to be heavy drinkers at Times 2 and 3 than HIV+ caregivers who were asymptomatic.

Unfortunately, the association between HIV symptomatology and heavy alcohol use could not be fully elaborated in this study, because only frequency and amount of alcohol consumption were assessed. Caregivers were not asked why they drink, or whether or not they experience problems because of their drinking, two important aspects of alcohol consumption (Pierce, Frone, Russell, & Cooper, 1996; Seeman, Seeman, & Budros, 1988). HIV+ symptomatic caregivers may have drunk alcohol to regulate or relieve stress, or drinking may have been a response to feelings of powerlessness.

AIDS Predispositions

AIDS alienation. Feelings of AIDS alienation importantly affected the mental health of HIV+ caregivers. High levels of AIDS alienation or increasing AIDS alienation were positively associated with depression, anxiety, anger, and heavy alcohol use among the continuing care subsample and the total HIV+ sample. Additionally, AIDS alienation was associated with the secondary stressor of financial worry at Time 1 among the continuing care. The magnitude of each of these associations was similar.

AIDS alienation measured aspects of AIDS stigma that caregivers perceived. Findings from this study indicated that AIDS alienation played a crucial role in determining how caregiver stress manifested in emotional distress. Caregivers who agreed with statements such as "no one outside the gay community really cares about people with AIDS," "if there were less prejudice against gays and I.V. drug users, more money would be spent on AIDS research," and "politicians are less interested in AIDS than in other diseases" were also likely to experience elevated levels of emotional distress. It is possible that some caregivers experienced AIDS alienation because they were depressed, anxious, and so forth, but the longitudinal nature of these data showed that even when controlling for prior levels of emotional distress AIDS alienation independently influenced mental health.

The independent effects of AIDS alienation on mental health differed somewhat between HIV+ and HIV– caregivers. Among the HIV–, AIDS alienation was not associated with depression or heavy alcohol use at the multivariate level. It appeared that AIDS alienation was more likely to produce a dysphoric response among the HIV+ than among the HIV–, but that both groups experienced anxiety and anger in response to AIDS alienation.

Close AIDS losses. Close AIDS losses had few independent effects on caregiver stress proliferation among HIV+ caregivers. The loss of close friends to AIDS was positively associated with heavy alcohol use among the continuing care at Time 1. Additionally, close AIDS losses and increasing losses were associated with increasing anger at Time 3, but only among the total HIV+ subsample (i.e., continuing care and bereaved). It appeared that the loss of close friends to AIDS was more likely to produce feelings of anger than the loss of the PLH. However, anger seems like a natural response to multiple bereavements. There were no similar effects of close AIDS losses on heavy alcohol use or anger among the HIV–.

The lack of extensive effects of close AIDS losses on caregiver mental health was somewhat surprising. Other studies found elevated levels of psychological distress in samples of gay men that may be attributable to multiple AIDS bereavements (e.g., Dew et al., 1997; Joseph et al., 1990). The average caregiver in this study had lost 7 close friends to AIDS, and HIV+ symptomatic caregivers had lost an average of 10 close friends at baseline and 3 additional close friends over the course of the study. Effects of baseline levels of AIDS losses on mental health could not be temporized, but the effects of increasing losses should have been detectable because they occurred proximal to the time of the interview. Still, increasing losses of close friends to AIDS was associated with only increasing anger. Multiple AIDS bereavements may have become somewhat normative for men in this study, obscuring its expected effects on depression and anxiety.

Gay Acceptance

The mental health of men in this study may have been independently affected by their homosexual orientation. That is, internalized homophobia may have produced adverse mental health consequences among these men if they harbored negative feelings about their own homosexuality.

Gay social comfort. There was only one small independent effect of gay social comfort in these analyses. At Time 3, anxiety was negatively associated with gay social comfort among continuing care and bereaved caregivers who were infected with HIV. Caregivers who were comfortable around other gays were less anxious than caregivers who were uncomfortable around other gays. There was no similar finding among the HIV–.

Outness. In contrast to gay social comfort, openness about homosexuality more often influenced caregiver mental health. Being "out" was independently associated with decreasing depression at Time 2 (among both the continuing care only, and the total HIV+ subsample), low anger at Time 1, and decreasing anger among those continuing to provide care at Time 3. "Outness" had a similar effect on depression at Time 2 among HIV– caregivers. Additionally, being "out" was associated with decreasing social constriction at Time 2 among those continuing to provide care, but only among the HIV+.

The independent effects of openness about homosexuality on depression were not pervasive, but they were similar for both HIV+ and HIV– caregivers. These findings indicate that being "closeted" potentially increased the risk for depression, regardless of the caregiver's own health status or care-related demands. Consistent with other studies (e.g., LaSala, 2000; Meyer, 1995), there appeared to be mental health benefits associated with being "out" that could apply to all gay men. Importantly, no negative mental health effects of being "out" were found.

Being "closeted" appeared to put HIV+ caregivers at risk for feelings of anger that persisted and increased over time. Men with HIV or AIDS often simultaneously inform members of their social network that they are gay and infected with HIV. Gay men who have internalized high levels of homophobia or whose friends and family are homophobic may have been angry because they felt forced to keep their HIV status a secret, or else their homosexuality would have been disclosed or presumed. HIV+ caregivers whose families and friends knew that they were gay benefited from this form of disclosure to the extent that it made them less angry.

Caregiving Assistance

ADL assistance. Among both HIV+ and HIV– caregivers, there was no direct effect of ADL assistance on well-being, consistent with previous research (e.g., Aneshensel et al., 1995). High ADL assistance was, however, independently associated with social constriction at Time 1 among the HIV+. Persisting and increasing levels of ADL assistance among these men were even more powerfully associated with further constriction of social activities at Times 2 and 3. Increasing social constriction, in turn, was independently associated with increasing depression and heavy alcohol use at Time 3. Thus, escalating social constriction was a potential mechanism through which ADL assistance influenced caregiver mental health. This mechanism was unique to HIV+ caregivers, because there was no indirect effect of ADL assistance on mental health among HIV− caregivers.

Therefore, the activities of caregiving—assistance with personal care, instrumental care, and affairs management—were not independently associated with emotional distress or heavy alcohol use, but they were not inconsequential. HIV+ caregivers who provided increasing levels of assistance to the PLH did so at the expense of their own social interests. The increasing inability to pursue social activities outside the confines of caregiving led to increasing depression and was associated with heavy alcohol consumption.

Role overload. Subjective perceptions of burden influenced caregiver mental health both directly and through the effects of secondary stressors. Among the HIV+, role overload was directly associated with depression and anxiety at Times 1 and 2. Role overload was also directly associated with financial worry and social constriction, which were in turn associated with depression. Among the HIV−, role overload was also directly associated with depression, anxiety, financial worry, and social constriction, but financial worry was not associated with depression.

SUMMARY OF RESULTS

Among statuses and resources, co-residence with the PLH as his significant partner most frequently influenced the caregiver stress proliferation process among HIV+ caregivers, but less so among the HIV−. The interpretation of these findings is difficult, however, because the associations were not consistent over time. Caregiver age was negatively associated with anger among both the HIV+ and HIV−, suggesting that young caregivers may be ill equipped emotionally to manage their situation. Caregiver income was negatively associated with financial worry for both groups, but increasing income was associated with increasing anxiety and anger among HIV+ caregivers. Unlike the HIV−, HIV+ caregivers who were unemployed and who had low education levels were prone to psychological distress. Minority status of the caregiver and PLH did not independently affect stress proliferation, and minimally affected mental health.

Poor or deteriorating caregiver physical health pervasively affected the proliferation of caregiving stress among HIV+ caregivers who continued to assist the PLH over time. Among these men, subjective perceptions of poor health more powerfully affected stress proliferation and mental health than objective measures of CD4+ counts or HIV symptomatology. In other words, it appeared that these caregivers' appraisals of their health may have been more strongly influenced by the meaning that they attached to bodily sensations than by their awareness of an underlying disease. This appraisal, in turn, influenced their perceptions of burden, financial worry, social constriction, and emotional distress. Similar effects of subjective health appraisals were not found among HIV– caregivers. Thus, the HIV+ may have been particularly attuned to and responsive to their physical health.

AIDS alienation more consistently influenced caregiver stress proliferation and mental health than multiple AIDS bereavements among HIV+ caregivers. This result may have arisen because these two constructs captured different aspects of AIDS-specific distress. That is, AIDS alienation was a marker for perceived AIDS stigma, whereas multiple AIDS bereavements were indicative of mourning, grief, and diminishing social support. Thus, AIDS stigma more pervasively affected both the experience of care-related stress and its mental health consequences than did the loss of potential supporters. Findings between HIV+ and HIV– caregivers were dissimilar in that the mental health manifestations of AIDS alienation were less pronounced among the HIV– and there were no independent effects of bereavement experiences on mental health among the HIV–.

Gay acceptance had varying levels of influence on the caregiving stress proliferation process and caregiver mental health. Being "out" was more important to mental health than being socially comfortable with other gay people. Additionally, "outness" was more likely to promote positive mental health among the HIV+ than among the HIV–.

As discussed above, caregiver stress arises out of both objective demands of care provision and subjective appraisals of burden. Findings here indicated that objective care-related demands (i.e., ADL assistance levels) were indirectly associated with caregiver mental health, whereas subjective appraisals of burden (i.e., feelings of role overload) were both indirectly and directly associated with caregiver mental health. Social constriction was an important mechanism by which ADL assistance influenced caregiver mental health. Additionally, among the HIV–, ADL assistance was less consequential to social constriction than it was among the HIV+. The effects of role overload on mental health, therefore, were more extensive than the effects of ADL assistance because role overload influenced several stress and mental health outcomes. Both HIV+ and HIV– caregivers who found it increasingly burdensome to meet caregiving role obligations were prone to emotional distress, as well as to increasing uncertainties about social affairs. These findings were not surprising, given the onerous nature of providing care to a dying friend or partner.

DISCUSSION

Unlike caregiving in other settings, AIDS caregivers are more likely to be drawn from the ranks of gay male partners and friends because of HIV infection patterns in the United States (Turner, Catania, & Gagnon, 1994). Many women occupy the AIDS caregiver role (see Wight, LeBlanc, & Aneshensel, 1998), but gay-identified men, unrelated by blood or marriage, have rallied in support of one another in unprecedented numbers (Pearlin et al., 1994). Gay men consider their partners and friends to be family and thus share much in common with caregivers in other contexts (LeBlanc & Wight, 2000). Yet, because these relationships fall outside of the traditional definition of family and gender roles, these men are faced with challenges associated with the general societal devaluation of homosexuality and negative attitudes towards AIDS. Until AIDS became a considerable social problem, gay-identified men and their relationships were somewhat invisible. AIDS has forced health care providers, social service agencies, parents, spouses, and siblings to come to terms with their own prejudices about homosexuality. This examination of AIDS caregiving among gay-identified men offered the opportunity to explore how caregiving stress, as it was first operationalized in a study of caregivers to persons with Alzheimer's Disease, was experienced and manifested within a segment of the population marginalized because of their homosexuality and their HIV status.

Sources of stress that are unique to AIDS caregiving—AIDS alienation, gay acceptance, young age, the caregiver's own poor health due to HIV infection—were, in fact, critical determinants of stress and mental health. Men who were themselves infected with HIV—"precursive" AIDS caregivers—were subject to bombardments from multiple sources of stress. Among HIV– men, the caregiving stress process was also impacted by these unique factors, but not to the same extent as among the HIV+. Still, the combined effects of these unique stressors and more traditional caregiving stressors (i.e., role overload, ADL assistance, financial worry, and social constriction) were quite consequential to the caregiver's mental health.

HIV+ AIDS caregivers were particularly vulnerable to reciprocal effects of role overload, ADL assistance, financial worry, social constriction, depression, anxiety, and anger. Co-residence with the PLH as his significant partner further compounded these effects. Support services that are targeted toward alleviating some or all of these factors are bound to have a rippling effect. For example, services that provide financial assistance to those infected with HIV are likely to influence the caregiver's feelings of financial worry, which in turn may influence depression. Services that provide practical assistance may allow caregivers the opportunity to pursue social activities, dampening the effect of caregiving on social constriction and on depression, especially among those who live with the PLH.

Effects of "outness" about homosexuality are important. At various time points, caregivers who were "out" were less likely to be emotionally distressed than caregivers who concealed their homosexuality. The lack of independent *positive* associations between "outness" and emotional distress is notable: Being open about homosexuality appeared to have no negative mental health consequences. Therefore, service providers should consider encouraging AIDS caregivers who are gay men, especially those who are also HIV+, to be open about their sexual orientation. Such openness may not only have mental health benefits, but may also facilitate their use of services that are targeted to the gay male community. However, because of wide variation in individual experiences and circumstances, it may not be practical for all caregivers to be "out" and future qualitative investigations might explicate how "outness" is relevant or not relevant to the experience of caregiving among gay men.

The effects of AIDS stigma on AIDS caregivers were extensive, especially among the HIV+. HIV+ caregivers who experienced AIDS alienation were prone to depression, anxiety, anger, and heavy alcohol use. Unfortunately, it is not realistic to suggest that AIDS stigma be eradicated. It is feasible, however, to advocate support for AIDS research, and AIDS education campaigns that aim to correct myths about AIDS and homosexuality and that encourage empathy for PLH. Such efforts may have no direct bearing on the mental health of AIDS caregivers, but they may help to alleviate some of the social distancing that caregivers and PLH experience. Healthcare providers, in particular, must continue to be educated about diversity in the medical care setting and gay men's health needs.

Results from this study indicated that, among the HIV+, the caregiver's own deteriorating health was one of the most important catalysts of stress proliferation. Therefore, it is crucial that health care professionals recognize the exacerbated effects of precursive caregiving when they prescribe home care that is undertaken by a partner or friend who may also be in poor health. Informal caregiving by partners and friends may save medical care costs, but it is not cost-free—as this research clearly documents. Homecare assistance services should be systematically provided to HIV+ caregivers to offset the synergistic negative impact of care-related stress to which they are prone.

The need for services from caregiving men remains high, even though combination drug treatments are extending the lives of PLH. The decline in AIDS deaths, combined with an estimated 35 to 40 thousand new HIV infections each year in the United States, means that the prevalence of AIDS cases is very high. Still, thousands of individuals continue to die from AIDS in the United States, the overwhelming majority of whom were men infected with HIV through same-sex contact (CDCP, 2000), and the sustenance of persons who provide informal care to these individuals is crucial. New HIV treatments have extended the survival of PLH, but their lives are now focused on complicated medication regimens and the ultimate specter of treatment failure (Wight, Aneshensel, & Wongvipat, 2000), creating an especially arduous scenario when the caregiver is also HIV+ and taking similar medications to survive. Thus, it does not seem likely that resources directed to alleviating stress and promoting well-being among AIDS caregivers and PLH are duplicative or unnecessary. Such resources may help to sustain caregivers by alleviating worries about their own health and their concerns about the PLH's well-being.

REFERENCES

Aneshensel, C. S. (1992). Social stress: Theory and research. *Annual Review of Sociology, 18*, 15–38.

Aneshensel, C. S., Pearlin, L. I., Mullin, J. P., Zarit, S. H., & Whitlatch, C. J. (1995). *Profiles in caregiving: The unexpected career.* San Diego, CA: Academic Press.

Aneshensel, C. S., Rutter, C. M., & Lachenbruch, P. A. (1991). Social structure, stress, and mental health: Competing conceptual and analytic models. *American Sociological Review, 56*, 166–178.

Benjamin, A. E. (1989). Perspectives on a continuum of care for persons with HIV illnesses. *Medical Care Review, 46*(4), 412–437.

Cass, V. (1996). Sexual orientation identity formation. In R. P. Cabaj & T. S. Stein (Eds.), *Textbook of homosexuality and mental health* (pp. 227–251). Washington, DC: American Psychiatric Press.

Centers for Disease Control and Prevention (2000). *HIV/AIDS Surveillance Report, 12*(1).

Derogatis, L. R., Lipman, R. S., Rickels, K., Uhlenhuth, E. H., & Covi, L. (1974). The Hopkins Symptom Checklist (HSCL): A self-report symptom inventory. *Behavioral Science, 19*, 1–15.

Dew, M. A., Becker, J. T., Sanchez, J., Caldararo, R., Lopez, O. L., Wess, J., Dorst, S. K., & Ganks, G. (1997). Prevalence and predictors of depressive, anxiety, and substance use disorders in HIV-infected and uninfected men: A longitudinal evaluation. *Psychological Medicine, 27*, 395–409.

Folkman, S. (1993). Psychosocial effects of HIV infection. In L. Goldberger and S. Breznitz (Eds.), *Handbook of stress*, (2nd ed., pp. 658–681). New York: Free Press.

Folkman, S., Chesney, M. A., Cooke, M., Boccellari, A., & Collette, L. (1994). Caregiver burden in HIV positive and HIV negative partners of men with AIDS. *Journal of Consulting and Clinical Psychology, 62*(4), 746–756.

Gluhoski, V. L., Fishman, B. A., & Perry, S. W. (1997). The impact of multiple bereavement in a gay male sample. *AIDS Education and Prevention, 9*(6), 521–531.

Gonsiorek, J. D. (1995). Gay male identities: Concepts and issues. In A. R. D'Augelli & C. J. Patterson (Eds.), *Lesbian, gay, and bisexual identities over the lifespan: Psychological perspectives*. Oxford: Oxford University Press.

Griffin, K. W., Rabkin, J. G., Remien, R. H., & Williams, J. B. (1998). Disease severity, physical limitations and depression in HIV infected men. *Journal of Psychosomatic Research, 44*(2), 219–227.

Herek, G. M. (1995). Psychological heterosexism in the United States. In A. R. D'Augelli & C. J. Patterson (Eds.), *Lesbian, gay, and bisexual identities over the lifespan: Psychological perspectives*. Oxford: Oxford University Press.

Herek, G. M., & Glunt, E. K. (1988). An epidemic of stigma: Public reactions to AIDS. *American Psychologist, 43*(11), 886–891.

Joseph, J. G., Caumartin, S. M., Tal, M., Kirscht, J. P., Kessler, R. C., Ostrow, D. G., & Wortman, C. B. (1990). Psychological functioning in a cohort of gay men at risk for AIDS. *Journal of Nervous and Mental Disease, 178*(10), 607–615.

Katz, M. M., & Lyerly, S. B. (1963). Methods for measuring adjustment and social behavior in the community. *Psychological Reports, 13*(2), 503–535.

Kessler, R. C., McConagle, K. A., Zhao, S., Nelson, C. B., Hughes, M., Eshelman, S., Wittchen, H., & Kendler, K. S. (1994). Lifetime and 12 month prevalence of DSM-III-R psychiatric disorders in the United States. *Archives of General Psychiatry, 51*, 8–19.

Kubler-Ross, E. (1969). *On death and dying*. New York: Macmillan.

LaSala, M. C. (2000). Gay male couples: The importance of coming out and being out to parents. *Journal of Homosexuality, 39*(2), 47–71.

Lawton, M. P., Lipton, M. B., & Kleban, M. H. (1969). A checklist for use in treatment, training, and program evaluation. *Pennsylvania Psychiatric Quarterly, 9*(3), 5–14.

LeBlanc, A. J., & Wight, R. G. (2000). Reciprocity and depression in AIDS caregiving. *Sociological Perspectives, 43*(4), 631–649.

Los Angeles County Department of Health Services HIV Epidemiology Program. (2000). *Advanced HIV Disease (AIDS) Surveillance Summary*.

Martin, J. L., Dean, L., Garcia, M., & Hall, W. (1989). The impact of AIDS on a gay community: Changes in sexual behavior, substance use, and mental health. *American Journal of Community Psychology, 17*(3), 269–293.

Meyer, I. H. (1995). Minority stress and mental health in gay men. *Journal of Health and Social Behavior, 36*, 38–56.

Mullan, J. T. (1998). Aging and informal caregiving to people with HIV/AIDS. *Research on Aging, 20*(6), 712–738.

Pearlin, L. I. (1989). The sociological study of stress. *Journal of Health and Social Behavior, 30*(3), 241–256.

Pearlin, L. I., Aneshensel, C. S., & LeBlanc, A. J. (1997). The forms and mechanisms of stress proliferation: The case of AIDS caregivers. *Journal of Health and Social Behavior, 38*, 223–236.

Pearlin, L. I., Mullan, J. T., Aneshensel, C. S., Wardlaw, L., & Harrington, C. (1994). The structure and function of AIDS caregiving relationships. *Psychosocial Rehabilitation Journal, 17*(4), 51–67.

Pearlin, L. I., Mullan, J. T., Semple, S. J., & Skaff, M. M. (1990). Caregiving and the stress process: An overview of concepts and measures. *The Gerontologist, 30*, 583–594.

Pearlin, L. I., & Radabaugh, C. (1985). Age and stress: Processes and problems. In B. B. Hess & E. W. Markson (Eds.), *Growing old in America: New perspectives on old age.* Brunswick, NJ: Transaction.

Perkins, D. O., Leserman, J., Stern, R. A., Baum, S. F., Kiao, D., Golden, R. N., & Evans, D. L. (1995). Somatic symptoms and HIV infection: Relationship to depressive symptoms and indicators of HIV disease. *American Journal of Psychiatry, 152*(12), 1776–1781.

Pierce, R. S., Frone, M. R., Russell, M., & Cooper, M. L. (1996). Financial stress, social support, and alcohol involvement: A longitudinal test of the buffering hypothesis in a general population survey. *Health Psychology, 15*(1), 38–47.

Raveis, V. H., & Siegel, K. (1991). The impact of caregiving on informal and familial caregivers. *AIDS Patient Care,* Feb., 39–43.

Rothblum, E. D. (1994). I only read about myself on bathroom walls: The need for research on the mental health of lesbians and gay men. *Journal of Consulting and Clinical Psychology, 62*(2), 213–220.

Seeman, M., Seeman, A. Z., & Budros, A. (1988). Powerlessness, work, and community: A longitudinal study of alienation and alcohol use. *Journal of Health and Social Behavior, 29*, 185–198.

Turner, H. A., & Catania, J. A. (1997). Informal caregiving to persons with AIDS in the United States: Caregiver burden among central cities residents eighteen to forty-nine years old. *American Journal of Community Psychology, 25*(1), 35–59.

Turner, H. A., Catania, J. A., & Gagnon, J. (1994). The prevalence of informal caregiving to persons with AIDS in the U. S. *Social Science and Medicine, 38*(11), 1543–1552.

Vedhara, K., & Nott, K. H. (1996). Psychosocial vulnerability to stress: A study of HIV positive homosexual men. *Journal of Psychosomatic Research*, 41(3), 255–267.

Wardlaw, L. (1994). Sustaining informal caregivers for persons with AIDS. *Families in Society*, June, 373–384.

Weitz, R. (1989). Uncertainty and the lives of people with AIDS. *Journal of Health and Social Behavior*, 30, 270–281.

Wight, R. G. (2000). Precursive depression among HIV-infected AIDS caregivers over time. *Social Science & Medicine*, 51, 759–770.

Wight, R. G., Aneshensel, C. S., & Wongvipat, N. *Emerging Issues in AIDS Caregiving Stress Among Midlife and Older Women*. Presented at the Annual Meetings of the American Public Health Association, Boston, MA, November 2000.

Wight, R. G., LeBlanc, A. J., & Aneshensel, C. S. (1998). AIDS caregiving and health among midlife and older women. *Health Psychology*, 17, 130–137.

The Voices of Husbands and Sons Caring for a Family Member With Dementia[1]

9

Phyllis Braudy Harris

Caregiving for older adults has been defined as "woman's work." This chapter advocates moving beyond this paradigm to redefine caregiving as a "gendered" experience. Such a paradigm shift openly acknowledges men's roles and responsibilities in elder care, and leads to a better understanding of the needs and concerns of *all* family caregivers. In addition, this perspective doesn't negate or lessen the contributions of wives, daughters, daughter-in-laws, or nieces who have been the mainstay of family caregiving (Abel, 1991; Brody, 1990; Horowitz, 1985), but it allows us to carefully listen to the voices of husbands and sons caring for an impaired family member. It assists us in identifying that men, as well as women, come to the caregiving experience with certain strengths and certain shortcomings. Using an inductive analysis of 60 interviews, this study seeks to broaden our understanding of son and husband caregivers, with the goal of articulating some of the common strengths and concerns, as well as some differences, which husbands and sons experience in taking on this non-normative role.

Husbands as Caregivers

Most of the studies of male caregivers have focused on the role of husband caregivers, who according to Stone, Cafferata, and Sangl (1987) comprise

[1] The author gratefully acknowledges the support and assistance of Joyce Bichler and the Cleveland Area Alzheimer's Association. The research on which this chapter is based was supported in part by grants from The Cleveland Foundation and John Carroll University.

13% of all caregivers. Qualitative research on husbands has expanded our understanding of the caregiving process of men and demonstrated more variability among husband caregivers than previously assumed. This research found that men oriented to the caregiving process in different ways: out of their role of work, out of a sense of duty, out of love, or as a team with their ill wife (Harris, 1993; Harris & Bichler, 1997). Husbands felt a sense of satisfaction, personal achievement, and pride in their ability to care for ill wives, but there was also a sense of despair (Harris, 1993; Motenko, 1988). Husbands experienced social isolation and loss on multiple levels: loss of companionship and sexual intimacy, loss of former identity, and loss of control (Harris, 1993; Harris & Bichler, 1997; Motenko, 1988; Vinick, 1984). Caregiver stress was felt strongly by some men, particularly those in a "transition phase" of caregiving—husbands whose wives had been recently diagnosed with dementia or who were moving into a new stage of the disease (Harris, 1995; Harris & Bichler, 1997). Some studies found men adapt a stereotypic stoic demeanor while others found men experience a fuller range of emotions caring for an ill wife such as love, despondency, frustration, and anger (Davies, Priddy, & Tinklenberg, 1986; Harris & Bichler, 1997; Motenko, 1988; Vinick, 1984).

Previous quantitative research had presented a unidimensional, less complex picture of husband caregivers, indicating that they fare better emotionally than women, having lower caregiver burden (Barusch & Spaid, 1989; Fitting, Rabins, Lucas, & Eastham, 1986; Horowitz, 1985; Ingersoll-Dayton, Starrels, & Dowler, 1996), higher morale (Gilhooly, 1984), and were motivated more out of a sense of obligation (Fitting, Rabins, Lucas, & Eastham, 1986; Pruchno & Resch, 1989). Kramer and Lambert's quantitative study (1999) is one of the few exceptions in this unidimensional view of husband caregivers. These results supported the findings of qualitative research that showed that the experience of husband caregivers was not a benign one. Husbands in this study reported a decline in happiness, an increase in depression, and a decline in emotional support and marital satisfaction.

Sons as Caregivers

Focusing on son caregivers, studies that make the distinction between primary and secondary caregivers have found that sons comprise 10–12% of primary caregivers to the elderly and 52% of secondary caregivers (Stone et al., 1987; Tennstedt, McKinlay, & Sullivan, 1989). Research on sons, though, has been limited, and survey research has focused primarily on gender task differences between sons and daughters. Horowitz (1985), among a sample of 32 sons, found that sons became caregivers only in the absence of available female caregivers; that sons were more likely than daughters to rely on the instrumental and emotional support of their spouses; and that sons provided less overall assistance, especially hands-on assistance, to their parents. Sons, though, are just as likely as daughters to provide financial and emotional support to their parents and to share their home with a parent. Montgomery and Kamo's (1989) study of 64 sons, Stoller's (1990) study of 60 sons, and Dwyer and Coward's (1991) large multivariate comparison of 13,000 sons and daughters all found that sons provided intermittent assistance with occasional tasks and were less involved in routine household chores than daughters. As the parent's level of functioning worsened over time, sons dropped out of the caregiving role. Chang and White-Mean's (1991) findings also supported the differences in the type of care provided by gender, but in contrast to the other studies, did not conclude that men took on the caregiving role primarily because no one else was available. Based on the Informal Caregivers Survey data of the 1982 to 1984 Channeling Study, Chang and White-Mean concluded that male and female caregivers on the average had the same number of other caregivers to help them on a regular basis. In a study of Puerto Rican sons and daughters as primary caregivers to elderly parents, Delgado and Tennstedt (1997) found that besides proximity to their parents and emotional attachment, the sons more than the daughters cited filial responsibility as a motivation to assume caregiving, and the sons were less likely to use formal services. Overall the Puerto Rican sons provided similar amounts of informal care as the daughters, pointing to the importance of ethnic differences in caregiving. Lee, Dwyer, and Coward (1993), in one of the few studies on adult children caregivers that goes beyond the gender role expectations in discussing reasons for task differences, examine same-gender preferences of the older adult and strength of kinship ties as possible explanations for why sons generally provide less care. They proposed that mothers do not select their sons as primary caregivers because of their own concern for modesty. These studies illustrate well task differences between sons and daughters as caregivers, but do not provide us with an in-depth understanding of a son's caregiving experience.

As with the qualitative research on husbands, qualitative research on sons provides a more in-depth, diverse, and complex understanding of son caregivers than what has been previously reported. Harris's (1998) study of 30 sons caring for parents with dementia, found that sons were committed to caring for their ill parents and were motivated out of a sense of love or obligation that did not depend upon the availability of a sister. These sons were the ones providing the care, and they oriented to the caregiving role in different ways. The role of most of the sons' wives were to support them emotionally. Matthews and Heidorn's (1998) study of 49 paired brothers without sisters whose parents were 74 years of age or older, found brothers were in regular contact with their parents and performed "masculine" type services, except during times of crises and transitions. The brothers defined their parents as self-sufficient, which was often congruent with their parents wishes, but not reality, and they acted to assist their parents in maintaining that goal.

THE STUDY

A qualitative research approach was chosen to gain insights into the daily issues and concerns husband and son caregivers face. This in-depth method aids in identifying commonalities and differences between the two groups. Findings from such a study can identify issues that need to be further evaluated by larger caregiver studies or can lay the foundation for new directions future research may take.

Sample (N = 60)

A nonrandom, purposive sample insured the inclusion of a range of different types of husband and son caregivers. Efforts were made to recruit caregivers who varied on the following demographic characteristics: race-ethnicity, socioeconomic status, urban-rural settings, number of years of caregiving, stage of dementia based upon their descriptions of symptoms and behavior, work status, and specifically for sons, marital status, only children or sons with siblings, and living arrangement of parent. The sample included 30 husbands and 30 sons. The son sample included sons, who were the primary caregiver ($N = 13$), as well as sons who were helping a well parent care for their ill spouse ($N = 17$). The term "secondary caregiver" does not accurately reflect the extent of this latter group's commitment and level of care. They were secondary because the well parent was still living with the ill parent, or the ill parent had moved into a nursing home; but these sons often saw their ill parent on a daily basis to assist in their care. For that reason, the terms primary or secondary caregivers were not used but were described as sons actively involved in their parent's care. Six of the son's parents had died within the last year, but they vividly recalled the active roles they took in their parent's care.

The local Alzheimer's Association chapter provided access to families for this study. Caregivers were recruited through ads in their bimonthly newsletter, from helpline call records, and support groups and other services. A total of 30 husbands and 30 sons caring for a spouse or parent with dementia comprised the final sample. The sample ranged from men who had made one call to the Alzheimer's Association Helpline or just received the Newsletter to one husband and one son who were Board of Trustees Members.

Demographic Profile

The demographic characteristics of husbands are shown in Table 9.1. Husbands ranged in age from 41 to 91, with a mean age of 72. Occupations were very diverse, from truck driver to physician. Education levels differed, with 7% having less than a high school education, 38% were high school graduates, and over 50% had a college education. Income was quite varied with 27% having income under $10,000 and 27% having income over $40,000. The men were in long-term marriages, married for an average of 43 years. The length of time these husbands had been caregiving was 5 years on average. The majority lived alone with their wives; two had recently placed their wives in nursing homes.

The demographic characteristics of sons are shown in Table 9.2. The mean age of the son caregivers was 50 years old. They ranged from a 32-year-old White stock broker, who had cared for his mother with Alzheimer's disease at home for 10 years, to a 71-year-old semiretired African American real estate agent whose 96-year-old mother had just entered a nursing home after a major stroke. The majority of the sons were college graduates; 26% were blue-collar workers. Reflective of their educational level, only 7% of the sample had incomes of $10,000 or under. It was predominately a middle-class sample, with much variation within that group. Occupations included construction worker, postman, teacher, artist, college professor, salesman, business executive, and entrepreneur. One son was unemployed and on disability leave. Twenty-three percent of the sons were retired.

The majority of sons (77%) had siblings; 57% had sisters, of whom 43% lived locally. The sample contained relatively equal proportions of only, oldest, middle, and youngest sons. Sixty percent of the sample were married. The average age of the parent with dementia was 77 years old, with a range of 63 to 96 years. The average length of time the sons had been caregiving was 3.5 years. Twenty-three percent of the parents were living with their sons and 23% were living in nursing homes.

Data Collection

An interview schedule was developed using a general interview guide approach derived from the research questions and the literature review. In this type of approach, the researcher outlines a set of major issues to be explored in each interview, but the order and exact wording of the question varies depending on the context of the interview (Patton, 1980). The topics included in the interview schedule were divided into four main categories: (a) role as caregiver, which included such topics as caregiver history, tasks performed, commitment, new roles learned, difficulties, satisfactions,

TABLE 9.1   Characteristics of Husband Caregivers (*n* = 30)

	n	%
Age in years		
Mean	72.6	
Range	41–91	
Age of wife in years		
Mean	71.3	
Range	43–88	
No. of years married		
Mean	44.3	
Range	13–69	
Race		
Caucasian	24	80
African American	6	20
Level of education*		
Less than high school	2	7
High school	11	38
College	16	55
Occupation		
Blue collar	12	40
Sales/middle management	3	10
Professional/business exec.	15	50
Employment status		
Working	4	13
Retired**	26	87
Household income		
Under $10,000	8	27
$11,000–$20,000	7	23
$21,000–$30,000	6	20
$31,000–$40,000	1	3
Over $40,000	8	27
Religion*		
Catholic	9	30
Jewish	2	7
Protestant	19	63
Living arrangement		
Lives with wife alone	21	72
Lives with wife and children	6	21
Lives separately	2	7

TABLE 9.1 *(Continued)*

	n	%
No. of years wife had dementia		
Less than 1 year	7	23
1–5 years	7	23
5 years or more	16	53
Mean	5.6	
Range	25–15	
Stage of dementia of wife***		
Early	12	40
Middle	8	27
Late	10	33
Children in town		
Yes	18	60
No	9	30
No children	3	10

* *n* will vary due to missing data.
** No respondent retired to take care of his wife.
*** Based on husbands' descriptions.

losses, affect on life style, and work; (b) stress and coping, which included the areas of caregiver burden, coping strategies, social supports, financial and caregiver health issues, and formal service usage; (c) interpersonal and marital-family relationships with wife or parent(s), and sibling(s), the impact of illness on these relationships, and the role of their children; and (d) motivations for taking on a caregiver role, meanings derived from experience, and personal growth. The interview guide was pretested on two husbands and two sons, one of whom suggested adding the topic of the responsiveness of service providers to male caregivers.

The data was collected through in-depth personal interviews from Spring 1991 to January 1996. The interviews lasted on the average an hour and a half to two hours at locations selected by the caregivers. The majority of the sons chose locations other than their homes, such as the author's university office, their offices, restaurants, and libraries. The husbands most often met in their homes because they did not want to leave their wives alone. All the interviews were taped and then transcribed and compared with the field notes for accuracy of the transcriptions. Caregivers were recontacted by phone if there were inconsistencies.

Data Analysis

The content analysis consisted of a six-step process completed by the author and a colleague (who was not involved in the data collection) with

TABLE 9.2   Characteristics of Son Caregivers (*n* = 30)

	n	%
Age in years		
Mean	50	
Range	32–71	
Marital status		
Married	18	60
Not married	12	40
Race		
Caucasian	25	83
African American	5	17
Level of education		
High school	8	27
College	16	53
Advanced degree	6	20
Employment status		
Working	23	77
Retired*	7	23
Occupation		
Blue collar	8	27
Middle management/sales	6	20
Professional	8	27
Entrepreneur/business exec.	8	27
Income		
Under $10,000	2	7
$11,000–$20,000	0	0
$21,000–$40,000	9	30
$41,000–$60,000	7	23
Over $60,000	12	40
Religion		
Catholic	17	57
Jewish	3	10
Protestant	8	27
No affiliations	2	6
Siblings in family		
Son only child	7	23
Has sisters	8	27
Has brothers	6	20
Has sisters and brothers	9	30
Geographic location of siblings		
Son only child in town	15	50
Sister(s) in town	6	20
Brothers(s) in town	2	7
Both in town	7	23

TABLE 9.2   *(Continued)*

	n	%
Birth order		
Only	7	23
Oldest	5	17
Middle	9	30
Youngest	9	30
Sex of parent		
Male	10	33
Female	20	67
Age of parent		
Mean	77	
Range	63–96	
No. of years parent has dementia		
Less than 1	5	16
1–4	17	57
5 or more	8	
Mean	3.5	
Range	.5–11	
Parents stage of dementia**		
Early	11	36
Middle	8	27
Late	5	17
Deceased	6	20
Living arrangements of parent		
Own home alone	2	7
Own home with spouse	6	20
With son	7	23
Other relatives' home	2	7
Nursing home	7	23
Deceased	6	20

* One respondent retired to take care of mother.
** Based on husband's descriptions.

extensive clinical social work experience working with Alzheimer's patients and their families. The author and clinician separately read the transcripts in their entirety then re-read the transcripts a second time to develop substantive codes for each of the 60 narratives, as suggested by Glaser and Strauss (1967). The codes were then grouped into themes that emerged from the codes, such as sense of duty and taking charge. Then a master list was developed of themes from each interview that allowed for easy cross-interview examination. During the fourth step, the author and clinician reexamined each narrative, looking for quotations that summarized the essence of each man's experience as a caregiver. These quotations were compared for consistency with themes that had been developed for that caregiver. In the fifth step of the analysis, the author and clinician met together and compared their separate findings. In areas of disagreement, portions of the transcripts were re-read and discussed until agreement was reached. The final step was a content analysis of the transcripts using features of the WordPerfect software program.

Study Limitations

This study has many limitations. The information is based only on interviews of 30 husbands and 30 sons who have accepted the responsibility for caring for a family member with dementia. These men stated that they were involved in the caregiving process; they indeed may represent a unique group of men. Also, the sample is biased toward service users. This study uses a cross-sectional collection of data to examine a dynamic process such as caregiving, and as a preliminary investigation, it did not conduct repeated interviews to verify participants' perceptions. Yet the voices of these husband and sons caregivers emerge from this qualitative research. This chapter provides a more in-depth diverse and complex understanding of male caregivers than has been previously reported.

FINDINGS

Commonalities (Common Themes that Emerged from the Data)

Problem-Solving Approach

One of the strengths that these men brought to caregiving, as noted by other researchers (Miller, 1987; Zarit, 1982), is a problem-solving approach they used in the world of work. Both husbands and sons often used this coping strategy as they learned the new roles and tasks, which fashioned them into caregivers and added another facet to their identities. They felt comfortable taking control of or supervising their relatives' care. It was a natural extension of their male role in our society. It was best exemplified by a 77-year-old husband caring for a wife in the end stages of Alzheimer's.

> I wish somehow or other that the knowledge over the years had been available in capsule form in the beginning. It is, to a degree, if you know what to

read. But there are the little things that you have to do, at least I do, just kind a lumber along until I finally stumble on the answers. I presume what works for one doesn't work on another patient in many cases. It's been an interesting challenging situation.

Problem solving was also a major coping strategy that sons talked about in their efforts to handle the emotional and physical demands of caring for a parent with dementia. Using a problem-solving approach helped the sons to focus on the immediate issues, gather information and strategize ways to find acceptable solutions, although as one son admitted, "The biggest frustration is there are no clear-cut solutions or answers." The men wanted to be prepared. Many sons used a search-and-seek method, best described by a 50-year-old son sharing the care of his father with his older brother:

> I think what we have tried to do is to get as much information available. Seek out and search and talk with as many people as you can. Get as much information as is available on the disease to learn about it. Learn about the course of events about what to expect. I think education is the primary key. We have done a lot of research. I think we know what to expect. Things don't always happen in the way we think they're going to happen, but at least I don't think there has to be what I call any major surprises.

Limited Caregiving Skills

For the most part, neither husbands nor sons were prepared to take on the role of a nurturer or caregiver. The gender roles to which they were socialized did not include caring for an impaired family member or good communication skills, so they struggled to learn the necessary skills of personal care and household management. They needed to learn about female hygiene, cooking, grooming, and which clothes were easiest to put on. They also had to learn how to negotiate the service delivery system and how to hire respite and chore workers.

A 73-year-old African American man stated that for him getting his wife dressed was the most difficult task; however, he has learned the "tricks of the trade."

> Forget about stockings. Forget about skirt. Forget about blouses. Just give her some decent slacks to put on and it comes in handy if you take her to the john. If she got all that fancy stuff on, I guarantee you the next day you will do it differently.

He has also had to take over balancing the checkbook, which he had never done in his life. As he said, "That was her job. I'd come home and put the money on the table and say, 'Here.' Now I have to pay the bills."

One son talked about men's communication patterns that made caregiving more difficult.

> The one thing a son really needs is to learn how to communicate. Men don't talk, and that's a big crisis. It's a crisis in their lives even without somebody being sick. So they go into this [caregiving] with no talking skills, and they're not able to verbalize. I think that's what they need up front is some skills in verbalization, which would make life better for them all the way around.

Another 53-year-old son reflected similar concerns based upon his own caregiving experience with his father and his experiences as a clinical psychologist.

> I really do think men tend to isolate themselves. We do believe this myth that we are suppose to be the *strong silent types* and be able to do everything all on our own.

Commitment

The most prevalent similarity between the husbands and sons in this study is their overriding sense of commitment and duty to care for their ill family members. They accepted this responsibility as "theirs," an acceptance, which for many came with great emotional, social, and financial costs. The commitment of the husbands in caring for their wives was a dominant feature of the relationships described in the interviews. They felt a strong sense of spousal obligation. One 71-year-old man caring at home for his wife with end stage Alzheimer's expressed his commitment this way, "Why do I do it? It goes back to my basic philosophy of life. This is part of life and she would have done the same thing for me. I will never abandon her."

Another 71-year-old African American man caring for his wife in the early stages of Alzheimer's shared his thoughts about commitment:

> This is a challenge. Can you be good now? Has she been good to you? I got a car outside. If three tires are going all right and one goes flat, you don't say the car should be dumped. Fix the tire. I've told her, "I've known you a lifetime almost, so I ain't goin' jump ship now, honey"; it doesn't work that way.

Sons too were committed. The most common theme among the 30 sons was their sense of duty to care for their ill parent; their sense of filial obligation was paramount in the interviews. It was expressed most clearly by a 53-year-old son who had just moved his father with early stage Alzheimer's from Florida to live with him. He explained, "It's my responsibility, that's all. I'm the one to do it."

Other sons expressed similar feelings, but with variations. But, perhaps it was a 60-year-old son, whose mother died a year ago who said it most poignantly:

> What kept me going was my devotion to her. I saw how they [his parents] treated me over my life time, the loyalty they felt. I learned. I learned that that's what you do with family. You don't moan and groan about them; you take care of them. You do what you have to do.

An African American son expressed his commitment in another way. He talked about a promise he had made to his mother many years ago.

> As a kid of four, I made a commitment to her that I would always take care of her. And when I started hearing about all of her weird behavior from family and neighbors [his mother lived out of town] I jumped into the car and went down and got her. I got a grave responsibility.

Losses

These men experienced multiple losses. For husbands this meant loss of a companion and confidant, loss of meaningful sexual intimacy, loss of one's former identity, loss of control, and loss of future plans and dreams. The loss of female companionship added to the husbands' feelings of social isolation. One 68-year-old husband, who had been caring for his wife for 10 years stated, "Women look at things differently; I'm not talking about sex now, but I miss having a conversation with women. I found that whenever I go to the grocery store, I try to strike up casual conversations with the female shoppers and the checkout clerks."

A 64-year-old caregiver poignantly voiced another loss alluded to by other caregivers, a loss of their former sense of identity (how one defines who one is); in this man's case, his sense of manliness.

> After being in this [caregiving] for a while, you begin to lose your male identity. A woman is used to everything in the house, so the role comes as probably a routine. Now you reverse the situation and a man has to learn all this. Now where does he go for the answers? It's very confusing. You're going to have to do some cooking, cleaning, washing, dusting, spots on clothes, this, that. It is a whole new learning process. I've been in construction all my life. To go from that to this was quite a transition, yes. Your whole psychological outlook on things changes. You don't view things as you did before. You begin to question who you are.

Loss was also a common theme expressed by sons. For some sons, it was the loss of a person they loved. For other sons, it was a loss of personal space and freedom, and for others it meant lost job opportunities and putting their careers "on hold." Some experienced all of these things and struggled to overcome a compounded sense of loss. One son described what he felt was the most difficult thing for him to deal with in the process of his mother's Alzheimer's disease: "I miss the person she was; she was somebody you could confide in—you could be yourself."

Studies have shown that, in general, men do have fewer friends and no confidants, especially after the loss of a spouse (Allen, 1994; Barer, 1994; Dulac & Kosberg, 1994; Solomon, 1982). Both husbands and sons in this study, especially sons who were not married, expressed this lack of support in their daily struggles to care for a family member. A 76-year-old husband talked about it this way, as he spoke of his wife who was in the middle stages of Alzheimer's disease.

> I used to be able to come home from work, and I could have had the world's worst day. I would sit down in the kitchen, where my wife would be cooking, and I would sound off and go through my day. It might take a half an hour, but I would really bare my soul. And think back on it and what she would do was listen. She didn't advise me; she never said she would help me or anything like that. She truly listened. And that was really all that was necessary. We've always been best of friends.

A 42-year-old son, caring for his mother and then his father with Alzheimer's, also discussed his feelings about "going it alone" and his limited social support network.

> My ability to have relationships is very limited. I have lots of professional relationships because of the nature of the work I do, but not in my personal life. I had a very, very small circle of friends. People don't understand it. My peers don't understand it because most of them have not gone through this. I have no one to talk to. I don't feel a support system. Romantic relationships don't last.

So husbands as well as sons shared many common experiences in their "new" caregiving role. They both demonstrated a commitment to caregiving and experienced multiple losses as well as a lack of a confidant. Their problem-solving approach helped them cope, but they needed to learn new communication skills and caregiving skills of personal care and household management.

Differences

However, the similarities between sons and husbands were sometimes overshadowed by the differences. The differences reflect both the relationship differences as well as generational differences.

Impact of Dementia on Their Lives

The husbands' lives were profoundly and deeply altered by their wives' illness. The sense of utter loss and unanticipated change in their lives was clearly evidenced in their narratives. As a 61-year-old husband caring for his wife with early onset dementia concluded about his situation, "I realized my life was changed forever and I began the first day of the rest of my life." Another husband echoed these words. He stated:

> I'll tell you, I am not the sweetest guy in the world. I've got to be one of the hardest people to live with because—up until recently, my job came first then my family, because without a job, I wouldn't have a family. So, now it's the opposite. It's my family then my job. My biggest priority is to make her happy, because only God knows how much more time I'm going to have with her, and I want it to be happy.

The sons' reactions to their parents' illness were much more complex and contradictory. Although the sons were emotionally involved in the caregiving experience, they evidenced less overall intensity of emotion than the husbands. They were able to approach the caregiving more objectively and accept it more quickly than the husbands. One African American son who cared for his mother in his home until she died expressed it this way.

> You can look at your mother and you can look at the disease, they're entirely different. You remember how sweet and how compassionate your mom was, and you look at the disease over here and it's totally out of character, so you have to try to find a balance. You might as well come out of this denial you're in and recognize the fact that she has a serious problem and begin to help her and yourself by dealing with it.

However, as horrendous as the sons' situations were, their lives would not be forever altered. True, these were their parents, whom many sons loved, and seeing the parent in this condition was very sad. Nevertheless, a parent's growing old and becoming ill was somewhat expected. After their parents' deaths, sons would continue on with their work and families. Their lives would go on much like before the illness, unlike the husband caregivers, and the sons knew this. They talked about life after their parents deaths, having more time for themselves, spending more time with their wives and children, returning to old hobbies that they sorely missed.

Yet the sons' pain, anguish, frustration, and anger were ever present. Many sons lived with an overwhelming feeling of guilt that they had not done enough. As one 46-year old son said about assisting his mother with his father who had Alzheimer's,

I operate out of a principle of fairness, and I did not shoulder a fair amount of the responsibility. There never was enough time to do what I felt I should have done. I let my mother carry too much of it because she is strong. She picked up the slack. I should have picked up more of the slack. And I sit here and sound like, gee, I've had this tough time. I mean I've seen what other people who have dealt with this disease for 10 years. They had loved ones who didn't know them and screamed. You know I've looked down that abyss and thankfully I didn't have to go down it. But I did not live up to my model of what a good son should be .

Sons also were more willing than husbands to verbalize their caregiver stress and burden they were feeling. More than half the sons, unlike the husbands, used terms "stress" and "burden" to describe their emotional experiences with caregiving. One 35-year-old African American son stated, "I'm putting so much in here that I am losing myself, you know? I'm really losing myself. I'm so stressed out."

Setting Limits on Caregiving

Sons, unlike the husband caregivers, were able to set boundaries and time limits on the caregiving. Often, when a parent reached the stage beyond which the son felt he was no longer able to provide the care, he looked for other options. Most often these options were nursing home placements. Sons much sooner than husbands were willing to consider a nursing home placement as a very real possibility; however, this did not mean that they were no longer involved in their parents' care. On the other hand, most husbands cared for their wives longer than their physical health should have allowed. The following quotes from sons and husbands reflects this difference.

On one of his visits home, it became apparent to a 55-year-old son that his mother was gradually getting worse, more confused and forgetful. He called a family meeting to discuss the situation.

The reaction of the other locals [children] was, "It's not our problem." They weren't even helping out my sister on weekends [who had her parents living with her]. As they did not want any responsibility and I was use to getting things done. I said, "Fine." That's when I became captain. On the advice of the physician, we started discussing nursing homes; we formed a little task force and looked at 15 nursing homes in the area.

When his mother moved into a nursing home, the son moved back to his hometown and visited her daily.

The following quote from a 75-year-old husband, reflective of most of the husbands' perspectives, demonstrates the different attitudes:

As long as these two weak knees can move one step in front of another, I will care for her. I made a vow to this woman and I intend to keep it. Don't matter if she would do it for me. I know what I need to do, and so does the man upstairs.

Satisfaction with Formal Services

Sons, on the whole, were much more critical and demanding of services for their family members and themselves. They were more politically sophisticated and more active in patient and family advocacy programs, and their expectations were higher, a key generational difference. One son voiced his concerns with the service delivery system this way:

The system didn't facilitate helping me try to get things under control. It absolutely exacerbates what a disease does to a family. I tried to speak to my family internist [to learn more about his father's other terminal illness] so I could guide the medication treatment if there was any, and make conscious decisions, knowledgeable decisions. And I would get answers like, "You don't have to worry about it." When he [his father] was transferred to the nursing home, I wanted to know if there were decisions we should be making about pain management. I just wanted to know, as part of the care and treatment of my father. And I would get a response, "Don't worry about this, we'll manage it. Why do you want to know?" And I said, "Because we have financial decisions to make. We have care decisions to make. We have living wills and all those decisions to make." I mean the whole thing just beats the family up terribly, the not knowing, the having to run around to talk to the social workers to try to access the system. I wanted to hold my father's hand and go through this last phase with him. And they really didn't let you. You know, the system didn't let you. You had to fight for whatever time you could.

Husbands were less questioning of the health care professionals and accepting of the services they received. They did not discuss issues of service delivery, except at the time of diagnosis. Then they complained about the lack of compassion some physicians showed for their situations, and that they often left their physician's offices without a clear understanding of the diagnoses.

Gratification from Caregiving

Sons more than husbands, came away with a feeling of gratification from their caregiving experience. Their parents' illness gave them an opportunity to "pay them back" for the years of love, care, and attention they had received, an opportunity that many sons believed they might never otherwise have had. "Paying back" was the exact words that reoccurred many times in the dialogues with sons. As one 60-year-old son caring for his mother said:

It's just that I was pleased that I was able in some small way to be able to pay her back. I think if she had died of a heart attack, I would have never had the chance to say to myself in some small way I repaid her for what she did. Not that she ever made me feel like I had to, but *I* had to.

For husbands, it was not so much a sense of gratification in being able to help their wives. It can best be understood from a different viewpoint, that of spousal obligation. As one husband insightfully stated, "It all boils down to the two V's, vows and values," living up to a promise made many years earlier.

Thus the husbands and sons in the study also experienced differences in their experiences of caregiving. Most notable were the impact of dementia on their lives, setting limits on their caregiving, service satisfaction, and gratification.

CONCLUSION AND SERVICE IMPLICATIONS

From listening to the voices of these husbands and sons, the "gendered" experience of caregiving can be heard. Husbands and sons bring to their caregiving some common elements and with it some strengths, as well as some shortcomings because of the way men are socialized in our society. Husbands and sons shared a commitment to care for their family member with dementia, be it from a sense of spousal obligation, a sense of filial duty, or love. They both shared a deep sense of loss due to the compound misfortunes of losing a companion or someone they could rely on for advice, as well as a loss of freedom, dreams, and a sense of control over their own destiny. From their experiences in the world of work, they brought with them a problem-solving approach that helped them cope and seek out needed information and services. However, socialized to the masculine gender role, husbands and sons had few friends and often lacked a confidant. Many also lacked the communication skills needed for caregiving, as well as the nurturing skills of cooking, household management, and personal care. Negotiating the formal and informal service delivery systems was difficult. With practice, they were able to learn the needed skills, but it took time.

There were also meaningful differences, however; which husbands and sons experienced in caring for an ill spouse or parent. For a husband, the change in his wife's cognitive status meant that his life would be changed forever. Every aspect of the husband's lifestyle was profoundly and deeply altered by his wife's illness. The impact of a parent with dementia on a son's life can be tremendous, but parents growing old and often becoming ill is somewhat expected. Sons would eventually continue on with their lives as they were, so the impact was less severe. The son's emotional involvement for the most part was less intense, but more ridden with guilt and feelings of caregiver burden, which they willingly expressed. Sons set limits on their caregiving beyond which they would or could not continue, and they had greater expectations of the service delivery system. Husbands went well beyond the expectations of physical and mental endurance in their effort to provide care to their wives. Yet, sons expressed greater gratification about the experience, in that it gave them a chance to repay their ill parent for their concern and care for them throughout their own lives.

In comparing the service needs of caregiving husbands and sons, it becomes clear that there are not only many similarities but also many contrasts. Both husbands and sons needed information about the disease, caregiver education, and information on how to hire help, but husbands wanted more on the "how-to's" of hands-on personal care while sons wanted information on navigating the service delivery system. Sons saw caregiving as a temporary task that they wanted to do well and efficiently. They wanted up-to-date information on all types of formal services, including nursing homes.

Both husbands and sons needed to expand their support networks with meaningful relationships with people in whom they could confide, and who in turn would understand their situations. They both needed to work on communication skills. However, husbands expressed more emotional needs than did the sons. The disease disrupted the entire lifestyle of husbands, and they were seeking services that would help them adjust to this change. Husbands wanted to talk to other men in similar situations, and they wanted to understand how others dealt with this new phase of their life. Sons were not interested in long-standing traditional support groups. They wanted short-term educational workshops.

Service providers need to recognize that there are men actively involved in elder care, and though some of the needs of husbands and sons are similar, there are also differences in terms of their needs to provide quality care as well as differences in their expectations of service providers. As more men enter into caregiving roles, there will be an increasing need to provide service to this population. Because caregiving is a "gendered" experience, it is essential to understand the needs of these men, their similarities and differences, so that a service system that is truly helpful to *all* family caregivers can be developed.

REFERENCES

Abel, E. K. (1991). *Who cares for the elderly: Public policy and experiences of adult daughters*. Philadelphia: Temple University Press.

Allen, S. M. (1994). Gender differences in spousal caregiving and unmet need for care. *Journal of Gerontology: Social Sciences, 49*(4), S187–S195.

Barer, B. M. (1994). Men and women aging differently. *International Journal of Aging and Human Development, 38*(1), 29–40.

Barusch, A., & Spaid, W. (1989). Gender differences in caring: Why do wives report greater burden? *The Gerontologist, 29,* 667–676.

Brody, E. M. (1990) *Women in the middle.* New York: Springer.

Chang, C. F., & White-Means, S. I. (1991). The men who care: An analysis of male primary caregivers who care for frail elderly at home. *The Journal of Applied Gerontology, 10,* 343–356.

Davies, H., Priddy, J. M., & Tinklenberg, J. R. (1986). Support groups for male caregivers of Alzheimer's Patients. *Clinical Gerontologist, 5*(3/4), 385–395.

Delgado, M., & Tennstedt, S. (1997). Puerto Rican sons as primary caregivers of elderly parents. *Social Work, 42,* 125–134.

Dulac, G., & Kosberg, J. I. (1994). *Elderly men in North America: Changes and challenges.* Paper presented at the 43rd Annual Scientific Meeting of the Gerontological Society of America, Atlanta, Georgia.

Dwyer, J. W., & Coward, R. T. (1991). A multivariate comparison of the involvement of adult sons versus daughters in the care of impaired parents. *Journal of Gerontology, 46*(5), S258–S269.

Fitting, M., Rabins, P., Lucas, M. J., & Eastham, J. (1986). Caregivers of dementia patients: A comparison of husband and wives. *The Gerontologist, 26,* 248–252.

Gilhooly, M. L. M. (1984). The impact of caregiving in caregivers: Factors associated with the psychological well-being of people supporting a dementing relative in the community. *British Journal of Medical Psychology, 57,* 35–44.

Glaser, B., & Strauss, A. (1967). *The discovery of grounded theory.* Chicago: Aldine.

Harris, P. B. (1993). The misunderstood caregiver?: A qualitative study of the male caregiver of Alzheimer's disease victims. *The Gerontologist, 33*(4), 551–556.

Harris, P. B. (1995). Differences among husbands caring for their wives with Alzheimer's disease: Qualitative findings and counseling implications. *Journal of Clinical Geropsychology, 1,* 97–106.

Harris, P. B. (1998). Listening to caregiving sons: Misunderstood realities. *The Gerontologist, 38*(3), 342–352.

Harris, P. B., & Bichler, J. (1997). *Men giving care: Reflections of husbands and sons.* New York: Garland.

Horowitz, A. (1985). Family caregiving to the frail elderly. *Annual review of gerontology and geriatrics, 5,* 194–246.

Ingersoll-Dayton, B., Starrels, M. E., & Dowler, D. (1996). Caregiving for parents and parents-in-law: Is gender important? *The Gerontologist,* *36*(4), 483–491.

Kramer, B. J., & Lambert, J. D. (1999). Caregiving as a life course transition among older husbands: A prospective study. *The Gerontologist, 39*(6), 658–667.

Lee, G. R., Dwyer, J. W., & Coward, R. T. (1993). Gender differences in parent care: Demographic factors and same gender preferences. *Journal of Gerontology: Social Sciences, 48*(1), S9–S16.

Matthews, S. H., & Heidorn, J. (1998). Meeting filial responsibilities in brothers-only sibling groups. *Journal of Gerontology: Social Sciences, 53*(5), S278–S286.

Miller, B. (1987). Gender and control among spouses of the cognitively impaired: A research note. *The Gerontologist, 32*(4), 498–507.

Montgomery, R., & Kamo, Y. (1989). Parent care by sons and daughters. In J. A. Mancini (Ed)., *Aging parents and adult children* (pp. 213–230). Lexington, MA: Lexington Books.

Motenko, A. K. (1988). Respite care and pride in caregiving: The experience of six older men caring for their disabled wives. In S. Reinhatz & G. Rowles (Eds.), *Qualitative gerontology* (pp. 104–126). New York: Springer.

Patton, M. Q. (1980). *Qualitative evaluation and research methods.* Newbury Park, CA: Sage.

Pruchno, R. A., & Resch, N. L. (1989). Husbands and wives as caregivers: Antecedents of depression and burden. *The Gerontologist, 29*(2), 159–165.

Solomon, K. (1982). The older man. In K. Solomon & N. B. Levy (Eds.), *Men in transition* (pp. 205–240). New York: Plenum Press.

Stoller, E. P. (1990). Males as helpers: The role of sons, relatives, and friends. *The Gerontologist, 30*(2), 228–235.

Stone, R., Cafferata, G., & Sangl, J. (1987). Caregivers of the frail elderly: A national profile. *The Gerontologist, 29,* 677–683.

Tennstedt, S. L., McKinlay, J. B., & Sullivan, L. M. (1989). Informal care for frail elders: The role of secondary caregivers. *The Gerontologist, 29*(5), 677–683.

Vinick, B. H. (1984). Elderly men as caregivers of wives. *Journal of Geriatric Psychiatry, 17*(1), 61–68.

Zarit, J. M. (1982). *Predictors of burden and distress for caregivers of senile dementia patients.* Unpublished doctoral dissertation, University of Southern California, Los Angeles.

Brothers and Parent Care: An Explanation for Sons' Underrepresentation[1]

10

Sarah H. Matthews

This chapter draws on a study of older families in which pairs of siblings were interviewed about their parents to offer an explanation for why a subcategory of men—brothers—provides less parent care than a subcategory of women—sisters. Most research that explores gender differences in the provision of services to older parents compares sons to daughters without taking into account their status as siblings. Regardless of the way care is measured, as a category, daughters, with few exceptions, are found to provide more services and to spend more time providing them than sons (Martin-Matthews & Campbell, 1995; Stoller, 1994). Although it has been suggested that the magnitude of the gender difference may be exaggerated due to the specific tasks about which questions are asked (Horowitz, 1992; Rosenthal & Martin-Matthews, 1999), no one has argued that it is solely an artifact of measurement.

Scholars have sought to explain what the variable "gender" indexes that might account for this difference. Finley (1989) tested four hypotheses about factors that might explain daughters' overrepresentation among caregiving adult children. She concluded, "Regardless of the time available, the attitudes of obligation, or the external resources, women provide more care for their mothers than do males. In addition, males are not more likely to specialize in care managing than are females" (p. 84; see also Martin-Matthews & Campbell, 1995). Lee, Dwyer, and Coward (1993)

[1] Research was supported by a grant from the National Institute on Aging (AG03484). Ideas for this paper were developed while the author was the Petersen Visiting Scholar in Gerontology and Family Studies, Department of Human Development and Family Sciences, Oregon State University, 1998.

suggest another explanation. They reason that mothers more often than fathers are widowed and, therefore, more likely to require personal care from their children. As a result, daughters *should* be overrepresented because of the embarrassment that would ensue from a son's providing hands-on care to his mother (see also, Arber & Ginn, 1995; Connidis, Rosenthal, & McMullin, 1996; Montgomery & Kamo, 1989; Ungerson, 1983). However, they found only limited support for the hypothesis that fathers prefer sons and mothers prefer daughters to provide their care. For the most part, then, the finding that daughters provide a great deal more care than sons continues to be a "fact in search of a theory" (Lee, 1992).

The case made here is that disaggregating adult children into categories based on gender composition and size of their siblings group is an important first step toward explaining brothers' poor showing in the research literature on parent care. Because the meaning of gender relies on context (Risman, 1998), the gender composition of the sibling group affects how gender is enacted. Following a brief review of the research literature in which findings about brothers are identified, the research design and informants for the study are described. Evidence is then presented that brothers and sisters have distinct ideas about how best to meet their parents' needs. These different ideas about "best practice" account for sons' lower level of involvement. Within the context of a sibling group where siblings negotiate who should do what for parents, brothers with sisters are at a disadvantage.

LITERATURE REVIEW

In this chapter the argument is made that at least part of the explanation for the consistent finding of gender differences in the provision of parent care lies in the gender composition of the sibling group. Including siblings as part of the explanation shifts attention from the individual to the family system. In most research on intergenerational caregiving, the unit of analysis is the individual adult child who is the primary caregiver. For only children, this is appropriate. When there is more than one child in a family, however, relationships among family members affect how parents' needs are met and the way each child is involved.

Most researchers now distinguish between sons and husband caregivers, recognizing that "male" is too encompassing a category to be useful. Similarly, research findings suggest that only children and those with siblings differ with respect to tasks and time devoted to caregiving (Logan & Spitze, 1996; Spitze & Logan, 1990). Only-sons and brothers may be the same gender, but their family relationships are far from equivalent.

Furthermore, the gender of brothers' siblings also is an important factor (Wolf, Freedman, & Soldo, 1997). Brothers of brothers and brothers of sisters experience family ties and parent care differently.

Reviewing the research literature to discover how brothers are involved in caring for old parents is not straightforward, because men typically are treated as sons rather than as brothers. A growing number of studies, however, uses size and gender composition of sibling group as variables. Coward and Dwyer (1990) found that sons who had at least one sister were slightly more likely than sons who only had brothers to provide help with activities of daily living (ADL) tasks; 7.7% compared with 6.9%. Daughters who only had sisters were also slightly more likely than daughters who had at least one brother to provide help with ADL tasks; 28.0% compared with 24.6%.

Similarly, Spitze and Logan (1990) found that parents reported that having a sister increased the amount of both face-to-face interaction and the time spent helping parents for both sons and daughters. They also found that in dyadic sibling groups, brothers with a sister reported helping their parents on average 1.46 hours per week, while brothers with a brother reported helping only 55 minutes per week. Sisters with a brother reported providing 2.3 hours of help per week, and sisters with a sister reported providing 3.21 hours of help per week. Again, the presence of a sister in a sibling dyad elevated the amounts of time both brothers and sisters reported assisting parents.

Focusing on adult children who reported providing at least one hour of help to their mothers, fathers, or both parents, Connidis, Rosenthal, and McMullin (1996, p. 424) found in a study of employed caregivers that "having more sisters increases the likelihood of shared help and decreases the probability of being the primary helper to mothers for men and women. This trend is also evident for fathers only and both parents, although these models are not significant." Again, they conclude that the presence of a sister in the sibling group increased siblings' contributions to their parents. Martin-Matthews and Campbell (1995) reported an exception to this general finding. They found that men who had siblings were significantly less likely to provide personal care if the men had sisters but no brothers. The focus on "personal care" rather than a more global measure of care may account for this difference.

Coward and Dwyer (1990) also found that sisters who had at least one brother reported significantly higher levels of burden and stress (see also Mui, 1995). This finding receives support in qualitative studies in which primary caregivers often complain bitterly about absence of support from siblings. Reviewing this literature is difficult because distinctions between brothers and sisters are not routinely made. Merrill (1997), for example, reports that 40 of the 50 primary caregivers recruited through Alzheimer's support groups and an adult day care center were siblings. Slightly less than one-third of them reported receiving help from siblings (p. 52). Sisters had little positive to say about their brothers. Some viewed their brothers as not competent to provide assistance. One sister, for example, said, "I wouldn't leave my worst enemy with my brother. He is more than irresponsible. It doesn't even begin to describe it" (p. 56). Another said,

Once when my mother's ankles were swollen and she couldn't walk, I called my brother over and asked him what he thought we should do. He said, "Leave her with me for the night, and I will take care of her with a pillow." I thought, "Great, why am I asking him for help?" (p. 36)

Others thought that their brothers were simply the wrong gender to provide personal services to their mothers:

Well, I am the caregiver because I am the only girl. I know that sounds chauvinistic, but my brothers are uncomfortable. They don't know how . . . They wouldn't even know how to take off her bra! (p. 37)

Sisters in Merrill's study also complained that their siblings did not support them more:

My brother comes on Friday night to cook their dinner and then again on Sunday to spend the day. But he says that he can't do more *to help me*. . . . I have no one else to help. (p. 55, emphasis added)

My brother and sister say that they feel sorry for me and what can they do. So I tell them that it would help if they would come over and spend the night sometimes so that *I could sleep* or the evening so that *I could go out*. But they aren't willing to do it. (p. 57, emphasis added)

Having siblings who will not help in the way that the sisters would like appears to add to the strain of providing care.

This brief review of the literature highlights what an explanation for brothers' poor representation in the parent-care literature must address. First, it must account for the brothers doing less than sisters. Second, it must account for brothers' higher level of help when they have at least one sister. Last, it must account for the increased level of stress experienced by sisters who have brothers.

RESEARCH DESIGN

The chapter draws on qualitative interviews that were conducted with 149 pairs of siblings who described how their parents' needs were met. The goal of the study is to understand the effects of gender composition and size on how the family labor of meeting the needs of old parents is divided among siblings. Siblings whose parents were at least 75 years old and not living in a nursing home were recruited for the study. Age rather than need or health status of parents was used as a criteria to insure that a range of older families was included rather than only those with a very needy parent.

Adult children were not asked to participate in research on caregiving but in research on older families with specific gender compositions. The initial 50 families included two sisters; one employed, one not employed. Advertisements were placed in local campus and community newspapers. Various community groups and agencies that had women as participants or clients—excluding caregiver-support groups—were contacted and asked if recruitment fliers could be posted or distributed. Usually, the first sister to make a contact indicated that she already had spoken with her sister or that she would. Sisters with more than one sister, then, chose the one who would participate. Subsequently, lone-sister families (those comprising only one sister and one or more brothers) and brothers-only families (those with at least two brothers and no sisters) were recruited, initially using the same tactics. In lone-sister families, sisters called and volunteered a brother, whom they usually preferred to contact themselves. Again, if a sister had more than one brother, she chose the one who would participate. Brothers-only families were not forthcoming. Almost all of the men in brothers-only families, therefore, were recruited through their parents. A colleague who recently had interviewed community-dwelling elders over the age of 85 had included a question about the gender of their children. Parents in her study who had two or more sons were identified and asked for permission to contact their children. Some of the sister-brother pairs were recruited this way as well. In addition, a registry of elders who had volunteered to participate in research on a university campus was tapped. Calls were made to find out whether their families met the criteria; if they did, parents were asked for permission to contact their children. They were also asked if they knew anyone whose family might qualify and, if they did, for permission to call them. The elders typically were very helpful and very few of the sons who were contacted said "no" to the request to participate in the study.

Siblings completed a written questionnaire about all living members of their original family. The researchers then interviewed each member of a pair of siblings, either in person (70%) or over the telephone, each by a different interviewer, and asked to respond to 18 open-ended questions, the first of which asked that they describe the current situation of the parent(s). Questions focused on what each sibling was doing for their parent(s), how they decided who would do what, and whether they thought the division of labor was fair. Interviews lasted approximately an hour and the interviewer recorded the answers as near to verbatim as possible.

To facilitate qualitative analysis, data collected through the open-ended interviews were typed into 149 family files juxtaposing the responses of the two siblings that were triggered by each question. Family files were read many times as various ideas for analysis were pursued. For a specific code, the entire interview rather than only answers to specific questions was coded. Analysis entailed moving back and forth between coded segments and the interviews to gauge the validity of the argument presented as it was developed inductively (Lofland & Lofland, 1995).

The 149 families consisted of 403 siblings of whom 176 were sisters and 227 were brothers. In 99 of the families brothers were interviewed. These included 50 brothers who had only one sister, whom they also interviewed (Matthews, 1995), and 49 pairs of brothers who had no sisters (Matthews & Heidorn, 1998). In an additional 21 of the families, pairs of sisters described their brothers' contributions. Twenty-nine of the families consisted of only sisters (Matthews & Rosner, 1988). The siblings ranged in age from 33 to 78. Seventy-seven percent of the adult children were married, with more brothers than sisters being married. More than half of the siblings had graduated from college. Seventy-one percent were employed at the time of the interview, with more brothers than sisters employed. Fifty-two percent of the informants lived no more than 10 miles from their parent(s), and 75% lived within 150 miles.

The 204 parents in these 149 families ranged in age from 71 to 97, with a median age of 79. Almost two thirds were mothers. In half of the families ($n = 75$) only the mother was living while in 12% ($n = 18$) only the father was living. Most of the parents lived in their own households—alone if they were widowed ($n = 63$), or together if they were married ($n = 50$ [100]). In two cases, one spouse was in a nursing home and the other lived alone. Eleven widowed mothers and four couples shared a household with one of their children (10 with daughters, 5 with sons). One couple and eight widowed mothers had live-in helpers, and one widowed father and one widowed mother had moved to the assisted-living section of a retirement community in which they had lived for a number of years. Respondents rated their parents' health status on a 4-point scale from excellent to poor: 28.5% of the sibling pairs agreed that their parent's health was excellent or good; 17.6%, that it was good or fair; and 37.2%, that it was fair or poor. For only 3% of the parents ($n = 6$) did the sibling pairs rank a parent differently by more than one level on the scale.

GENDERED APPROACHES TO MEETING PARENTS' NEEDS

An implicit assumption in the caregiving literature is that there is a "best practice" for meeting parents' needs. Disagreement among family members about whether to institutionalize a frail parent is sometimes noted, but that there is a variety of ways to meet the needs of a parent is largely ignored. Furthermore, more help is generally viewed as better than less help (Silverstein, Chen, & Heller, 1996). Analysis of the 298 qualitative interviews with pairs of siblings indicated that brothers and sisters have different ideas about the best way to meet their parents' needs, that is, about what constitutes "best practice." Like all gender dichotomies, this one is too strongly drawn. With that caveat, three major differences emerged from analysis that differentiated broadly the approaches of brothers and sisters.

First, brothers responded to parents' requests for assistance. They expected their parents to tell them when they needed help and what to do. They provided services when asked rather than offering advice and assistance. Sisters, on the other hand, not only responded to requests but also monitored their parents and routinely offered unsolicited services and advice. Contrast the words of the following informants, the first a brother with two brothers, the second a sister with one sister:

> If she needs to go someplace and she doesn't have transportation, one of us will always take her, or arrange for transportation. There's no set schedule. It's as the need arises. When I go to work in the morning and my mother seems more depressed, I'll call my sister and tell her to get in touch with Mom. She'll come over, all the way from the other side of town, and visit with my mother or take her out. She's very supportive.

Brothers were "on call" while sisters "monitored" and intervened when they saw a need.

Even during major transitions, brothers were likely to see their parents as self-sufficient. Note the difference in the following responses of a brother and a sister to their respective mother's widowhood. A brother with one brother said,

> When my father died 8 years ago, my mother went on to independent living. I don't think she started leaning on us for more support.

A sister with one sister described her mother's situation after her father's death 5 years earlier:

> She felt very lost. Their generation, their social life was their family, and after my father died, she didn't know how to make friends or how to project herself. That's why she's working [in a job that her daughters had found for her and encouraged her to take]. She has a social life there as a waitress. This summer I think she's a little better than she had been. Last Sunday we gave a dinner party and it was the first time she's enjoyed doing this since my father died. I think she's finally getting over it; but if you've never made friends in your life, it's hard to start at age 75.

Brothers regarded their parents (unless they were seen as mentally incompetent) as capable of making decisions about how to include them in their lives. Sisters responded to parents' requests but they also monitored their parents, gave them advice, and attempted to intervene when they thought it was appropriate.

Second, brothers made contributions to their parents exclusively in their role as sons except when crises brought siblings together to consult with one another to solve a problem. Siblings were not seen as particularly relevant to their ongoing relationships with their parents except in times of crisis. A brother with one brother explained:

> I'll call my mother and ask, "Have you heard from them [brother and wife]?" At times she'll say "not in months" at times it'll be "yesterday." I think my mother probably has had some dry spells, doesn't hear from either of us. Other times she has feast times, hears from both of us. It's not something we schedule, and maybe we should. We haven't sat down and said, "Call then, so a week doesn't go by."

Brothers, then, did not routinely discuss with their siblings what they were doing with and for their parents but acted independently.

In contrast, sisters saw their own contributions to their parents in relation to their siblings. They viewed themselves simultaneously as daughters and sisters. They expected to share responsibility with their siblings and to be part of a coordinated effort to meet parents' needs. A sister with one sister explained:

> My sister and I talk every day. We find Mother colors what she tells us; so we find it best to communicate daily. Absolutely we discuss her medical problems. You can't go blind into these things. We do talk about it.

Unlike brothers, when sisters talked about doing things for their parents, they also talked about what they did for their siblings. A sister with one sister said:

> I can't provide long-term residence as well as my sister can, but I can get my mother out of the house on Saturday. That's my contribution to my sister's mental health when my mother is visiting from Florida.

Sisters viewed themselves as part of a family system in which being a daughter and being a sister were interdependent, while brothers viewed their ties to each family member as independent. Sisters took into account not only their parents' circumstances but their siblings' as well. In short, brothers saw their duty as *filial* while sisters saw it as *familial*.

Third, the brothers' goal in providing assistance was to enable their parents to maintain or reestablish self-sufficiency. They saw as legitimate their parents' use of both formal and informal support networks to accomplish this. Their goal was to maintain the parent-adult child relationship as one between equals, albeit with the attendant deference that such a relationship entails. Brothers found frustrating parents who refused to act to regain self-sufficiency, thereby undermining the egalitarian nature of their adult relationship with their parents. A brother with one brother explained:

> The day-to-day things of looking after her I do. I've done a lot of yard work for her, but I'm really trying to encourage her to run her own life. I try to encourage her to be more active, less dependent than she already is. I go there two or three times a week. I try to avoid a regular calling schedule.

Sisters' response as their parents became more needy was to increase their own level of services. They accepted their parents' increased dependence on them as appropriate. A sister with one sister explained what would happen to her relationship with her father if her mother were to die, "I'd want to be there and see he's eating right, wash his clothes, clean his house, take over the wifely duties." Sisters found frustrating finding enough time and the appropriate services to supplement their own contributions to their parents. When they arranged formal services, they monitored them closely.

BROTHERS' POORER SHOWING EXPLAINED

In this section the case is made that these gendered approaches to parent care may provide the "theory" to explain the "fact" (Lee, 1992) that daughters are more involved in parent care than sons. They also explain why brothers with sisters are generally more involved with their parents than brothers with brothers, and why sisters with brothers feel more burdened than sisters with sisters. How gendered approaches explains each of these findings is discussed in turn.

Brothers Do Less than Sisters

The gendered approaches to meeting parents' needs were derived inductively from interviews with siblings, but the approaches are those of individuals. If they apply to only-sons and only-daughters, and there is no reason to believe that they should not, they would account for sons' under representation in the parent-care literature. A consistent finding, for example, is that daughters interact more than sons with their parents on the telephone (Logan & Spitze, 1996). In order to monitor, daughters must check on their parents. Responding primarily to requests, as sons are more likely to do, requires contact only when a need arises and consequently will occur less frequently. Hence, sons are less likely to be in contact with their parents as often as daughters. Likewise, accepting a parent's dependence leads to more interaction than encouraging a parent to remain self-sufficient. This would explain the finding that sons are more likely than daughters to "drop out" as parents' needs increase (Montgomery & Kamo, 1989) or to be "case managers" rather than provide hands-on care. Different ideas about what constitutes "best practice" explain differences in sons' and daughters' involvement in parent care.

Enacting these approaches to "best practice" in a group of siblings, depending on its gender composition and other factors, may further reduce sons' involvement. Gender differences in what is considered the appropriate way to assist older parents means that brothers and sisters are unlikely to agree on solutions to their parents' problems or even that their parents have problems. In a contest between sisters and brothers over whose approach to implement, sisters have the advantage, although the word advantage may be a poor choice to describe their situation.

Winning the dispute over what constitutes "best practice" means that sisters will take on more responsibility. Their advantage stems, first, from families being the domain of women. In the nineteenth, twentieth, and now twenty-first centuries, women are considered to be experts on family matters (Cowan, 1983). When it comes to "doing family," women know the standard, in this case, for what constitutes *appropriate* care for parents. Sisters, then, have no reason to listen to brothers who have different ideas about how best to meet their parents' needs. A sister in the study who had one sister and one brother said, "Daughters end up with the mothers, not the boys. We would call my brother after the fact, but never ask his opinion." After all, sisters know best. In sisters' view, brothers should recognize their authority and act accordingly, by following their example and injunctions, and doing "what needs to be done."

Sisters are likely to win the contest with their brothers for another reason. They want to do *more* for their parents while brothers want to do *less*. This means that when sisters institute their own plans, their brothers are precluded from implementing their ideas. A sister who is willing to take her lonely, frail mother into her household, for example, prevents her brother from helping his mother move to an assisted living apartment where she would be less dependent on her children.

Having a Sister Increases Brothers' Participation

Whether brothers have sisters or brothers is consequential for their participation in parent care. Brothers who only have brothers are likely to share an approach. Each brother, as a son, is able to do for their parents what he views is required. Each responds to his parents' requests independently. No attempt is made to coordinate actions unless there is a crisis, in which case brothers come together to institute a plan on which it is relatively easy to agree because their ideas about what is appropriate are likely to be quite similar. Because brothers opt to maintain their parents' independence rather than encourage dependence, they do less for their parents than sisters do. This is captured in the research literature by the term "case management," something brothers are reputed to do more often than sisters who opt for providing care themselves. In addition, for brothers to view themselves as "caregivers" is a sign that they have failed to reach their goal of maintaining an egalitarian relationship with their parents. This accounts for the fact that brothers tend to downplay what they do for their parents, describing their contributions as "little" and of little consequence even though from an objective standpoint what they do for them is quite significant (Matthews, 1995; Matthews & Heidorn, 1998).

Brothers who have sisters must deal with someone who expects them to behave *familially* rather than *filially*. Brothers may not live up to their sisters' expectations, but if brothers wish to remain on good terms with a sister there is some pressure to comply with her approach. This would explain the consistent findings that brothers who have at least one sister are reported by parents and report themselves to do more with and for their parents than brothers who have only brothers. Brothers who have sisters are drawn into sisters' ideas of "best practice" and as a consequence participate in ways that they might forego if left to implement their own approach.

Sisters Burdened with Brothers

Because they have different approaches to "best practice," brothers and sisters are more likely than same-gender siblings to have difficulty agreeing about the best approach. This would account for the finding (Coward & Dwyer, 1990; Mui, 1995) that sisters who had at least one brother reported significantly higher levels of burden and stress than those who had no brothers. In addition to solving a parent's problems, sisters may also be dealing with brothers who do not support their approach. This was precisely the complaint voiced by sisters cited above who were interviewed by Merrill (1997). These sisters' complaint is that their siblings see their responsibility as filial not as familial, something brothers are more likely than sisters to do. For a brother to participate as his sister instructs he would need to see himself not only as a son but also as a brother, to allow his ties to his parents to be mediated by his sister.

The size of a sibling group comes into play as well. The 50 sisters included in this study who had at least one brother but no sisters expressed the most unhappiness with their siblings. Pairs of sisters who had brothers were less critical of their brothers because they had a sister with whom they shared an approach and could more easily tolerate a brother's unwillingness to be a team player. It is important to remember that brothers have a perspective as well. A brother with two sisters would have little chance of implementing his approach and would be in greater danger of being excluded from decision making by his sisters who may support one another at his expense.

Factors that Mitigate Against Implementing Gendered Approaches

There are, of course, situations in which brothers who have sisters provide parent care using their own approach. One obvious factor that works against sisters' winning a contest with brothers is when brothers but not sisters live near their parents (Stoller, Forster, & Duniho, 1992). Under those conditions, brothers are less likely to be thwarted. The extreme form of this occurs when brothers live *with* their parents while sisters do not. Sisters may disapprove of brothers' approach, but the fact that their brothers are in residence hinders sisters' doing things their way. Other situational factors that privilege brothers over sisters include such things as health status and competing family responsibilities (Campbell & Martin-Matthews, 2000). These factors are difficult to capture as variables in quantitative studies but are taken into account by siblings as they negotiate the provision of services to parents.

Even when brothers and sisters are in close proximity to their parents, they may not compete with one another over the issue of implementing approaches if parents do not require a great deal of support to maintain independence. Sisters may monitor their parents, brothers respond to requests, but the needs of their parents are easily met so that conflict between their approaches is not obvious. A sister and brother may assume that they agree with one another and, because their parents' needs are relatively minor and their contributions orchestrated by their parents, the assumption need never be tested. Most qualitative research on caregiving adult children focuses on those giving care to very needy parents, typically to parents who have Alzheimer's disease or some other cognitive impairment. When parents require a great deal of assistance, differences of opinion among siblings about how much or what to do for parents are more difficult to ignore.

The qualitative literature provides evidence that some sons do provide care, in some cases extraordinary care (Harris & Bichler, 1996; Kaye & Applegate, 1990; Merrill, 1997). Although some sons are caregivers "by default" (Arber & Ginn, 1995; Campbell & Martin-Matthews, 2000; Horowitz, 1985) in that they have no sisters to assume this role, others provide such care even when sisters are available. At least some sons, then, are capable of providing care. Nevertheless, respondents who participate in qualitative research rarely have kind things to say about their brothers' involvement in parent care. They complain, often bitterly, that siblings in general and brothers in particular are not supportive of their efforts to meet parents' needs. These denounced brothers and sisters rarely have the opportunity to present their view, a perennial problem with research in which one member is privileged to speak for an entire family.

CONCLUSION

This chapter is based on an inductive analysis of interviews with 149 pairs of siblings who independently answered questions about how they and their siblings met the needs of their parents. Gendered approaches to "best practice" in the provision of services to parents were identified. The argument was made that these approaches account for brothers' apparent underrepresentation in parent care. Central to the argument is that any explanation of adult children's involvement in parent care must take into account the size and gender composition of their sibling group. Researchers should differentiate only-children from brothers and sisters in analysis of parent care. They may feel overwhelmed by what they may perceive as their sole responsibility, but their experience is different enough from siblings to warrant treating only-sons and brothers (and only-daughters and sisters) as separate populations.

Brothers' participation in the provision of services is a function of the number of sisters in their families. If they have none, they are in a position to carry out their own views of how best to meet their parents' needs. This approach includes responding to parents' requests rather than monitoring; viewing their responsibility as filial rather than familial; and seeking to preserve an egalitarian relationship with their parents by maintaining their parents' self-sufficiency. When brothers have sisters, their approach is eclipsed by their sisters' approach. Sisters not only consider themselves (and are considered by others) to be the experts on parent care but also believe that it is important to monitor their parents and to accept their parents' dependence on them. Brothers who have sisters but still are able to implement their own approach have sisters who have abdicated by living farther away from the parents than their brothers or for some other reason such as poor health or other family obligations.

These approaches to parent care were derived inductively from a nonprobability sample. As such, they are hypotheses that should not be accepted without additional research to test them. As with any gender dichotomy, the one presented in this paper is too bold. There were brothers in these 149 families whose approach to parent care was familial rather than filial and there were sisters who promoted their parents' self-sufficiency and discouraged dependency. Furthermore, other family ties also affected siblings. Many of the siblings were married. Given that spouses are different genders, they are unlikely to share a view of "best practice." It is not surprising that daughters-in-law rather than sons-in-law are credited with helping their parents-in-law.

Perhaps the most important insight to emerge from the analysis is the notion of "best practice." Gerontologists who study the family may have become so inured in their thinking that the lived experiences behind such concepts as "intimacy at a distance," "filial responsibility," and "parent care," as well as the implicit assumption that daughters rather than sons know best what should be done for parents, limit the kinds of question that are asked. One goal of this chapter, then, is not so much to convince readers that there are gendered approaches but to encourage researchers to raise new questions that take into account relationships among members of older families rather than continuing to seek explanations that view family members solely as individuals.

REFERENCES

Arber, S., & Ginn, J. (1995). Gender differences in informal caring. *Health and Social Care in the Community, 3,* 19–31.

Campbell, L. D., & Martin-Matthews, A. (2000). Caring sons: Exploring men's involvement in filial care. *Canadian Journal on Aging, 19,* 57–79.

Connidis, I., Rosenthal, C. J., & McMullin, J. (1996). The impact of family composition on providing help to older parents: A study of employed adults. *Research on Aging, 18,* 402–419.

Cowan, R. Schwartz. (1983). *More work for mother.* New York: Basic Books.

Coward, R. T., & Dwyer, J. W. (1990). The association of gender, sibling network composition, and patterns of parent care by adult children. *Research on Aging, 12,* 158–181.

Finley, N. J. (1989). Theories of family labor as applied to gender differences in caregiving for elderly parents. *Journal of Marriage and the Family, 51,* 79–86.

Harris, P. B., & Bichler, J. (1997). *Men giving care: Reflections of husbands and sons.* New York: Garland.

Horowitz, A. (1985). Sons and daughters as caregivers to older parents: Differences in role performance and consequences. *The Gerontologist, 25,* 612–617.

Horowitz, A. (1992). Methodological issues in the study of gender within family caregiving relationships. In J. W. Dwyer & R. T. Coward (Eds.), *Gender, families, and elder care* (pp. 132–150). Newbury Park, CA: Sage.

Kaye, L. W., & Applegate, J. S. (1990). *Men as caregivers to the elderly.* Boston: Lexington.

Lee, G. R. (1992). Gender differences in family caregiving: A fact in search of a theory. In J. W. Dwyer & R. T. Coward (Eds.), *Gender, families, and elder care* (pp. 120–131). Newbury Park, CA. Sage.

Lee, G. R., Dwyer, J. W., & Coward, R. T.(1993). Gender differences in parent care: Demographic factors and same-gender preferences. *Journals of Gerontology: Social Sciences, 48,* S9–S16.

Lofland, J., & Lofland, L. H. (1995). *Analyzing social settings: A guide to qualitative observation and analysis.* Belmont, CA: Wadsworth.

Logan, J. R., & Spitze, G. D. (1996). *Family ties: Enduring relations between parents and their grown children.* Philadelphia: Temple University Press.

Martin-Matthews, A., & Campbell, L. D. (1995). Gender roles, employment and informal care. In S. Arber & J. Ginn (Eds.), *Connecting gender and ageing: A sociological approach* (pp. 129–143). Bristol, PA: Open Uni-versity Press.

Matthews, S. H. (1995). The division of filial responsibility in lone-sister sibling groups. *Journal of Gerontology: Social Sciences, 50B,* S312–S320.

Matthews, S. H., & Heidorn, J. (1998). Meeting filial responsibilities in brothers-only sibling groups. *Journal of Gerontology: Social Sciences, 53B,* S278–S286.

Matthews, S. H., & Rosner, T. T. (1988). Shared filial responsibility: The family as the primary caregiver. *Journal of Marriage and the Family, 50,* 185–195.

Merrill, D. J. (1997). *Caring for elderly parents: Juggling work, family, and caregiving in middle and working class families.* Westport, CT: Auburn House.

Montgomery, R. J. V., & Kamo, Y. (1989). Parent care by sons and daughters. In J. Mancini (Ed.), *Aging parents and adult children* (pp. 213–230). Lexington, MA: Lexington Books.

Mui, A. (1995). Caring for frail elderly parents: A comparison of adult sons and daughters. *The Gerontologist, 35,* 86–93.

Risman, B. J. (1998). *Gender vertigo.* New Haven, CT: Yale University Press.

Rosenthal, C., & Martin-Matthews, A. (1999). *Families as care-providers versus care-managers? Gender and type of care in a sample of employed Canadians.* SEDAP Research Paper No. 4, McMaster University, Hamilton, Ontario Canada.

Silverstein, M., Chen, X., & Heller, K. (1996). Too much of a good thing? Intergenerational social support and the psychological well-being of older parents. *Journal of Marriage and the Family, 58,* 970–982.

Spitze, G., & Logan, J. (1990). Sons, daughters, and intergenerational social support. *Journal of Marriage and the Family, 52,* 420–430.

Stoller, E. P. (1994). Teaching about gender: The experience of family care of frail elderly relatives. *Educational Gerontology, 20,* 679–697.

Stoller, E. P., Forster, L. E. & Duniho, T. S. (1992). Systems of parent care within sibling networks. *Research on Aging, 14,* 28–49.

Ungerson, C. (1983). Women and caring: Skills, tasks and taboos. In E. Gamarnikow, D. H. J. Morgan, J. Purvis, & D. Taylorson (Eds.), *The public and the private* (pp. 62–77). London: Heinemann.

Wolf, D. A., Freedman, V., & Soldo, B. J. (1997). The division of family labor: Care for elderly parents. *The Journals of Gerontology, 52B* (Special Issue): 102–109.

Fathers as Caregivers for Adult Children With Mental Retardation[1]

11

Elizabeth L. Essex
Marsha M. Seltzer
Marty W. Krauss

INTRODUCTION

This chapter examines a unique group of male caregivers, fathers of adult children with mental retardation. Family research has largely neglected fathers in studies of parents caring for adults with mental retardation. Much more attention has focused on mothers, who typically function as the primary caregiver. However, there is growing recognition of the important roles of fathers in all families, and an emerging literature on the similarities and differences between fathers and mothers in their experiences as parents of children with lifelong dependency. The focus of this chapter is on older fathers of adults with mental retardation, who differ in three major aspects from most older men who provide care to a family member. First, in contrast to older men who provide primary care to dependent wives or parents, these men provide care to *an adult dependent child*. Second, in contrast to older men who become primary caregivers, these men usually do not bear the full responsibility for the dependent's care and thus have *an adjunctive caregiving role*. Third, in contrast to men whose caregiving responsibilities are time-limited, these fathers have weathered *decades of caregiving* as a parent of a child with a lifelong disability. Although much

[1] Preparation of this chapter was supported by a grant from the National Institute on Aging (R01 AG08768) to the second and third authors. Support was also provided by the Waisman Center at the University of Wisconsin-Madison and the Starr Center on Mental Retardation at the Heller School at Brandeis University.

of the "care" that a father provides to his son or daughter with mental retardation is indistinguishable from typical parenting, when the child becomes an adult this care becomes increasingly non-normative. Adults with retardation who continue to live with their parents vary enormously, but all share a common characteristic: continued dependency on the parents beyond the time that children ordinarily become independent. It is at this point that *parenting* takes on the features of *caregiving*.

It is important to recognize that family-based care is the norm rather than the exception for persons with mental retardation. Less than 15% of those with mental retardation, estimated to be between 1% and 3% of the general population, ever live in a licensed residential facility (Fujiura & Braddock, 1992). Rather, most live with or under the supervision of their parents throughout their lives. The tableau of father and mother caring for a child with retardation throughout the parents' adult and older years is a familiar one for thousands of families. Since the late 1950s, there has been an accumulation of knowledge about families of children with mental retardation (Farber, 1959; Keltner & Ramey, 1993). Although early research focused on the unique and common stresses experienced by such families, particularly during the early childhood period, there is recognition that, over the life course, families with a child with a disability manifest the same range of patterns of adaptation as "typical" families (Ramey, Krauss, & Simeonsson, 1989).

There has been little research on older fathers of adults with mental retardation, although fathers of young children with disabilities have been studied in a number of investigations. We review this research to identify trends regarding paternal roles within the family, impacts on paternal well-being, and sources of support for fathers. Next, we describe our study and summarize the findings from our research on paternal roles and well-being based on a dozen years of longitudinal research on older families of adults with mental retardation who live at home with their aging parents.

PAST RESEARCH ON FATHERS OF CHILDREN WITH MENTAL RETARDATION

Researchers have found that despite the extra caregiving needs of young children with mental retardation, fathers do not take on a larger share of child care or housework than fathers of children without handicaps (Barnett & Boyce, 1995; Erickson & Upshur, 1989). Many have concluded that families of children with mental retardation tend to have quite traditional family task allocations, with fathers being the breadwinner and mothers providing the daily nurturance, guidance, and coordination of care for the children (Schilling, Schinke, & Kirkham, 1988). There is also evidence that the low level of paternal instrumental assistance is a lifelong pattern, with mothers continuing to provide the bulk of direct care even after their child with a disability reaches adulthood (Heller, Hsieh, & Rowitz, 1997; Holmes & Carr, 1991).

A small number of researchers have examined factors that might influence the level of instrumental involvement of fathers with their children with disabilities. There is some evidence that unemployed fathers have greater involvement with their son or daughter than employed fathers (Cooke & Lawton, 1984; Hirst, 1985). On the other hand, whether or not the wife is employed tends not to be related to the amount of paternal assistance provided (Bristol, Gallagher, & Schopler, 1988; Hirst, 1985; Willoughby & Glidden, 1995). A study of families of young adults with developmental disabilities reported that fathers provided significantly more assistance to sons than daughters (see Hirst, 1985).

Only a few researchers have investigated the relationship between fathers' assistance to the son or daughter with mental retardation and maternal well-being. No association was found between the father's level of assistance to the son or daughter and the mother's level of depressive symptoms or caregiving burden (Bristol et al., 1988; Heller et al., 1997), although greater paternal assistance may increase marital satisfaction for both parents (Willoughby & Glidden, 1995).

Other evidence suggests that providing emotional support for their wives is an important role of fathers of children with disabilities (Floyd, Gilliom, & Costigan, 1998; McKinney & Peterson, 1987). In a study of parents of young boys with autism or communication impairments, Bristol et al. (1988) found that the level of expressive support from the husband for his wife was a significant positive predictor of quality of maternal parenting. This finding concurs with the general literature on fathers, which indicates that the father's relationship with the mother has a significant indirect effect on the children (Lamb & Meyer, 1991).

A second area of research on fathers focuses on their psychological well-being. Compared with mothers, fathers of children with disabilities have reported fewer depressive symptoms (Beckman, 1991), higher self-esteem (Trute, 1995), lower subjective burden (Heller et al., 1997), and less of a sense of role restriction (Krauss, 1993). These differences in distress between fathers and mothers of children with disabilities may reflect their different roles in the family. Studies have found a relationship between degree of caregiving demands and distress for mothers but not for fathers of children with disabilities, presumably because fathers are much less involved in the day-to-day care of the child with disabilities (Beckman, 1991; Roach, Orsmond, & Barratt, 1999). Mothers also define themselves more in terms of child rearing, and may be more apt to feel emotional turmoil related to their child's disability (Nadler, Lewinstein, & Rahav, 1991). Moreover, fathers have more opportunity to escape the home situation through employment, and therefore can define themselves in terms of their work role as well as their role as parent (Mardiros, 1985). Alternatively, these findings of greater distress in mothers than fathers may reflect the general findings of greater parenting stress and higher levels of dysphoria and anxiety among women than men (Cleary, 1987; Krauss, 1993).

However, these seeming advantages for fathers may create certain disadvantages as well. Because of their lower involvement, fathers have fewer opportunities than mothers to feel close to the child with a disability and to develop feelings of parental competence (Roach et al., 1999). In addition, fathers may have particular difficulty defining a role for parenting a child with a disability (Lamb & Meyer, 1991). While mothers typically tend to the child's needs for basic care and nurturance, fathers' traditional roles have been physical playmate and achievement role model, guiding the child to eventual independence, particularly for sons (Lamb & Meyer; Nydegger & Mitteness, 1996). Children with disabilities are often less responsive and more difficult to play with and teach than the typical child. In addition, the extent to which they can emulate their father's achievement patterns is compromised. Because child rearing is seen as more essential to the role of mothers, fathers of children with disabilities may not receive as much support from friends, family, self-help groups, and professionals as mothers receive (Davis & May, 1991). In a study comparing fathers and mothers of young children with disabilities, fathers reported more problems than their wives in attachment with their child and viewed the child as less adaptable, moodier, and less reinforcing to them as parents (Krauss, 1993). In another study (Roach et al., 1999), fathers of children with mental retardation perceived more difficulties with parental competence than fathers of typically developing children. The strains fathers experience in relating to their son or daughter may persist into later phases of the family life course. In a study comparing fathers and mothers of adults with chronic disabilities, the fathers reported poorer relationships than mothers with their adult child and perceived the child more negatively, reporting more maladaptive behavior and lower functional skills (Pruchno & Patrick, 1999).

A salient source of stress for fathers of a child with disabilities is concern about the future. Fathers' concerns and related anxiety about the future for their children with disabilities have been reported in studies of parents of young children (McLinden, 1990), adolescents (Hornby, 1995), and adults (Brubaker, Engelhardt, Brubaker, & Lutzer, 1989). In a study of older caregivers of adults with mental retardation (Brubaker et al.), fathers indicated more concern than mothers about their physical ability to care for the child in the future.

Contemporary stress theorists (e. g., Lazarus, 1999) emphasize the importance of social and personal resources in determining the extent to which
an experience is stressful for an individual. Research on the general population suggests that married men tend to rely on their wives for support
in times of stress, while women tend to turn to a wider social network
(Belle, 1987). In her study of parents of young children with disabilities,
Krauss (1993) found evidence for this general pattern. Specifically, the
helpfulness of their social network reduced stress for mothers but not for
fathers, while family cohesion and adaptability were more prominent in
reducing stress for fathers than for mothers.

The few studies of coping by parents of children with mental retardation suggest similarity in the overall patterns for fathers and mothers. In
their study of families of young children with disabilities, Frey, Greenberg,
and Fewell (1989) found that for both fathers and mothers, avoidance and
wishful thinking as coping strategies were related to greater psychological distress, while problem-focused coping was associated with lower
parenting stress and psychological distress. Knussen, Sloper, Cunningham,
and Turner (1992) reported similar findings in a study of fathers and
mothers of school-age children with Down syndrome.

The majority of the research reviewed above pertains to fathers of
minor children with disabilities. Our own research study provided the
opportunity to investigate family patterns later in the life course. We
expected that some of the earlier patterns of paternal roles and well-being
would be modified by later life experiences, such as retirement, declining
health and, in some cases, the adult child's move from the family home to
an alternate living arrangement. Research on caregivers of older adults in
the general population has found a hierarchy of caregiving roles, with a
co-resident spouse (whether husband or wife) to become the initial caregiver, with an adult child taking over parental care when the spouse caregiver
dies (Dwyer & Coward, 1992). We were particularly interested in whether
a similar pattern would apply to families of adults with mental retardation, that is, whether co-resident fathers take over the role of primary
caregiver after the mother dies or becomes incapacitated.

AGING FAMILIES OF ADULTS WITH
MENTAL RETARDATION: FATHERS
IN THE CAREGIVING CONTEXT

Our longitudinal research on 461 families with an adult son or daughter
with mental retardation began in 1988 (Seltzer & Krauss, 1989). The study
has been guided by several theoretical perspectives. First, theories of the
stress process (Lazarus & Folkman, 1984; Pearlin, Mullan, Semple, & Skaff,

1990) have informed many studies of family caregiving (e.g., Aneshensel, Pearlin, Mullan, Zarit, & Whitlatch, 1995), including ours. Three domains of variables are considered in stress process theory: sources of stress, resources that can lessen the effects of stress, and the manifestations or outcomes of stress (Pearlin, 1989). In our investigation of aging caregivers of adults with mental retardation, we have applied stress process theories to the analysis of the sources of stress experienced by fathers and mothers, the extent to which resources such as coping, social support, and marital satisfaction can ameliorate stress, and whether the manifestations or outcomes of stress differ in fathers and mothers.

We have also been informed by life course and life span development theories (Featherman & Lerner, 1985). Exposure to stress at various points in the life course has been shown to have long-term consequences for well-being (Wheaton, Roszell, & Hall, 1997). As parenthood is a role from which one does not exit, difficulties experienced by children may have a lifelong impact on how the parent's life course unfolds (Ryff, Schmutte, & Lee, 1996). In our research, we have applied a life course perspective by tracking change prospectively over more than a decade during the later years of the family life course and across various transitions of caregiving, and by investigating the conditions under which fathers and mothers of adults with mental retardation evidence a pattern of resilience in the face of the stresses of non-normative and lifelong parenting.

In addition, we have incorporated theories of intergenerational solidarity (Bengtson & Roberts, 1991; Lawton, Silverstein, & Bengtson, 1994; Rossi & Rossi, 1990) in our research. In the normative context, parents and children exchange varying levels of affection throughout the life course, and this contributes to the individual well-being of both parent and child. Past research has shown, however, that the patterns are different for fathers and mothers. In general, father-adult child relationships have been found to be conditioned by multiple factors (such as conflict during the child's adolescence and the father's current marital happiness), whereas mother-child relationships tend to be more unconditional (see Lawton et al.; Rossi & Rossi). We have applied theories of intergenerational solidarity in our research through investigation of the affective relationship between parents and their adult child with mental retardation and the factors that account for heterogeneity in these bonds of affection.

Study Description

Parents of adults with mental retardation face a unique dual challenge: continuing caregiving responsibility for their son or daughter with mental retardation and dealing with the manifestations and consequences of their own aging. In 1988, we began our investigation of 461 families of adults with mental retardation. Our goals were to elucidate how the families have responded to the unique stresses they encountered and how their divergent life course may have affected their psychological well-being in midlife and old age. When the study began, all the adults with mental retardation co-resided with a mother aged 55 or older. In 307 of the families, the adult lived with both a mother and a father. In most of the other families, the father was deceased (27.3%) or the parents were no longer married (5.0%).

The members of our sample lived in Massachusetts and Wisconsin. The study encompassed eight waves (called Time 1 through Time 8 in this chapter) of data collection between 1988 and 2000, each spaced 18 months after the previous one. At each point of data collection, the mother (who was the primary respondent for the family) was interviewed in her home and completed a self-administered set of standardized measures. We also collected data from the fathers and the non-disabled siblings via self-administered questionnaires. The sample included families from all sized cities and towns who had a wide range of economic and social resources. Nearly all were non-Hispanic Caucasian. Therefore, the findings should not be generalized to other ethnic groups. Characteristics of the 307 families in which there was both a father and a mother at Time 1 are presented in Table 11.1.

At Times 5, 6, and 7, we expanded our data collection protocol with the fathers by conducting telephone interviews that were supplemented by self-administered questionnaires. This expansion afforded us opportunities to probe further into the roles and functioning of fathers in the families and provided rich qualitative data.

Families continued to participate in our research even after the death or incapacitation of the mother. In such instances, and if the father survived the mother, the father became the primary respondent. This subsample provided us with insight into how the family managed the transmission of caregiving responsibility from the mother to the father, who generally had been in an adjunctive caregiving role while his wife was alive or in good health.

Thus, we have multiple waves of data about parental social, physical, and mental health, family relations, use of services, and provision of care. This methodology has afforded a longitudinal view on the unfolding of later-life family caregiving, spanning more than a decade. It also has revealed multiple perspectives in each family, making it possible to ask and answer questions that expose the within-family diversity of experience. This chapter focuses on one axis of diversity: how the fathers' experience of later-life caregiving for a son or daughter with mental retardation is distinct from the experience of mothers.

In this chapter, we summarize the findings of multiple analyses about fathers in our sample. These analyses have been published as journal articles

TABLE 11.1   Characteristics of the Families with Married Parents at Time 1 (n = 307)

I. Parents	Fathers	Mothers
Age		
mean	66.35	64.12
range	52–84	55–83
Education		
less than high school	13.3%	16.3%
high school graduate	27.8%	40.4%
more than high school	58.9%	43.4%
Race (Caucasian)	98.5%	99.0%
Employment status (employed)	46.9%	26.1%
Health status		
poor	4.3%	2.9%
fair	19.1%	13.7%
good	48.0%	54.7%
excellent	28.5%	28.7%
Family income (median category)	$20,000–29,999	

II. Sons and Daughters with Mental Retardation		
Gender (male)	56.4%	
Age		
mean	32.4	
range	15–58	
Level of mental retardation		
severe/profound	23.7%	
mild/moderate	76.3%	
Diagnosis (Down syndrome)	37.1%	
Number of behavior problems[a]		
mean	1.86	
range	0–8	

[a] The data about behavior problems are from Time 2, since the behavior problems measure was not included at Time 1.

or chapters (Essex, Seltzer, & Krauss, 1999; Gordon, Seltzer, & Krauss, 1997), presented as papers at professional conferences (Essex, Seltzer, & Krauss, 1993; Seltzer, Krauss, & Hong, 1995), and formed the basis of a doctoral dissertation (Essex, 1998). The analyses were conducted using data from multiple points throughout the study period and addressed the following questions:

1. What roles do fathers have in providing care to their adult son or daughter with mental retardation who lives at home? What factors predict variation in fathers' caregiving roles?
2. How do these roles change during and after transitions in the family, either due to the move of the son or daughter to a nonfamily setting or due to the incapacitation or death of the mother?
3. Do fathers and mothers of adults with mental retardation differ in their psychological well-being? What factors are experienced as stressful by fathers and mothers and how do these factors differentially affect their well-being? What coping and social support resources are helpful to fathers and mothers in buffering the stresses of caregiving and maintaining psychological well-being?

OUR RESEARCH FINDINGS

Fathers' Family Caregiving Role

Our research has shown that fathers of adults with mental retardation in two-parent families are involved in a variety of activities, all of which are components of their role as family caregivers. These include providing direct care and assistance to the son or daughter, participating in shared social activities with the son or daughter, and providing support to their wife. In general, fathers play a distinctive caregiving role as compared with mothers, although there are also areas of similarity.

Caregiving assistance. Our findings show that although most fathers provide some care to their son or daughter with the disability, the mothers are the primary caregivers. We explored the division of labor within the family regarding who provides care to a co-resident adult child with mental retardation (Essex et al., 1993). Of 31 possible personal and instrumental activities of daily living for which an adult child might need assistance, fathers helped with an average of 4 caregiving tasks, significantly fewer than the average of 11 caregiving tasks that mothers helped with. In addition, fathers were less likely to provide help than mothers with 27 of the 31 tasks, and were more likely to provide help with only one task—simple home repairs, a traditional male domain. The three tasks for which fathers and mothers were equally likely to provide help included helping adult children with ambulation difficulties to walk indoors, to use stairs, and to move in and out of an automobile.

We also investigated the factors that might influence the amount of assistance provided by a father to his son or daughter, including circumstances of the father's life (employment, health, and age), circumstances of the mother's life (employment, health, and age), and characteristics of the adult with retardation (level of retardation, gender, and age) (Essex et al., 1993). We found that neither the wife's needs nor the father's availability determine whether fathers provide assistance to their adult child with retardation. Overall, a father was no more likely to help when he was retired than employed, healthy or in declining health, over or under 65 years of age, when his wife was employed or not, when his wife was healthy or in declining health, when his wife was over or under 65 years of age, or when his child was a minor or had reached the legal age of adulthood.

Rather, significantly more help was provided by the father when the adult had severe or profound retardation (IQ < 40) than when the adult had mild or moderate retardation (IQ 40–70). Also, fathers were significantly more likely to help a son with mental retardation than a daughter. Of the 31 tasks for which the father could provide help to an adult child who needed assistance, fathers of sons were more likely to help than fathers of daughters with 13 tasks. While many of the tasks for which fathers were found to provide more help to sons than daughters involve personal care (e.g., dressing, bathing), for which gender similarity would support social norms of privacy, other such tasks are gender neutral—such as running errands, doing laundry, and managing finances. It is noteworthy that there was no task for which fathers were more likely to help daughters than sons. This pattern of parental assistance was characteristic only of fathers. Mothers' assistance was not related to the adult child's gender, with one exception: mothers were more likely to help their daughters than their sons with bathing.

Shared social activities.   Parents with a son or daughter with mental retardation engage in many kinds of activities with their adult child in addition to providing direct care, such as going to a restaurant or movie and taking vacations. We found that fathers were just as involved with their adult child in these types of shared social activities as mothers (Essex, 1998) and were equally likely to be involved with daughters as sons. Indeed, for many of the fathers we interviewed, the adult child was an integral part of their social life and enhanced their quality of life, as well as the life of the son or daughter. Regarding affective closeness, fathers were less close than their wife was with their adult child, but the child's gender made no difference in fathers' feelings of closeness.

Thus, we found that, compared with mothers, fathers provided less direct care to their adult child and were less close affectively, but fathers were equally likely as mothers to participate in social activities that included the son or daughter with the disability. Fathers were more likely to provide care to a son than a daughter but did not differentiate between sons and daughters in affective closeness or participation in social activities.

Spousal support. A third way that fathers might enhance the care provided to the son or daughter with mental retardation is by supporting
the well-being of their wives, who are the primary caregivers (Essex et
al., 1993). One perspective on spousal support comes from comparison
of the married mothers in our sample to those who were widowed or
divorced. If married mothers had better well-being than mothers who
were widowed or separated-divorced, these differences might be an indicator of the support that husbands provide to their wives. We found that
married mothers had significantly better health and morale than mothers who were not currently married. However, a primary reason for the
difference was the extra income that the father provides. With income
controlled, there was no difference in well-being between the married
and the unmarried mothers.

Another indicator of spousal support among the currently married
mothers is the emotional support provided by husbands to their wives.
Mothers who felt that their husbands provided personal support to them
reported significantly better health and better morale than mothers who
did not view their husbands as a source of support. A third indicator of
fathers' support for their wives is division of caregiving labor in the family. We found that mothers whose husbands provided at least some care
for the son or daughter had significantly better morale than those whose
husbands did not help at all. However, in all these analyses, there was no
relation between paternal support and the level of caregiving stress and
burden experienced by mothers.

Thus, three types of spousal support enhance the well-being of mothers caring for adults with retardation: additional income, emotional support, and assistance with caregiving. Although fathers play a secondary
direct caregiving role, they contribute to family functioning by supporting the general well-being of their wives, who are the primary caregivers.

Changes in Fathers' Caregiving Role Over Time

Guided by a life course perspective, our longitudinal study tracked changes
in family composition during the parents' elder years and examined concomitant shifts in caregiving patterns. The two most common changes
experienced by the families in our study were the placement of the son or
daughter with mental retardation in an out-of-home residential setting
and the death or incapacitation of one or both parents. These family life
transitions offer the opportunity to investigate how the fathers' caregiving role changes over time.

When an adult with mental retardation moves to an out-of-home residential setting, the responsibility for daily care shifts naturally to the formal service sector. Nevertheless, parents continue to provide some care.

We found that the prior division of labor between fathers and mothers maintains after placement, with fathers continuing to provide less assistance than mothers (Gordon et al., 1997).

However, when the mother dies or becomes incapacitated through illness or frailty, the family must make choices regarding who will become the primary caregiver—the father, adult siblings in the family, or the formal service sector. This is a turning point in family life, particularly for those families in which the adult still lives at home. We found that in all cases in which the adult child co-resided with both parents prior to the mother's death or incapacitation, the father took over the role of primary caregiver, providing assistance with a full array of activities of daily living. Siblings' involvement in caregiving also increased, but was considerably less than the fathers' (Gordon et al., 1997).

Thus, although fathers generally play an adjunctive caregiving role, the level of care they provide is conditioned by later-life changes in family composition. We found that the adult's place of residence is consequential, with hands-on care diminishing after the period of co-residence ends. We also found that fathers assume the primary caregiving role when their wives no longer can do so due to death or incapacitation, which is consistent with previous findings about the hierarchy of caregiving within families (Dwyer & Coward, 1992). Thus, although the provision of care by fathers to their adult child with retardation is stable for several decades, the role becomes fluid again following changes in family composition during the later years of the life course.

Psychological Well-Being of Fathers

An additional focus of our research is the psychological well-being of caregiving fathers in two-parent families, as manifested in both their global well-being and their affective reactions to the caregiving role. We examined three research issues: the extent to which fathers differ from mothers in psychological well-being, the factors fathers and mothers find stressful, and the coping and social support resources that are helpful to fathers and mothers in buffering the stresses of caregiving.

Level of well-being.   Based on past research on the general population, which suggests that older men report less depression and caregiving burden than women (Miller & Cafasso, 1992; Nolen-Hoeksema, 1990), we expected the fathers in our sample to have superior well-being to mothers. In fact, we found that fathers and mothers do not differ in morale, depressive symptoms, or subjective burden (Essex et al., 1993, 1999). Therefore, we explored why fathers and mothers were similar in well-being, even though past research led us to expect fathers to have an advantage. For this analysis, we compared fathers and mothers with respect to the factors that they experienced as stressful, which potentially could account for their unexpected similarity in well-being.

Sources of stress.   A major source of stress for this population of older parents is pessimism or worry about the future care of their son or daughter with mental retardation, who will always have some dependency on others for meeting their basic needs (Krauss & Seltzer, 1999). At the outset of our study, when all the adult sons and daughters co-resided with their parents, there were no differences between fathers and mothers in their level of pessimism about the adult child's future. Later in the course of the study, after some of the adults moved away from home, we did find gender differences in parental pessimism (Essex, 1998). Mothers whose son or daughter had moved to a nonfamily residence were less pessimistic about the adult's future than other mothers, but for fathers, placement did not have this salutary effect. Thus, one reason why fathers in our sample might not have better psychological well-being than their wives is because they remain pessimistic about their adult child's future even after long-term plans are implemented.

Fathers in our study also differ from their wives in the characteristics of the adult child that they experience as stressful. In a longitudinal analysis (Essex et al., 1999), we found that for fathers, having a son was associated with increasing depressive symptoms, but gender of the adult child did not have this effect for mothers. Conversely, we found that for mothers, having a child with Down syndrome (as compared with other types of mental retardation) was associated with less subjective burden, but had no similar advantage for fathers. Thus, the gender of the child is a source of stress experienced by fathers but not by mothers, while the type of mental retardation is a protective factor against stress for mothers but not for fathers.

Fathers and mothers react differently to the functional deficits and behavior problems of their adult child. Functional deficits are more likely to provoke psychological distress in fathers, whereas behavior problems are more strongly related to distress in mothers (Essex, 1998; Essex et al., 1999). Another difference between fathers and mothers concerns their reactions to participation in the workforce. For mothers, holding paid employment is related to higher subjective caregiving burden, but for fathers, employment has no relationship to psychological distress (Essex et al., 1999).

Thus, fathers and mothers experience stress differently, with fathers stressed particularly by having sons and their adult child's functional limitations, and mothers stressed by their adult child's behavior problems and by outside employment. Mothers, but not fathers, are advantaged (i.e., less stressed) if their adult child is placed away from the home or has Down syndrome.

Coping and social support. Coping and social support have been conceptualized as resources that can lessen the impact of stress and enhance well-being (Pearlin et al., 1990). Problem-focused coping strategies are intended to alter the sources of stress, whereas emotion-focused coping includes attempts to reduce emotional distress (Lazarus & Folkman, 1984). In general, research suggests that problem-focused coping is associated with lower levels of distress, while emotion-focused coping has the opposite effect (Billings & Moos, 1981; Kramer, 1997).

In longitudinal analyses, we found evidence that for mothers but not fathers, coping buffers the impacts of caregiving stress on psychological well-being (Essex et al., 1999). Under stressful conditions (such as having an adult child with more behavior problems or fewer functional skills), mothers who used adaptive coping strategies (higher levels of problem-focused coping and lower levels of emotion-focused coping) experienced declining levels of depressive symptoms, caregiving burden, and pessimism about the adult child's future. For fathers, no buffering effects were detected. Overall, we found very little relation between coping and well-being for fathers. Refraining from using emotion-focused coping predicted lower burden for fathers, but there was no relation between problem-focused coping and psychological well-being for fathers.

In addition to these gender differences in coping, we found that fathers and mothers of adults with retardation make differential use of social support. Marital satisfaction was negatively associated with both depressive symptoms and caregiving burden for fathers, and with depressive symptoms for mothers (Essex, 1998; Seltzer et al., 1995). On the other hand, satisfaction with wider sources of social support (i.e., the social support network of family members and friends) buffered caregiving stress for mothers but had no effect on well-being for fathers (Essex, 1998).

We have an emerging understanding as to why fathers of adults with mental retardation do not have lower levels of distress than their wives, contrary to the pattern reported in the general population. Mothers in our study benefit from using problem-focused coping, from having a satisfying marriage, and from social support, all of which are associated with elevated levels of psychological well-being. In contrast, the fathers in our study draw on comparatively fewer resources, benefiting only from marital satisfaction in reducing distress. Hence, even though older women in general, and female caregivers in particular, are at risk for psychological distress, mothers of adults with retardation are advantaged in their coping and social support resources, and thus may surpass their age-peers with respect to psychological well-being. Fathers draw on fewer resources and thus may be disadvantaged as compared with their age peers who do not have lifelong caregiving responsibility.

SUMMARY

Our research on older fathers as caregivers for adult children with mental retardation provides a much more nuanced portrait of the dynamics of family-based care than would be seen if we had focused solely on mothers in these families. Rather than being a figure in the background of the family tableau, fathers are active caregivers (even if less involved instrumentally than mothers), socially engaged with their sons and daughters, and providers of critical emotional and financial support to their wives. The fact that there is far less research on fathers' roles in families of children with disabilities than on mothers' roles should not obscure the reality that fathers are an integral part in the day-to-day functioning of these families. Clearly, research in the future needs to continue to investigate the variability in paternal roles, the effects of different roles on the social and emotional development of their children with disabilities (and their wives), and the factors that sustain paternal involvement and well-being. Our data point to several promising areas for future research.

First, a greater understanding of the development of the affective relationship between fathers and their children with mental retardation over the life course is needed. Second, we need to elucidate why fathers and mothers of adults with mental retardation may differ in the aspects of their situation they find stressful and in their use of resources for coping with lifelong caregiving. Third, investigations (both qualitative and quantitative) into how having a child with mental retardation alters the parental experience for fathers would be helpful in identifying aspects of their atypical parenting careers that are rewarding (and thus potentially worthy of supportive engagement by service providers) and stressful. Theoretical models that help organize studies of the stress and adaptation process among caregivers have been based largely on women. More focused research on male caregivers may reveal different processes than currently conceptualized. Finally, investigation should be extended to fathers from diverse cultural and ethnic backgrounds, which set the context for particular family and caregiving experiences.

We note, in conclusion, that our research began, as is the case for most research in this area, with a primary focus on older mothers as caregivers for their adult child with mental retardation. The expansion of our focus to include fathers has yielded a much more complete and informed portrayal of the resilience of families and of the human capacity to transform initial disappointments into opportunities for lifelong learning.

REFERENCES

Aneshensel, C. S., Pearlin, L. I., Mullan, J. T., Zarit, S. H., & Whitlatch, C. J. (1995). *Profiles in caregiving: The unexpected career.* New York: Academic Press.

Barnett, W. S., & Boyce, G. C. (1995). Effects of children with Down syndrome on parents' activities. *American Journal on Mental Retardation, 100*, 115–127.

Beckman, P. J. (1991). Comparison of mothers' and fathers' perceptions of the effect of young children with and without disabilities. *American Journal on Mental Retardation, 95*, 585–595.

Belle, D. (1987). Gender differences in the social moderators of stress. In R. C. Barnett, L. Biener, & G. K. Baruch (Eds.), *Gender and stress* (pp. 75–95). New York: The Free Press.

Bengtson, V. L., & Roberts, R. E. L. (1991). Intergenerational solidarity in aging families: An example of formal theory construction. *Journal of Marriage and the Family, 52*, 856–870.

Billings, A. G., & Moos, R. H. (1981). The role of coping responses and social resources in attenuating the stress of life events. *Journal of Behavioral Medicine, 4*, 139–157.

Bristol, M. M., Gallagher, J. J., & Schopler, E. (1988). Mothers and fathers of young developmentally disabled and nondisabled boys: Adaptation and spousal support. *Developmental Psychology, 24*, 441–451.

Brubaker, T. H., Engelhardt, J. L., Brubaker, E., & Lutzer, V. D. (1989). Gender differences of older caregivers of adults with mental retardation. *The Journal of Applied Gerontology, 8*, 183–191.

Cleary, P. D. (1987). Gender differences in stress-related disorders. In R. C. Barnett, L. Biener, & G. K. Baruch (Eds.), *Gender and stress* (pp. 39–72). New York: The Free Press.

Cooke, K., & Lawton, D. (1984). Informal support for the carers of disabled children. *Child: Care, Health, and Development, 10*, 67–79.

Davis, P. B., & May, J. E. (1991). Involving fathers in early intervention and family support programs: Issues and strategies. *Children's Health Care, 20*, 87–92.

Dwyer, J. W., & Coward, R. T. (1992). Gender, family, and long-term care of the elderly. In J. W. Dwyer & R. T. Coward (Eds.), *Gender, families, and elder care* (pp. 1–17). Newbury Park, CA: Sage.

Erickson, M., & Upshur, C. C. (1989). Caretaking burden and social support: Comparison of mothers of infants with and without disabilities. *American Journal on Mental Retardation, 94*, 250–258.

Essex, E. A. (1998). *Parental caregivers of adults with mental retardation: The experience of older mothers and fathers.* Doctoral dissertation, University of Wisconsin-Madison, 1998. *Dissertation Abstracts International, 59*–68.

Essex, E. L., Seltzer, M. M., & Krauss, M. S. (1993). *Aging fathers as caregivers for adult children with developmental disabilities.* Paper presented at the National Institute of Aging Symposium on "Men's Caregiving Roles in an Aging Society," Rockville, MD.

Essex, E. L., Seltzer, M. M., & Krauss, M. W. (1999). Differences in coping effectiveness and well-being among aging mothers and fathers of adults with mental retardation. *American Journal on Mental Retardation, 104,* 545–563.

Farber, B. (1959). Effects of a severely mentally retarded child on family integration. *Monographs of the Society for Research in Child Development, 24* (2, Serial No. 78).

Featherman, D. L., & Lerner, R. M. (1985). Ontogenesis and sociogenesis: Problematics for theory and research about development and socialization across the lifespan. *American Sociological Review, 50,* 659–676.

Floyd, F. J., Gilliom, L. A., & Costigan, C. L. (1998). Marriage and the parenting alliance: Longitudinal prediction of change in parenting perceptions and behaviors. *Child Development, 69,* 1461–1479.

Frey, K. S., Greenberg, M. T., & Fewell, R. R. (1989). Stress and coping among parents of handicapped children: A multidimensional approach. *American Journal on Mental Retardation, 94,* 240–249.

Fujiura, G. T., & Braddock, D. (1992). Fiscal and demographic trends in mental retardation services: The emergence of the family. In L. Rowitz (Ed.), *Mental retardation in the year 2000* (pp. 316–338). New York: Springer.

Gordon, R. M., Seltzer, M. M., & Krauss, M. W. (1997). The aftermath of parental death: Changes in the context and quality of life. In R. L. Schalock (Ed.), *Quality of life: Vol. 2. Application to persons with disabilities* (pp. 25–42). Washington, DC: American Association on Mental Retardation.

Heller, T., Hsieh, K., & Rowitz, L. (1997). Maternal and paternal caregiving of persons with mental retardation across the lifespan. *Family Relations, 46,* 407–415.

Hirst, M. (1985). Dependency and family care of young adults with disabilities. *Child: Care, Health, and Development, 11,* 241–257.

Holmes, N., & Carr, J. (1991). The pattern of care in families of adults with a mental handicap: A comparison between families of autistic adults and Down syndrome adults. *Journal of Autism and Developmental Disabilities, 21,* 159–176.

Hornby, G. (1995). Fathers' views of the effects on their families of children with Down syndrome. *Journal of Child and Family Studies, 4,* 103–117.

Keltner, B., & Ramey, S. L. (1993). Family issues. *Current Opinion in Psychiatry, 6,* 629–634.

Knussen, C., Sloper, P., Cunningham, C. C., & Turner, S. (1992). The use of the Ways of Coping (Revised) Questionnaire with parents of children with Down's syndrome. *Psychological Medicine, 22*, 775–786.

Kramer, B. J. (1997). Differential predictors of strain and gain among husbands caring for wives with dementia. *The Gerontologist, 37*, 239–249.

Krauss, M. W. (1993). Child-related and parenting stress: Similarities and differences between mothers and fathers of children with disabilities. *American Journal on Mental Retardation, 97*, 393–404.

Krauss, M. W., & Seltzer, M. M. (1999). An unanticipated life: The impact of lifelong caregiving. In H. Bersani, Jr. (Ed.), *Responding to the challenge: Current trends and international issues in developmental disabilities* (pp. 173–188). Cambridge, MA: Brookline Books.

Lamb, M. E., & Meyer, D. J. (1991). Fathers of children with special needs. In M. Seligman (Ed.), *The family with a handicapped child* (pp. 151–180). Boston: Allyn and Bacon.

Lawton, L., Silverstein, M., & Bengtson, V. (1994). Affection, social contact, and geographic distance between adult children and their parents. *Journal of Marriage and the Family, 56*, 57–68.

Lazarus, R. S. (1999). *Stress and emotion: A new synthesis.* New York: Springer.

Lazarus, R. S., & Folkman, S. (1984). *Stress, appraisal and coping.* New York: Springer.

Mardiros, M. (1985). Role alterations of female parents having children with disabilities. *Canada's Mental Health, 33*(4), 24–26.

McKinney, B., & Peterson, R. A. (1987). Predictors of stress in parents of developmentally disabled children. *Journal of Pediatric Psychology, 12*, 133–150.

McLinden, S. E. (1990). Mothers' and fathers' reports of the effects of a young child with special needs on the family. *Journal of Early Intervention, 14*, 249–259.

Miller, B., & Cafasso, L. (1992). Gender differences in caregiving: Fact or artifact? *The Gerontologist, 32*, 498–507.

Nadler, A., Lewinstein, E., & Rahav, G. (1991). Acceptance of mental retardation and help-seeking by mothers and fathers of children with mental retardation. *Mental Retardation, 29*, 17–23.

Nolen-Hoeksema, S. (1990). *Sex differences in depression.* Stanford, CA: Stanford University Press.

Nydegger, C. N., & Mitteness, L. S. (1996). In midlife: The prime of fathers. In C. D. Ryff & M. M. Seltzer (Eds.), *The parental experience in midlife* (pp. 533–559). Chicago: University of Chicago Press.

Pearlin, L. I. (1989). The sociological study of stress. *Journal of Health and Social Behavior, 30*, 241–256.

Pearlin, L. I., Mullan, J. T., Semple, S. J., & Skaff, M. M. (1990). Caregiving and the stress process: An overview of concepts and their measures. *The Gerontologist, 30,* 583–594.

Pruchno, R., & Patrick, J. H. (1999). Mothers and fathers of adults with chronic disabilities: Caregiving appraisals and well-being. *Research on Aging, 21,* 683–713.

Ramey, S. L., Krauss, M. W., & Simeonsson, R. J. (1989). Research on families: Current assessment and future opportunities. *American Journal on Mental Retardation, 94,* ii–vi.

Roach, M. A., Orsmond, G. I., & Barratt, M. S. (1999). Mothers and fathers of children with Down syndrome: Parental stress and involvement in childcare. *American Journal on Mental Retardation, 104,* 422–436.

Rossi, A. S., & Rossi, P. H. (1990). *Of human bonding: Parent-child relations across the life course.* New York: Aldine de Gruyter.

Ryff, C. D., Schmutte, P. S., & Lee, Y.-H. (1996). How children turn out: Implications for parental self-evaluation. In C. D. Ryff & M. M. Seltzer (Eds.), *The parental experience in midlife* (pp. 383–422). Chicago: University of Chicago Press.

Schilling, R. F., Schinke, S. P., & Kirkham, M. A. (1988). The impact of developmental disabilities and other learning deficits on the family. In C. S. Chilman, E. W. Nunnally, & F. M. Cox (Eds.), *Chronic illness and disability* (pp. 156–170). Newbury Park, CA: Sage.

Seltzer, M. M., & Krauss, M. W. (1989). Aging parents with adult mentally retarded children: Family risk factors and sources of support. *American Journal on Mental Retardation, 94,* 303–312.

Seltzer, M. M., Krauss, M. W., & Hong, J. (1995). *Marital quality and coping as stress-buffering resources for aging mothers of adults with mental retardation.* Paper presented at the 28th Annual Gatlinburg Conference on Research and Theory in Mental Retardation and Developmental Disabilities, Gatlinburg, TN.

Trute, B. (1995). Gender differences in the psychological adjustment of parents of young developmentally disabled children. *Journal of Child Psychology and Psychiatry, 36,* 1225–1242.

Wheaton, B., Roszell, P., & Hall, K. (1997). The impact of twenty childhood and adult traumatic stressors on the risk of psychiatric disorder. In I. H. Gotlib & B. Wheaton (Eds.), *Stress and adversity over the life course: Trajectories and turning points* (pp. 50–71). Cambridge, England: Cambridge University Press.

Willoughby, J. C., & Glidden, L. M. (1995). Fathers helping out: Shared child care and marital satisfaction of parents of children with disabilities. *American Journal on Mental Retardation, 99,* 399–406.

Differences Between Fathers and Mothers in the Care of Their Children With Mental Illness[1]

12

Jan S. Greenberg

Families who provide support and assistance to their relatives with mental illness often report costs associated with this care, whether financial, social, or psychological. Researchers and others designate these costs as family burdens. Regardless of the wide variation in the conceptualization and measurement of family burden research has consistently shown that families of persons with mental illness experience moderate levels of burden (Cook & Pickett, 1988; Fisher, Benson, & Tessler, 1990; Lefley, 1996; Lefley & Wasow, 1994; Seltzer, Greenberg, & Krauss, 1995; Solomon & Draine, 1995).

However, what is known about the burdens of mental illness and their consequences largely translates into what is known about the experiences of women, in particular mothers (Cook, 1988; Ryan, 1993). Early literature on families of adults with mental illness portrayed fathers as rejecting and emotionally absent at one extreme and intrusive at the other end of the continuum (Bowen, 1959; Gerard & Siegel, 1950; Lidz, Fleck, & Cornelison, 1965). Literature suggested that not only were mothers overprotective and domineering, but that fathers were weak and failed to fulfill their role in the family. Thus, studies implicated fathers as well as mothers as agents causing or at least contributing to their child's mental health problems.

[1] The author gratefully acknowledges the valuable contributions of Dorothy F. Edwards for her helpful comments on earlier drafts of this manuscript. Preparation for this chapter was supported by a grant from the National Institute of Mental Health (MH45988). Support was also provided by the Graduate School at the University of Wisconsin-Madison.

The emerging research portrays a very different picture of the involvement of fathers in the lives of their sons and daughters with mental illness. In a qualitative study on the experiences of 12 fathers of adults with mental illness, Howard (1998) found that fathers were very supportive of their adult children with mental illness by helping with finances, assisting during a crisis, and socializing with their son or daughter. In another small-scale qualitative study of married couples, Wintersteen and Rasmussen (1997) reported that fathers became more involved in all aspects of family life after their child's diagnosis, although their wives wanted them to take on a more active role in caregiving. Vine (1982) suggested that for men, retirement may be a turning point that marks their greater involvement in the day-to-day care of a son or daughter with mental illness. Thus, contrary to past portrayals of fathers of adults with mental illness as being distant and unresponsive to the needs of their children, recent empirical evidence indicates that many fathers actively engage in their child's life. However, this research on fathers of adults with mental illness has been qualitative in nature and based on small highly selected samples. Ultimately, little is known about the role of fathers in the care of their adult child with mental illness, how they differ from their female counterparts, and whether different factors are related to their experience of well-being. These are the issues addressed in this chapter.

To organize this investigation of how the experiences of fathers are similar to and different from those of their wives, I adopt a general stress-appraisal framework consisting of four broad domains: (a) background and contextual factors; (b) sources of stress (i.e., primary caregiving stressors and secondary strains, and other life stressors); appraisal of the caregiving role; and (c) psychological well-being (see Figure 12.1). The social location of individuals within the larger society, defined by such contextual characteristics as age, gender, and education affect the kinds and intensities of stressors to which families are exposed, their appraisal of the stressor, and the way stress is manifested (Lazarus & Folkman, 1984; Pearlin, Mullan, Semple, & Skaff, 1990). Of the many contextual variables that may affect the stress process, the gender of the adult child may loom large in understanding the experiences of fathers of adults with mental illness. Research on normative father-adult child relationships suggest that being a father to a son, compared with a daughter, are profoundly different experiences. Although fathers see their primary responsibility as guiding their sons toward independence, they view their role in their daughter's life as that of a provider and protectorate (Nydegger & Mitteness, 1996). Rossi and Rossi (1990) find that the father-son relationship is more responsive to current characteristics of the son and the earlier quality of the relationship between the two men than is the case for other parent-child dyads. There are many characteristics of mental illness such as the cyclical

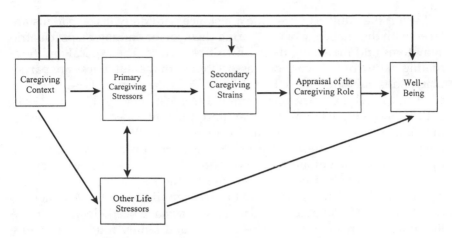

FIGURE 12.1   Conceptual model.

nature of the illness that are likely to strain the father-son relationship. Because schizophrenia occurs in late adolescence, this period is likely marked by tension in the quality of the father-son relationship that may have rippling effects on the relationship for years to come. Schwoon and Angermeyer (1980) found that fathers more closely identified with their sons but also rejected their sons more often than their daughters with mental illness. Similarly, Goldstein and Kreisman (1988) found that fathers were less tolerant of behavior problems in their sons than in their daughters with mental illness. Mother, however, did not differ in their tolerance of symptoms among their sons and daughters. Thus, due to fathers' socialization experiences, they may have higher expectations for a son's independent functioning, and experience greater distress when a son, rather than a daughter, violates these expectations.

The challenges of caregiving as well other major life events are conceptualized as stressors that have the potential to produce distress. Pearlin and his colleagues (1990) differentiate between primary stressors of caregiving and secondary caregiving strains. *Primary stressors* are the objective caregiving demands and hardships inherent in the caregiving situation. These demands are anchored in the daily care and supervision of the adult with mental illness, and include tasks such as monitoring medications, providing transportation, and helping with household chores and meal preparation. While some researchers report a positive relationship between the amount of hands-on care provided and feelings of subjective distress (Greenberg, Seltzer, & Greenley, 1993; Stueve, Vine, & Struening, 1997), others find no relationship between these caregiving demands and the family's level of distress (Anderson & Lynch, 1984; Jones, 1996).

Even if the adult requires little assistance with daily tasks, parents are faced with the challenge of monitoring their son or daughter's psychiatric symptoms and managing their difficult behaviors. The cyclical and fluctuating nature of the symptoms associated with mental illness are particularly stressful for families (Biegel, Song, & Chakravarthy, 1994; Coyne et al., 1987; Pruchno, Patrick, & Burant, 1996; Winefield & Harvey, 1993). Fathers and mothers, however, may find different aspects of the caregiving situation stressful. Tessler and Gamache (2000) found that whereas men show most distress when providing hands-on care, women show most distress when monitoring and controlling their child's behavior.

Stress proliferation occurs when the primary stressors of caregiving create *secondary strains* in the lives of these families (Pearlin, Aneshensel, & Leblanc, 1997). A range of secondary strains have been identified in the literature and include disruptions in sleep and family routines, a reduction in social activities, and stigma (Gubman & Tessler, 1987; Lefley, 1989, 1996; Maurin & Boyd, 1990). Hatfield (1978) found that approximately 20% of the families reported disruptions in their social or personal lives as a consequence of their relative's behavior. In a more recent study of relatives of people with schizophrenia, Winefield and Harvey (1993) found that almost half of the families reported that their family and social relationships had been disrupted.

Despite an increasing awareness of stigma and its negative consequences on persons with mental illness (Phelan, Bromet, & Link, 1998), there has been relatively little empirical research on the effects of stigma on family well-being. Greenberg, Greenley, McKee, Brown, and Griffin-Francell (1993a) found that higher levels of stigma related to poor physical health. Similarly, in a longitudinal survey of over 300 family respondents, Tessler and Gamache (2000) reported that feelings of stigma affected higher levels of emotional distress. Stueve, Vine, and Struening (1997) also found that stigma related to higher levels of family burden.

These primary stressors and secondary strains of caregiving increase the individual's vulnerability to experiencing distress. The amount of distress felt, however, depends in part on the individual's cognitive appraisal of the caregiving context. Based on the work of Lawton, Kleban, Moss, Rovine, and Glicksman (1989), I conceptualized subjective burden as a component of the appraisal process. In studies of families of adults with mental illness, subjective burden is often defined in terms of the caregiver's feelings about providing care and supervision (Fisher, Benson, & Tessler, 1990; Marsh, 1992; Maurin & Boyd, 1990) and has been most commonly investigated as the outcome of the stress process. Consequently, few investigators have examined the relationship between subjective burden and more general measures of distress. These studies provide preliminary evidence that the subjective burden associated with the care of a relative with mental illness has enduring effects on the general mental health of family members (Coyne et al., 1987; Noh & Avison, 1988; Noh & Turner, 1987).

The outcome of the stress process is typically conceptualized in terms of distress. There is a common conception that mothers of adult children with mental illness experience higher levels of distress than fathers. This is based on the assumption that mothers in general assume the primary burden of care which, in turn, leads to higher levels of distress. Cook (1988) did find that mothers showed significantly more measurable emotional distress, anxiety, depression, fear, and emotional strain than fathers. Similarly, in a study of support groups, Cañive et al. (1996) found that mothers had higher levels of anxiety and depression than fathers. However, Wintersteen and Rasmussen (1997) reported that fathers appear to experience more distress than their wives as indicated by more persistent difficulties with sleep, mood, or appetite. Similarly, Davis and Schultz (1998) found no difference between mothers and fathers in the intensity of their grieving over their child's psychiatric illness. Thus, the existing research is inconclusive as to whether coping with the challenges of mental illness takes a greater toll on fathers or mothers.

In summary, to date there is virtually no research on fathers of adults with mental illness, which may reflect the residual effects of past family theories of schizophrenia that implicated fathers in their child's illness by virtue of the father's absence or emotional detachment from the family. Several theories of normative family life similarly viewed fathers as being quite removed from the day-to-day lives of children because child care was viewed as the domain of women, with the primary roles of fatherhood being concerned with how the family interfaces with the larger community. In addition, the experience of fathers has remained poorly documented and understood because researchers have recruited their samples almost exclusively from the National Alliance for the Mentally Ill, an organization whose membership historically has been overwhelmingly female. Only recently have researchers turned their attention to understanding the unique role of fathers as caregivers to their sons and daughters with mental illness. The purpose of this chapter is to contribute to this emerging literature on fathers by contrasting their experiences with those of their wives with regard to both the types of challenges they face and the differential effects of these challenges on well-being. Two major research questions are the focus of this investigation:

1. Do fathers and mothers differ with respect to the challenges of caregiving, their appraisal of the caregiving context, and their psychological well-being?
2. Do these challenges of caregiving have differential effects on the well-being of fathers versus mothers?

DESIGN AND METHODS

This study involved a large cross-section of Wisconsin clients with serious mental illness and their families who lived in rural counties or counties with small urban centers (metropolitan centers of 50,000 or less). The counties studied were 32 of 68 such counties in Wisconsin. Counties were purposively sampled to capture the natural variation occurring across Wisconsin in terms of the different strategies for organizing and delivering mental health services.

In participating counties, researchers asked clients of the public mental health system to take part in the study. Clients were eligible for the study if they met the following criteria: (a) The client had a chronic mental illness as defined by the State of Wisconsin criteria; for example, a serious psychiatric diagnosis, such as schizophrenia, which results in substantial functional impairment; (b) the client was a county resident and lived in the community; and (c) the client had at least three face-to-face or telephone contacts with a family member during the past year.

Case managers approached each eligible client, explained the study, and asked if the client wished to participate. If the client consented, the case manager asked the client to list the three family members with whom the client had the most contact. From the list, the research staff selected and interviewed the family member with whom the client had the most contact. In cases where both parents were listed and lived together, each parent completed the Family Burden Questionnaire (Greenberg, Greenley, & Brown, 1997) in a 90-minute telephone interview conducted by professional interviewers at the Wisconsin Survey Research Laboratory. The analysis reported here is based on interviews with the 95 fathers and mothers who were living together and completed separate interviews about their experience of coping with their son's or daughter's mental illness.

Table 12.1 provides demographic characteristics on the 95 couples. The fathers and mothers averaged 63.9 and 61.4 years of age, respectively. The majority of parents had graduated high school and approximately 40% were still working. Fifty-five percent of the fathers were retired, with 33.7% of the mothers being retired and 25.3% having never worked outside the home. These couples had a median family income of approximately $25,000. Both fathers and mothers rated their health as good. About a fifth were living with their adult child, typically an adult son in his mid-30s. Adults not living with their parents had an average of about 9 hours of weekly face-to-face contact with their mothers and about 6 hours of contact with their fathers. About 20% of the parents were current members of the National Alliance for the Mentally Ill.

The adults with mental illness averaged 33.3 years of age and about two thirds were men. Diagnosis revealed the majority (57.9%) with

TABLE 12.1   Sample Background Characteristics

	Fathers	Mothers
Characteristics of parents		
Age	63.9	61.4**
Education		
(% high school graduates)	73.7%	84.2%
Employment (currently employed)	42.1%	37.9%
Income (median)	$25,000	$25,000
Health	2.9	2.9
Hours of weekly contact		
(non-co-resident)	5.9	9.1*
Characteristics of adult children		
Age (mean)	33.3%	
Gender (% female)	32.6%	
Diagnosis		
Schizophrenia	57.9%	
Bipolar disorder	14.7%	
Major depression	6.3%	
Dual diagnosis	14.7%	
Other	6.3%	
Employment (% in competitive jobs)	16.9%	
Currently married	3.2%	

*$p < .05$. **$p < .001$.

schizophrenia or schizoaffective disorder, 14.7% with bipolar disorder, and 6.3% with major depression. Only 15.8% had ever been married and only 3.2% were currently married. Approximately 17% of the adults with mental illness were employed in competitive jobs.

Measures

There is increasing recognition that mental health is not simply the absence of distress but also the presence of positive mood (Ryff, 1995). Furthermore, growing evidence suggests that positive and negative dimensions of mental health may be explained by different mechanisms (Kramer, 1997a; Lawton, Moss, Kleban, Glicksman, & Rovine, 1991). Thus, psychological well-being, the outcome variable in this study, was operationalized by measures of positive mental health (happiness) and psychological distress (depressive symptoms). *Happiness* was measured by a single item from the National Survey of Families and Households [NSFH] (Sweet,

Bumpass, & Call, 1988). Respondents were asked to rate their happiness along a 7-point scale, with 1 being very unhappy and 7 being very happy. *Depressive symptoms* was measured by a short version of the Center for Epidemiologic Studies Depression Scale [CES-D] (Radloff, 1977) also used in the NSFH. The NSFH version of the CES-D included the depressed mood (5 items) and psychomotor retardation (7 items) subscales of the CES-D. For each of the 12 depressive symptoms, the respondents indicated how many days (0 to 7) during the past week they experienced the symptom. Given the evidence that the CES-D forms a single second-order factor (Hertzog, VanAlstein, Usala, Hultsch, & Dixon, 1990), I calculated a total depressive symptoms score by summing across the 12 items. The Cronbach's alpha reliability of the CES-D in this sample was .79 and .93 for fathers and mothers, respectively.

The analysis included two indicators of primary stressors: (a) amount of care, and (b) psychiatric symptoms. The *amount of care* was measured using a slightly modified version of Tessler and Gamache's objective burden scale (Tessler & Gamache, 1995). For each of eight daily living tasks (e.g., personal hygiene, housework), we asked responents to indicate along a 4-point scale (1 = none, 4 = a lot) how much help they provided their son or daughter with mental illness during the past 30 days. The Cronbach's alpha reliability was .68 and .75 for fathers and mothers, respectively.

The child's *psychiatric symptoms* were operationalized using the General Psychopathology Scale (Katz & Lyerly, 1963). This scale has been widely used in mental health research on psychiatric patients and found to be a reliable and valid measure of psychiatric symptomatology (Goldberg, Schooler, Hogarty, & Roper, 1977; Greenberg, Greenley, McKee, Brown, & Griffen-Francell, 1993; Wallace, 1986). Respondents indicated along a 4-point scale, ranging from *almost never* (1) to *almost always* (4), how often their son or daughter had exhibited 24 specific symptoms and behaviors during the past 30 days. In this study, the scale had a Cronbach's alpha of .93 in both the sample of fathers and mothers. There was no difference between mothers and fathers in their independent reports of their child's symptoms (2.73 vs. 2.69 for fathers and mothers, respectively).

Pearlin's (1988) measure of life stressors, developed for a study of caregivers of persons with Alzheimer's disease, was used to measure *other life stressors* experienced by the family. The stressors included the death of a family member or close friend, major illness of a family member or close friend, divorce in the family, and an open-ended question asking the respondent to list any other major life stressors during the past year. The number of stressors these parents experienced ranged from 0 to 9, with a mean of 1.53 for fathers and 1.99 for mothers.

Secondary strains associated with caring for a relative with mental illness included measures of stigma, disruptions, and role engulfment. The measure of *stigma* consisted of 6 items about the extent to which family members avoided telling others about their relative's condition for fear of what others might think. This scale was adapted by Greenley (1979) from earlier work by Freeman and Simmons (1961) by modifying the items slightly to make them more specific to the stigma associated with mental illness across a range of situations. The Cronbach's alpha reliability was .83 and .87 for fathers and mothers, respectively.

Disruptions in the lives of parents caring for a child with mental illness were measured by items developed by Tessler and Gamache (1995) based on the earlier work of Platt, Hirsch, and Weyman (1983). The scale used in this study consisted of 3 types of disruptions: (a) sleep, (b) household and domestic routines, and (c) social and leisure activities. For each disruption, respondents indicated along a 7-point scale (0 = not at all, 6 = daily) how often in the last 30 days the son or daughter with mental illness had disrupted their lives in this way. The Cronbach's alpha reliability for this scale was .68 and .65 for fathers and mothers, respectively.

The measure of *role engulfment*, based on the work of Skaff and Pearlin (1992), consisted of three items asking how often, ranging from *never* (1) to *often* (4), respondents felt they had no time for themselves, had given up personal hobbies and other activities, and had reduced contact with family and friends because of their child's illness. The Cronbach's alpha was .76 and .77 for fathers and mothers, respectively.

The parent's appraisal of caregiving was measured by the Subjective Burden Scale (Greenberg et al., 1997). Respondents indicated on a 4-point scale, ranging from *never* (1) to *often* (4), how frequently they felt strain, tension, burden, resentment, appreciation, good, and enjoyment from their involvement with their son or daughter with mental illness. Positive items were recoded and summed with a higher score reflecting a more negative appraisal of their involvement in caregiving. The scale had a Cronbach's alpha reliability of .82 and .83 for fathers and mothers, respectively.

Three background characteristics of the parent (i.e., age, education, and parental health), and the gender of the adult son or daughter and whether the son or daughter lived with his or her parents were included in the model as control variables. The respondent's age was coded in years. Education was coded into one of 8 categories (1 = less than 8 years of school to 8 = some graduate school). The respondent's health was measured using a single item from the NSFH (Sweet et al., 1988), which asked the respondent to rate his or her health along a 4-point scale ranging from *poor* (1) to *excellent* (4). Parents who were co-residing with their son or daughter were coded 1, and 0 otherwise. Finally the adult child's gender was indicated by a dummy variable (male = 1; female = 0).

RESULTS

Our first research question examined mean level differences between fathers and mothers in the amount of care provided, their exposure to the secondary strains of caregiving, their appraisal of caregiving, and their psychological well-being. As shown in Table 12.2, there were few differences between fathers and mothers in the percent assisting their child with various activities of daily living. Fathers were just as likely as mothers to be helping with self-care activities, shopping, supervision of medications, money management, and helping their son or daughter find things to do with their free time. It was only in areas of housework, meal preparation, and transportation that fathers and mothers differed. Although mothers provided significantly more help with housework and meal preparation, there was a trend for fathers to assist their child more often with transportation. In total, 90% of the fathers helped their son or daughter with at least one daily living task, and more than half of the fathers helped with three or more tasks.

Even though these data indicate that fathers assume an active caregiving role in the life of their son or daughter, mothers reported overall higher levels of caregiving involvement and the fathers concurred with their assessment. Even though 84.2% of the mothers reported that they were "very or somewhat" involved in their child's care, 66.3% of the fathers reported a similar level of involvement. When asked about the level of their spouse's involvement, 79.1% of the fathers reported that their wives were "very or somewhat" involved, and 84.2% of the mothers reported that their husbands were "very or somewhat" involved in their son or daughter's care. Thus, there was general consensus among couples about the involvement of the mother in the care of the son or daughter with mental illness. However, wives were more likely to see their husbands as being involved as compared to their husbands' own perception of their level of involvement.

Next I examined mean differences in other life stressors, the secondary strains of caregiving, the appraisal of burden, and psychological well-being. As shown in Table 12.3, fathers and mothers did not differ in their level of stigma and frequency of disruptions. However, fathers reported fewer life stressors and lower levels of role engulfment, subjective burden, and depressive symptoms. Although statistically significant, the difference between fathers and mothers in perceptions of role engulfment and subjective burden was quite small. In contrast, the difference in level of depression was striking. Whereas fathers had a mean depression score of 6.4, mothers had a mean depression score of 12.2. Quite surprisingly, however, fathers and mothers did not differ in their overall level of happiness, with both groups reporting being happy with their lives.

TABLE 12.2   Percent of Parents Providing Care by Type of Caregiving Activity

Type of Caregiving Activity	Fathers (%)	Mothers (%)
Self-care	28.4	27.4
Housework	25.5	44.7
Cooking and meal preparation	20.0	49.5
Shopping	22.1	30.5
Transportation	47.9	37.2[+]
Medications	27.4	23.2
Money management	26.3	26.3
Making use of time	38.9	45.3

Note: Numbers represent percentage of parents providing any assistance with activity.
[+] $p < .10$.

In summary, fathers were quite similar to mothers in the amount of caregiving assistance to their adult son or daughter, and in their experience of other life strains related to caring for a son or daughter with mental illness. The majority of fathers were "very or somewhat" involved in their son's or daughter's care, and it was only in the traditional sex-link tasks (e.g., household chores and cooking) that mothers reported providing more assistance than fathers. Also, fathers and mothers reported similar levels of stigma and frequency of disruptions. Fathers were significantly less likely to report a sense of role engulfment but the absolute difference was small, less than a point on a 12-point scale. Consistent with prior studies (Cañive et al., 1996; Cook, 1988) fathers were less likely than mothers to appraise caregiving as burdensome and reported lower levels of depressive symptoms. Yet, paradoxically the groups did not differ in terms of their overall happiness.

Turning to our second research question, I investigated whether or not the challenges of caregiving had differential effects on the well-being of fathers and mothers. I first examined the factors predicting the parent's appraisal of their caregiving context, that is their level of subjective burden. The predictors were background and contextual variables (i.e., the parent's age, education, and health, the gender of adult with mental illness, and whether the adult co-resided with his or her parents), the primary stressors (i.e., amount of caregiving assistance and the son's or daughter's psychiatric symptoms), other life stressors, and secondary strains (i.e., stigma, disruptions, and role engulfment).

TABLE 12.3   Mean Level Differences in Secondary Strains, Other Life
Stressors, Appraisal of Caregiving, and Psychological Well-Being

	Fathers	Mothers
Secondary strains		
Stigma	8.84	9.22
Disruptions	1.33	1.33
Role engulfment	6.24	6.81*
Other life stressors	1.53	1.99*
Appraisal of caregiving		
Subjective burden	13.60	14.85*
Psychological well-being		
Depression	6.40	12.17**
Happiness	5.7	5.5

* $p < .05$. ** $p < .001$.

Next, I investigated the factors related to the parent's more general sense of well-being, with separate analyses predicting parental depression and happiness. For each measure of well-being, two predictive models were assessed. The first included the background and caregiving factors, and the second added the parent's subjective appraisal of caregiving to determine whether caregiving appraisal mediates the relationship between any of the primary stressors and secondary strains of caregiving and the parent's psychological well-being. Baron and Kenny's (1986) procedure for establishing a mediation effect was followed.

Prior to running these regression models, I conducted preliminary analyses to examine the distributions on the variables and to reduce the number of predictor variables given the small sample size. A square root transformation was applied to the depression score to correct for skewness in the variable. Stigma was excluded from the final analyses because it had no significant effect on any of the dependent variables and dropping it did not substantially change the findings. Also, I tested whether the gender of the adult child moderated the relationship between any of the primary stressors and secondary strains of caregiving and the three outcome measures. No significant interactions were found.

As shown in Table 12.4, there was a trend for more educated fathers and younger mothers to appraise their involvement as more burdensome. Both fathers and mothers who had a child with more psychiatric behavior problems and symptoms experienced higher levels of subjective burden, although the effect was considerably stronger for mothers than fathers. In regard to the secondary strains of caregiving, both fathers

TABLE 12.4   Predictors of Subjective Burden

Predictors	Fathers	Mothers
Background characteristics		
Age	−.15	−.17+
Education	.18+	−.01
Health	−.08	.02
Gender of adult child	.06	−.03
Co-residence	−.13	.14
Primary caregiving stressors		
Amount of care	.09	−.21+
Psychiatric symptoms	.31**	.43***
Other life stressors	−.14	−.07
Secondary caregiving strains		
Disruptions	.16	.20*
Role engulfment	.24*	.27*
R^2	.33	.50

$^+ p < .01.$ $^* p < .05.$ $^{**} p < .01.$ $^{***} p < .001.$

and mothers who experienced greater role engulfment were more likely to appraise caregiving as burdensome. Mothers also were more likely to appraise their involvement as burdensome when their lives had been more frequently disrupted by their child's behavior. Surprisingly, mothers who provided more care were less likely to appraise their involvement as burdensome (at the trend level). The model explained 50% of the variance in the mother's subjective appraisal of caregiving and 33% of the variance among fathers.

Next I investigated whether primary stressors, secondary strains, and the parent's appraisal of the caregiving context had more enduring effects on parental well-being, as indicated by depressive symptoms and happiness. Turning to the predictors of depression, the results in Table 12.5 (Step 2) indicate that fathers were less directly affected by the challenges of caregiving than mothers. Maternal depression was lower when she was in better health but higher when her adult child had more psychiatric symptoms and when she experienced greater role engulfment. In fact, feelings of role engulfment had the strongest effect on maternal depression. There was no evidence that the mother's appraisal of burden mediated the relationship between these challenges and depression.

Factors outside of the caregiving role played a more prominent role in predicting the father's level of depression. Younger fathers and those with less education reported higher levels of depression. It was the presence of

TABLE 12.5   Predictors of Parental Depression

	Fathers		Mothers	
Predictors	Step 1	Step 2	Step 1	Step 2
Background characteristics				
Age	−.24*	−.21*	.09	.10
Education	−.15	−.18$^+$	−.03	−.03
Health	.12	−.11	−.27**	−.27**
Gender of adult child	.04	.03	.05	.05
Co-residence	.16	.19$^+$	−.12	−.12
Primary caregiving stressors				
Amount of care	−.10	−.11	.01	.02
Psychiatric symptoms	.21*	.15	.29**	.27*
Other life stressors	.31**	.34***	.10	.11
Secondary caregiving strains				
Disruptions	−.06	−.09	.04	.03
Role engulfment	.11	.06	.34**	.32**
Appraisal of caregiving				
Subjective burden		.19$^+$		.05
R^2	.30	.33	.42	.42

$^+ p < .10.$ * $p < .05.$ ** $p < .01.$ *** $p < .001.$

other life stressors that led to increased levels of depression among fathers, and the strength of its effect was considerably greater than any other variable in the model. The stressors related to caregiving had few *direct* impacts on the father's level of depressive symptoms. Only trend level effects were found for the appraisal of caregiver burden and whether the son or daughter lived at home. Fathers living with their son or daughter reported higher rates of depression than fathers living apart from their child, and fathers who appraised their involvement as more burdensome also reported higher levels of depressive symptoms. The final model explained 32% of the variance in depression for fathers as compared with 42% of the variance in the model for mothers.

Notably, the father's appraisal of burden was found to mediate the relationship between behavioral problems and depression. As shown in Step 1 in Table 12.5, prior to entering the father's appraisal of burden, the adult child's psychiatric symptoms and behaviors significantly affected levels of depressive symptoms, but became nonsignificant upon entering the father's appraisal of burden in the second step. As shown previously (see Table 12.4), the adult child's psychiatric symptoms and behaviors significantly affected the father's appraisal of burden, and therefore, Baron and Kenny's (1986) three conditions for establishing a mediation effect were met. In other words, behavior problems had an indirect effect on depressive symptoms by influencing how fathers appraise their caregiving involvement.

Table 12.6 reports the effects of these caregiving challenges on parental happiness. As shown in the final model (Step 2), both fathers and mothers who reported better health expressed greater happiness. Again, mothers appeared more directly affected by the primary and secondary strains of caregiving, but the father's happiness was most strongly related to his overall appraisal of the caregiving context. Mothers reported less happiness when their adult child was more symptomatic (trend level) and perceived themselves tied to the caregiving role, without sufficient time for themselves and friends. Counter to our expectations, mothers reported greater happiness when they were providing more care to their son or daughter with mental illness.

Fathers who appraised caregiving as more burdensome reported less happiness in their lives. The father's appraisal of burden, however, did not mediate the relationship between any of the challenges of caregiving and positive well-being among fathers. Even though the effect of psychiatric symptoms on happiness is reduced substantially (Beta changes from .18 to .11) upon entering the father's appraisal in the model, the criteria for mediation are not met because the effect of behavioral problems on happiness was not significant in Step 1. The model predicting parental happiness explained considerably less of the variance than the model predicting parental depression. The final model explained only 20% of the variance in happiness for fathers and 27% for mothers.

DISCUSSION AND CONCLUSIONS

The findings from this study challenge the notion that it is only women who "mother" persons with mental illness (Cook, 1988). Over 90% of the fathers were involved in the care of their son or daughter with mental illness, and over 40% reported being "very involved." Except for housework and cooking, fathers were just as likely as their wives to be helping out with daily activities such as shopping, managing medications, and money management. In fact, fathers may underestimate their level of involvement, since their wives were more likely to report that their husbands were involved in the care of their son or daughter with mental illness. It may be that our assessment of caregiving activities does not adequately assess the caregiving that these fathers did. Further, there were no differences between fathers and mothers in their reports of stigma or the

TABLE 12.6 Predictors of Parental Happiness

	Fathers		Mothers	
Predictors	Step 1	Step 2	Step 1	Step 2
Background characteristics				
Age	.09	.05	.11	.12
Education	−.10	−.05	−.13	−.13
Health	.27*	.25*	.21*	.21*
Gender of adult child	−.03	−.01	.02	.02
Co-residence	−.15	−.19	−.04	−.05
Primary caregiving stressors				
Amount of care	.13	.15	.36**	.38**
Psychiatric symptoms	−.18	−.11	−.21+	−.24+
Other life stressors	.07	.03	−.03	−.03
Secondary caregiving strains				
Disruptions	.01	.05	−.05	−.06
Role engulfment	−.16	−.10	−.35**	−.37**
Appraisal of caregiving				
Subjective burden		−.25*		.09
R^2	.16	.20	.26	.27

$^+ p < .10.$ $^* p < .05.$ $^{**} p < .01.$

frequency of disruptions related to their son or daughter's problems. Though fathers reported significantly lower levels of role engulfment and subjective burden than mothers, the absolute differences were quite small.

Furthermore, several of the challenges of caregiving had similar effects on the parents' appraisal of burden. The adult child's psychiatric behavior was the most powerful predictor of subjective burden for both mothers and fathers, and feelings of role engulfment were significantly related to feelings of burden for both groups of parents. Both fathers and mothers were more likely to appraise their involvement as burdensome the more frequently their lives had been disrupted by their son's or daughter's behavior, although this effect was significant only for mothers. Thus, contrary to popular portrayal of fathers as playing a peripheral role in care of adults with mental illness, our findings indicate that the involvement of fathers as caregivers approaches the level of involvement of their wives and for the most part, fathers are no less likely than their wives to experience the primary and secondary caregiving strains as burdensome.

However, the different challenges of caregiving appear to have very different effects on the psychological well-being of fathers versus mothers.

The adult son's or daughter's psychiatric symptoms had only an indirect effect on the father's level of depression and no effect on his level of happiness, although these behaviors and symptoms had a direct effect on maternal depression and happiness. This finding may reflect the greater saliency of the parental role for the psychological well-being of women. Ryff, Schmutte, and Lee (1996) found that mothers gave greater importance to and felt more responsible for their children's adjustment than did fathers. This sense of responsibility may be particularly intensified for the mothers in our study because many of their children first became ill during the 1970s and early 1980s, a time period during which many in the mental health community believed that mothers were to blame for their child's condition. Thus, the child's behavior problems may be particularly likely to trigger in these mothers feelings of self-blame and guilt for their child's difficulties. We also know the presence of behavioral problems and psychiatric symptoms is likely to lead to a deterioration in the quality of the parent-adult child relationship (Pickett, Cook, Cohler, & Solomon, 1997). Umberson, Chen, House, Hopkins, and Slaten (1996) found that the quality of relationships with children had a greater impact on depression among mothers than among fathers. Thus, the strength of the negative effect of the son's or daughter's behavioral problems on maternal well-being is consistent with the more general research suggesting that women are more directly affected than men by parental role strains.

Recent literature on violence and mental illness provides an additional explanation on why the child's psychiatric symptoms and behaviors might have a direct and more profound affect on maternal psychological well-being. Estroff, Zimmer, Lachicotte, and Benoit (1994) found that mothers of adults with mental illness are the most likely family members to be targeted when a son or daughter acts out. Thus, these behavior problems and symptoms may pose a greater risk to mothers than fathers, which would further explain the strength of its effect on maternal well-being.

In addition, feelings of role engulfment had a major impact on the mother's well-being but had no significant effect on any of the outcomes for fathers. It was our underlying assumption that role engulfment, by reducing the opportunities for contacts with friends and family, leaves the parent with fewer sources of positive self-evaluation outside of the family, which in turn is likely to lead to a diminished sense of well-being (Skaff & Pearlin, 1992). However, men, particularly of the older generation represented in this sample, are less likely than women to confide in their friends, preferring to confide in their wives (Antonucci, 1990; Beckman, 1991; Essex, Seltzer, & Krauss, 1999). Also, men tend to have social relations primarily initiated and maintained by their spouse (Antonucci & Akiyama, 1995). Thus, what may be critical for men of this generation is their wives' experience of role engulfment because of the greater propensity of married men to rely on their spouse for intimacy, social participation, and support. This led us to explore whether role engulfment among mothers had a rippling effect on the well-being of fathers. We found support for this as fathers reported greater depression when their wives felt greater role engulfment. The effect was highly significant (Beta = .29, p < .01) and similar in magnitude to the effect of other life stressors. Thus, our findings indicate that feelings of role engulfment have a direct effect on the lives of mothers and possibly a rippling effect on the well-being of fathers. Though role engulfment has received some attention in studies of caregivers (Skaff & Pearlin, 1992), it has not been systematically studied in families of adults with mental illness. Given the broad effects of role engulfment on the well-being of mothers, and the possibility of its spillover effect on the lives of fathers, additional research is warranted on the underlying mechanisms by which role engulfment affects parental well-being.

The father's appraisal of his involvement as opposed to the actual stressors and strains of caregiving had the most consistent effect on his psychological well-being. Fathers who appraised their involvement as more burdensome reported more depressive symptoms and lower levels of happiness. This finding has important clinical implications for it highlights that a priority in working with fathers is to first understand how they appraise their caregiving involvement. It also suggests that the most effective interventions will be ones that aim to help fathers reframe caregiving in a more positive light.

It is noteworthy that other life stressors unrelated to the child's mental illness influenced fathers' depression, controlling for indicators of objective caregiving demands and subjective burden. In a study of spouses of persons with mental illness, Noh and Avison (1988) similarly found that other life stressors had a stronger negative effect on the well-being of husband caregivers than wife caregivers. In previous research on persons with mental illness, these life stressors have often gone unmeasured. Our findings indicate that focusing narrowly on the stressors associated with mental illness fails to capture the range of stressors that may influence the psychological well-being of fathers. In fact, among fathers of adults with mental illness, other life stressors may be as important a correlate of mental health as the challenges of caregiving. In studying the impact of mental illness on the lives of fathers, it becomes critical to investigate how the challenges of caregiving interact with other life stressors to increase their vulnerability to distress.

Furthermore, I did not find evidence for the hypothesis that fathers would be more burdened and distressed when a son rather than a daughter had a mental illness. This hypothesis was based on research on normative father-adult child relationships in which fathers have been found to see their role as guiding their sons toward independence, while viewing their role in their daughter's life as that of a provider (Nydegger & Mitteness, 1996). I suspect that if we had sampled fathers closer to the time that their son or daughter was first diagnosed with a mental illness, we would have found this expected gender effect. However, the majority of fathers in our study were in their 60s, and had been coping with their child's illness for more than a decade. Tessler, Killian, and Gubman (1987) find that family members move through various stages in the process of coming to terms with their child's illness. Through a process of self-reflection, advocacy, and education about the etiology and treatment of mental illness, many parents come to accept their child's condition as an illness over which their son or daughter has no control, much like a physical illness. In our culture, individuals who are ill are seen as deserving of care and support. After years of coping with the challenges of their child's condition, many fathers in our study likely came to attribute their child's condition to an illness. When an adult child develops a disability, therefore, the norms governing the responsibility of parents to care for their children during illness may replace gender-linked role expectations in shaping the father's response to their son's or daughter's behavior.

One of the most surprising findings was that mothers felt less burdened and greater happiness when they provided more care. One possible explanation is that the temporal ordering of the variables was mispecified. It may be that mothers provide more assistance when they feel less burdened and are more satisfied with their lives. Another explanation is that the caregiving role has its own rewards and gains (Kramer, 1997b). Greenberg, Seltzer, and Judge (2000) found mothers were more burdened from caregiving than fathers, but paradoxically also reported more gains from coping with its challenges. These gains included developing more self-confidence, learning new skills, and becoming closer to their family. Thus the gains realized through caregiving might have more than offset the burdens experienced.

There are several limitations of this research that should be noted. First, there are important limitations to the generalizability of the study. Only clients who were receiving public mental health services were eligible to participate, and therefore, the sample is not representative of those in the private sector. The sample was drawn from rural and small urban areas of Wisconsin, and consequently, the participants were all European Americans, reflecting the lack of ethnic diversity in rural Wisconsin. However, in several ways the sample is more representative of families of persons with mental illness than those sampled in previous research. Only 20% of the parents were members of the National Alliance of the Mentally Ill. The sample is diverse in terms of the parent's education, income, age, and the adult child's diagnosis. Nevertheless, caution must be exercised in generalizing the findings, and replication is needed on different samples of parents of persons with mental illness, in particular families of color and those living in large urban areas.

Second, because the present data are cross-sectional, it was not possible to address the issue of causality. A particular causal ordering of the variables was assumed based on a stress-appraisal model and a different theoretical perspective might have involved a substantially different ordering of the variables. Longitudinal research is required to further explore the temporal ordering of among the set of variables examined in this study.

Third, the measures available to assess depression and happiness were less than optimal. The CES-D consisted of only 12 items, which reduced the scale variance, in particular among fathers. This is evident by the sizeable difference in the reliability of the CES-D for mothers versus fathers (.93 vs. .79, respectively). Also, a single item was available in the data set to measure parental happiness. Thus, the failure to detect certain hypothesized effects may be due to limitations of the outcomes measures.

Finally, in the tradition of stress research, we relied on outcome measures that assess "internalized symptoms," such as depression, which are known to be more commonly the response of women to a stressful life event than men. Insofar as caregiving is shaped by an individual's location in the social structure, men and women may differ in how they manifest their stress. The research literature is inconclusive as to whether men and women express distress differently. Several researchers have found that stressful life events are related to substance abuse for men and psychological distress for women (Aneshensel, Rutter, & Lachenbruch, 1991; Horwitz & Davies, 1994; Seltzer, Greenberg, Floyd, Pettee, & Hong, 2001). However, in a large-scale longitudinal study, Umberson and her colleagues (1996) found little support for the assertion that men and women react to distress in gender-specific ways. Yet, Umberson et al. (1996) did find that for both men and women hours of caregiving positively associated with alcohol consumption over time. This emerging body of research suggests the importance of including a range of outcomes beyond measures of "internalized symptoms" that capture other forms of men's psychological reactivity to stress.

In conclusion, in contrast to earlier portrayal of fathers of adults with mental illness as distant and aloof, we found that fathers of adults with mental illness remain actively involved in the lives of their sons and daughters with mental illness and continue to assist them with a broad range of activities. Research has rarely acknowledged, and only recently studied, this role of fathers as caregivers to adults with mental illness. The community support system has done little to acknowledge the involvement of fathers as caregivers because of the prevailing myth that it is only "mothers" who care for persons with mental illness. It is only when we recognized the unique ways that fathers care for their sons and daughters with mental illness and validate their experience that fathers will be able to move out from the shadow of their wives and speak openly of their frustrations and gratifications of coping with their child's illness.

REFERENCES

Anderson, E., & Lynch, M. M. (1984). A family impact analysis: The deinstitutionalization of the mentally ill. *Family Relations, 33,* 41–46.

Aneshensel, C. S., Rutter, C. M., & Lachenbruch, P. A. (1991). Social structure, stress, and mental health. *American Sociological Review, 56,* 166–178.

Antonucci, T. C. (1990). Social supports and social relationships. In R. H. Binstock & L. K. George (Eds.), *Handbook of aging and the social science* (pp. 205–226). San Diego, CA: Academic Press.

Antonucci, T. C., & Akiyama, H. (1995). Convoys of social relations: Family and friendships within a life span context. In R. Blieszner & V. H. Bedford (Eds.), *Handbook of aging and the family* (pp. 355–371). Westport, CT: Greenwood Press.

Baron, R. M., & Kenny, D. A. (1986). The moderator-mediator variable distinction in social psychological research: Conceptual, strategic, and statistical considerations. *Journal of Personality and Social Psychology, 51,* 1173–1182.

Beckman, P. J. (1991). Comparison of mothers' and fathers' perceptions of the effect of young children with and without disabilities. *American Journal on Mental Retardation, 95,* 585–595.

Biegel, D. E., Song, Li-y, & Chakravarthy, V. (1994). Predictors of caregiver burden among support group members of persons with chronic mental illness. In E. Kahana, D. E. Biegel, & M. L. Wykle (Eds.), *Family caregiving across the lifespan* (pp. 178–215). Thousand Oaks, CA: Sage.

Bowen, M. (1959). The role of the father in families with a schizophrenic patient. *American Journal of Psychiatry, 115,* 1017–1020.

Cañive, J. M., Sanz-Fuentenebro, J., Vazquez, C., Qualls, C., Fuentenebro, F., Perez, I. G., & Tuason, V. B. (1996). Family psychoeducational support groups in Spain: Parents' distress and burden at nine-month follow-up. *Annals of Clinical Psychiatry, 8,* 71–79.

Cook, J. A. (1988). Who "mothers" the chronically mentally ill? *Family Relations, 37,* 42–49.

Cook, J. A., & Pickett, S. A. (1988). Feelings of burden and criticalness among parents residing with chronically mentally ill offspring. *Journal of Applied Social Sciences, 12,* 79–107.

Coyne, J. C., Kessler, R. C., Tal, M., Turnbull, J., Wortman, C. B., & Greden, J. F. (1987). Living with a depressed person. *Journal of Consulting and Clinical Psychology, 55,* 347–352.

Davis, D. J., & Schultz, C. L. (1998). Grief, parenting, and schizophrenia. *Social Science and Medicine, 46,* 369–379.

Essex, E. L., Seltzer, M. M., & Krauss, W. M. (1999). Differences in coping effectiveness and well-being among aging mothers and fathers of adults with mental retardation. *American Journal of Mental Retardation, 104,* 545–563.

Estroff, S. E., Zimmer, C., Lachicotte, W. S., & Benoit, J. (1994). The influence of social networks and social supports on violence by persons with serious mental illness. *Hospital and Community Psychiatry, 45,* 669–679.

Fisher, G. A., Benson, P. R., & Tessler, R. C. (1990). Family responses to mental illness: Developments since deinstitutionalization. In J. R. Greenley (Vol. Ed.), *Mental disorder in social context: Vol. 6. Research in community and mental health* (pp. 203–236). Greenwich, CT: JAI Press.

Freeman, H. E., & Simmons, O. G. (1961). Feelings of stigma among relatives of former mental patients. *Social Problems, 8,* 312–321.

Gerard, D. L., & Siegel, J. (1950). The family background of schizophrenia. *Psychoanalytic Quarterly, 24,* 47–73.

Goldberg, S. C., Schooler, N. R., Hogarty, G. E., & Roper, M. (1977). Prediction of relapse in schizophrenic outpatients treated by drug and social therapy. *Archives of General Psychiatry, 34,* 171–184.

Goldstein, J. M., & Kreisman, D. (1988). Gender, family environment and schizophrenia. *Psychological Medicine, 18,* 861–872.

Greenberg, J., Greenley, J. R., & Brown, R. (1997). Do mental health services to clients reduce family distress? *Psychosocial Rehabilitation Journal, 21,* 40–50.

Greenberg, J. S., Greenley, J. R., McKee, D., Brown, R., & Griffen-Francell, C. (1993). Mothers caring for adult children with schizophrenia: The effects of subjective burdens on parental health. *Family Relations, 42,* 205–211.

Greenberg, J. S., Seltzer, M. M., & Greenley, J. R. (1993). Aging parents of adults with disabilities: Gratifications and frustrations of later life caregiving. *The Gerontologist, 33,* 542–550.

Greenberg, J. S., Seltzer, M. M., & Judge, K. (2000). Another side of the family's experience: Learning and growing through the process of coping with mental illness. *The Journal of the California Alliance for the Mentally Ill, 11,* 8–10.

Greenley, J. R. (1979). Family symptom tolerance and rehospitalization experiences of psychiatric patients. *Research in community and mental health, 1,* 357–386.

Gubman, G. D., & Tessler, R. C. (1987). The impact of mental illness on families: Concepts and priorities. *Journal of Family Issues, 8*, 226–245.

Hatfield, A. (1978). Psychological costs of schizophrenia to the family. *Social Work, 23*, 563–569.

Hertzog, C., Van Alstine, J., Usala, P. D., Hultsch, D. F., & Dixon, R. (1990). Measurement of the Center for Epidemiological Studies Depression scale (CES-D) in older populations. *Psychological Assessment, 2*, 64–72.

Horwitz, A. V., & Davies, L. (1994). Are emotional distress and alcohol problems differential outcomes to stress? An exploratory test. *Social Science Quarterly, 75*, 607–621.

Howard, P. B. (1998). The experience of fathers of adult children with schizophrenia. *Issues in Mental Health Nursing, 19*, 399–413.

Jones, S. L. (1996). The association between objective and subjective caregiver burden. *Archives of Psychiatric Nursing, 10*, 77–84.

Katz, M. M., & Lyerly, S. B. (1963). Methods for measuring adjustment and social behavior in the community: I. Rationale, description, discriminative validity and scale development. *Psychological Reports, 13*, 502–535.

Kramer, B. J. (1997a). Differential predictors of strain and gain among husbands caring for wives with dementia. *The Gerontologist, 37*, 239–249.

Kramer, B. J. (1997b). Gain in the caregiving experience: Where are we? What next? *The Gerontologist, 37*, 218–232.

Lawton, M. P., Kleban, M. II., Moss, M., Rovine, M., & Glicksman, A. (1989). Measuring caregiving appraisal. *Journal of Gerontology, 44*, 61–71.

Lawton, M. P., Moss, M., Kleban, M. H., Glicksman, A., & Rovine, M. (1991). A two-factor model of caregiving appraisal and psychological well-being. *Journal of Gerontology: Psychological Sciences, 46*, P181–P189.

Lazarus, R., & Folkman, S. (1984). *Stress, appraisal and coping.* New York: Springer.

Lefley, H. P. (1989). Family burden and family stigma in major mental illness. *American Psychologist, 44*, 556–560.

Lefley, H. P. (1996). *Family caregiving in mental illness.* Thousand Oaks, CA: Sage.

Lefley, H. P., & Wasow, M. (Eds.). (1994). *Helping families cope with mental illness.* Newark, NJ: Harwood Academic.

Lidz, T., Fleck, S., & Cornelison, A. R. (1965). *Schizophrenia and the family.* New York: International Universities Press.

Marsh, D. T. (1992). *Families and mental illness: New directions in professional practice.* New York: Praeger.

Maurin, J. T., & Boyd, C. B. (1990). Burden of mental illness on the family: A critical review. *Archives of Psychiatric Nursing, 4*, 99–107.

Noh, S., & Avison, W. (1988). Spouses of discharged psychiatric patients:

Factors associated with their experience of burden. *Journal of Marriage and the Family, 50,* 377–389.

Noh, S., & Turner, R. J. (1987). Living with psychiatric patients: Implications for the mental health of family members. *Social Science Medicine, 25,* 263–271.

Nydegger, C. N., & Mitteness, L. S. (1996). Midlife: The prime of fathers. In C. D. Ryff & M. M. Seltzer (Eds.), *The parental experience in midlife* (pp. 533–560). Chicago: The University of Chicago Press.

Pearlin, L. I. (1988). *Caregiver's stress and coping study.* San Francisco: University of California, Human Development and Aging Programs.

Pearlin, L. I., Aneshensel, C. S., & Leblanc, A. J. (1997). The forms and mechanisms of stress proliferation: The case of AIDS caregivers. *Journal of Health and Social Behavior, 38,* 223–236.

Pearlin, L. I., Mullan, J. T., Semple, S. J., & Skaff, M. M. (1990). Caregiving and the stress process: An overview of concepts and their measures. *The Gerontologist, 30,* 583–594.

Phelan, J. C., Bromet, E. J., & Link, B. G. (1998). Psychiatric illness and family stigma. *Schizophrenia Bulletin, 24,* 118–126.

Pickett, S. A., Cook, J. A., Cohler, B. J., & Solomon, M. L. (1997). Positive parent/adult child relationships: Impact of severe mental illness and caregiving burden. *American Journal of Orthopsychiatry, 67,* 220–230.

Platt, S. D., Hirsch, S. R., & Weyman, A. (1983). *Social behaviour assessment schedule* (3rd ed.). Windsor, Berks, England: NFER-Nelson.

Pruchno, R. A., Patrick, J. H., & Burant, C. (1996). Aging women and their children with chronic disabilities. *Family Relations, 45,* 318–326.

Radloff, L. (1977). The CES-D scale: A self-report depression scale for research in the general population. *Applied Psychological Measurement, 1,* 385–401.

Rossi, A. S., & Rossi, P. H. (1990). *Human bonding. Parent-child relations across the life course.* New York: Aldine de Gruyter.

Ryan, K. A. (1993). Mothers of adult children with schizophrenia: An ethnographic study. *Schizophrenia Research, 11,* 21–31.

Ryff, C. (1995). Psychological well-being in adult life. *Current Directions in Psychological Science, 4,* 99–104.

Ryff, C., Schmutte, P. S., & Lee, Y. H. (1996). How children turn out: Implications for parental self-evaluation. In C. Ryff & M. M. Seltzer (Eds.), *The parental experience in midlife* (pp. 383–422). Chicago: The University of Chicago Press.

Schwoon, D. R., & Angermeyer, M. C. (1980). Congruence of personality assessments within families with a schizophrenic son. *British Journal of Medical Psychology, 53,* 255–265.

Seltzer, M. M., Greenberg, J. S., Floyd, F. J., Pettee, Y., & Hong, J. (2001). Life course impacts of parenting a child with a disability. *American Journal of Mental Retardation, 106,* 282–303.

Seltzer, M. M., Greenberg, J. S., & Krauss, M. W. (1995). A comparison of coping strategies of aging mothers of adults with mental illness versus mental retardation. *Psychology and Aging, 10,* 64–75.

Skaff, M. M., & Pearlin, I. (1992). Caregiving: Role engulfment and the loss of self. *The Gerontologist, 32,* 656–664.

Solomon, P., & Draine, J. (1995). Subjective burden among family members of mentally ill adults: Relation to stress, coping, and adaptation. *American Journal of Orthopsychiatry, 65,* 419–427.

Stueve, A., Vine, P., & Struening, P. (1997). Perceived burden among caregivers of adults with serious mental illness: Comparison of Black, Hispanics, and White families. *American Journal of Orthopsychiatry, 67,* 199–209.

Sweet, J., Bumpass, L., & Call, V. (1988). *The design and content of the national survey of families and households* (Working Paper NSFH-1). Madison, WI: University of Wisconsin, Center for Demography and Ecology.

Tessler, R., & Gamache, G. (1995). *Toolkit for evaluating family experiences with severe mental illness.* Cambridge, MA: Human Services Research Institute.

Tessler, R., & Gamache, G. (2000). *Family experiences with mental illness.* Westport, CT: Auburn House.

Tessler, R. C., Killian, L. M., & Gubman, G. D. (1987). Stages in family response to mental illness: An ideal type. *Psychosocial Rehabilitation Journal, 10,* 3–16.

Umberson, D., Chen, M., House, J. S., Hopkins, K., & Slaten, E. (1996). The effect of social relationships on psychological well-being: Are men and women really so different? *American Sociological Review, 61,* 837–857.

Vine, P. (1982). *Families in pain: Children, siblings, spouses, and parents of the mentally ill speak out.* New York: Pantheon Books.

Wallace, C. J. (1986). Functional assessment in rehabilitation. *Schizophrenia Bulletin, 12,* 604–630.

Winefield, H. R. & Harvey, E. J. (1993). Determinants of psychological distress in relatives of people with chronic schizophrenia. *Schizophrenia Bulletin, 19,* 619–625.

Wintersteen, R. T., & Rasmussen, K. L. (1997). Fathers of persons with mental illness: A preliminary study of coping capacity and service needs. *Community Mental Health Journal, 33,* 401–413.

Husbands Caring for Wives With Cancer

13

Desirée Ciambrone
Susan M. Allen

Cancer is one of the most challenging of illnesses, often called the "dreaded disease." The need for caregiving support is crucial at the time of diagnosis and throughout treatment. Support needs may ease following treatment, or they may escalate with the progression of the disease and impending death. The morbidity associated with cancer treatment often requires ongoing assistance. Further, the potentially fatal nature of the disease combined with the difficulties of cancer treatment often result in anxiety and depression. For married people with cancer, their primary source of support is their spouse.

In this chapter we discuss spousal caregiving to women with cancer. To illustrate what caregiving among this population entails, we describe women's need for both instrumental and emotional support. We focus on men's caregiving experiences, including the nature of the assistance they provide, their perception of caregiver burden, and barriers to optimal care provision. We also address how the nature of the marital relationship is tied to positive caregiving outcomes. Finally, we discuss the challenges facing husband caregivers, including competing social roles and gendered expectations.

Although research has focused on older men caring for their wives (e.g., Chang & White-Means, 1991; DeVries, Hamilton, Lovett, & Gallagher-Thompson, 1997; Kaye & Applegate, 1990; Rose-Rego, Strauss, & Smyth, 1998), with the exception of Alzheimer's disease, less attention has been given to men caring for wives with a specific illness. In this chapter we broaden our view of men as caregivers by investigating husbands' experiences as caregivers to women with cancer. We focus on breast cancer because it is by far the most common cancer among women (National Cancer Institute, 2000). It is estimated, for example, that approximately one in eight women in the United States will develop breast cancer during her lifetime (American Cancer Society, 2000). In addition, unlike diseases prevalent among particular age groups, such as Alzheimer's disease, cancer affects working age and older women and, thus, has implications for both young and old spousal caregivers. Although the risk of developing breast cancer increases with age, nearly one quarter of diagnosed cases are in women under the age of 50 (ACS, 2000). Treatment advances have extended the period of breast cancer survivorship; approximately 85% of women diagnosed with breast cancer are alive 5 years postdiagnosis, 71% are alive 10 years postdiagnosis, and 57% are alive 15 years postdiagnosis (ACS, 2000). Thus, breast cancer is a chronic illness that impacts women and their husbands at all stages of the adult life course.

SPOUSAL SUPPORT AND THE QUALITY OF THE MARITAL RELATIONSHIP

Meeting Wives' Practical Needs

The need for practical assistance may be quite substantial among women with cancer. Despite gains in survival for breast cancer, especially for younger women (Bailar & Gornik, 1997), surgical treatment, adjuvant chemotherapy, and radiation are likely to exacerbate the negative impact of the disease through their potentially substantial side effects, including pain, severe fatigue, nausea, loss of sensation, stiffness, and lymphedema (Goodman, 1989; Knobf, 1990; Love, Leventhal, Easterling, & Nerenz, 1989; Moyer & Salovey, 1996; Paci et al., 1996). These problems may be intermittent or persist over the course of treatment; thus, women may require assistance with a range of ADLs (activities of daily living; such as eating and bathing) and IADLs (instrumental activities of daily living; such as grocery shopping and house cleaning). Insufficient instrumental assistance may lead to unmet daily living needs that can interfere with condition management and ultimately compromise health status (Allen & Mor, 1997).

Married women with impairment typically turn to their spouses for assistance when they are unable to fill the homemaker role alone (Thompson & Pitts, 1992), and husbands are called upon to assume tasks they may not have had responsibility for prior to their wives' illness. Compared to non-caregiving husbands, caregiving husbands appear to take an active role in traditionally female household labor tasks (Kramer & Lambert, 1999). Several respondents in a study of psychosocial issues among younger women with breast cancer discussed the help they receive from their husbands with household tasks (Allen, Petrisek, & Ciambrone, 2000). For example, one woman explained how her husband takes over her chores in times of need, using her pregnancy and breast cancer as analogous examples:

[He helped] at the beginning with the surgery and not being able to move your arm and stuff like that. But no more so than when I had kids, because when I had kids I had c-sections, so he would still come home and help me with the laundry and the vacuuming, so it was really like another one of those deals . . . so it's like anytime Mom wasn't doing okay for a few weeks, he would just assume all that.

Interestingly, another respondent noted that her ex-husband was a great source of assistance, helping with childcare as well as household chores:

When I got sick the first person called was my ex-husband, and he flew out and moved in and took care of us. My children are not his, they act like they're his but, in fact, they're not. And he moved in for four or five months—living with us, feeding us, cleaning, cooking, laundry . . . [He] was always there through everything, and I'm very, very happy that he was.

Some husbands also offered consolation and advice to their wives, making it easier for them to ponder important medical decisions. As one respondent said regarding her partial mastectomy: "I just knew it had to be done. Fortunately, I had a very helpful husband, who agreed that that was the best thing to do."

For some husbands, however, assuming traditionally female roles may be problematic because husbands may not have experience in performing household tasks (Lamanna & Riedmann, 1997). Indeed, wives have historically been the family manager, responsible for ensuring that the household runs smoothly. When husbands are suddenly given this role, they may be surprised and overwhelmed by the extent of the planning and labor involved (Pederson & Valanis, 1988).

Research on populations of people with physical impairments has indicated that married women may be at risk for inadequate practical support (Allen, 1994; Morgan, Patrick, & Charlton, 1984). For example, Allen examined gender differences in spousal caregiving in a sample of married people with cancer who were undergoing outpatient treatment. Consistent with past research, she found that husbands were less likely than wives to help their sick spouses with household tasks, and husbands who helped were more likely to have other helpers, whereas wives tended to be sole caregivers. In fact, wives provided approximately twice the hours of care that husbands provided (4.9 hours vs. 2.9 hours, respectively). Women undergoing treatment who experienced high levels of morbidity received more hours of help with household tasks from nonspousal sources than men with comparable levels of morbidity, thus compensating for the deficit in hours of care provided by their husbands. At lower levels of morbidity, however, compensatory help to women was not sufficient to fill the gap in care. In fact, women were more likely than men to report unmet need for assistance with household tasks (30.7% vs. 16.2%, respectively).

Although many husbands, especially older men, appear to adjust well to the caregiving role, it is not surprising that some husbands may have difficulty assuming traditionally female tasks as men and women are socialized into distinct social roles, and these gender-typed roles are especially evident in the context of marriage (Shelton & John, 1993). Husbands may feel uncomfortable assuming roles outside of the male-typed tasks they are more accustomed to performing. For example, a study of 148 male participants in caregiver support groups (the majority of whom were spousal caregivers) found that men felt less competent in household management and personal care tasks than in more "masculine" tasks such as financial management and providing transportation (Kaye & Applegate, 1990). Personal care tasks (e.g., ADLs) may be especially challenging because they are more time consuming, require a high level of hands-on contact, and are tasks typically allocated to women.

Relative to older husbands, younger husbands may have a particularly hard time assuming the role of primary caregiver because they have greater obligations outside of the private realm. Faced with increasing illness demands in addition to the duties of "everyday life," these men may have a more difficult time assuming traditionally female domestic roles because of their multiple obligations (Northouse, 1994).

Women, feeling they are better suited than their partners to perform household chores, may also present barriers to effective spousal caregiving. That is, women may perceive their spouses' attempts as inadequate because of their reluctance to relinquish domestic responsibilities to their husbands (Dempsey, 1997), rather than based primarily on the nature of their spouses' contributions.

Husbands' Response to Wives' Emotional Distress

Women with cancer grapple with psychosocial concerns throughout the course of their illness. At initial diagnosis, psychological distress appears to be particularly acute and worries arise concerning functional decline, abandonment, and death (Moyer & Salovey, 1999). In the case of breast cancer, many undergo disfiguring full or partial mastectomies. In addition, treatments may result in hair loss and weight fluctuation. These side effects are at odds with cultural standards of femininity and are often a blow to women's self-esteem. Physical manifestations of cancer are often accompanied by psychosocial morbidity, including fear of recurrence, anger, anxiety, depression, and denial (Irvine, Crooks, & Browne, 1991; Moyer & Salovey, 1996). Issues regarding sexuality and body image also loom large for these women (Cameron & Horsburgh, 1998). In later stages, particularly when the medical management of their disease subsides, some of these issues may be less pressing, but women still grapple with an uncertain illness trajectory, the fear of recurrence, and fear of passing on the disease to their daughters.

Thus, throughout their illness women with cancer can benefit greatly from an emotionally close relationship (Rose, 1990). For individuals without difficulties with physical functioning, such as most long-term cancer survivors, emotional support appears more critical to psychological well-being than instrumental support. Previous research has noted the importance of positive relationships to adequate informal care provision. Having someone to confide in about personal issues appears to be the "simplest and most powerful measure of social support" (Smith, Redman, Burns, & Sagert, 1986; Thoits, 1995, p. 64).

Theoretically, husbands are in an ideal position to provide both instrumental and emotional support due to their internalized commitment, and close proximity, to their spouses (Messeri, Silverstein, & Litwak, 1993). Marital norms and values generally prescribe that partners will care for and comfort each other "in sickness and in health." Thus, in a sense spouses are obligated to help one another if one partner becomes ill. Therefore, couples who perceive their marriages to be emotionally close may be more comfortable both seeking assistance for and providing assistance to their spouses than those whose marriages are emotionally distant (Vinokur & Vinokur-Kaplan, 1990).

Research supports these claims, suggesting that the emotional support provided by husbands has a marked impact on how their wives cope with chronic, disabling conditions. Studies among couples with cancer, like other illness populations, consistently show that the spouse is the most important source of support (Lee, 1997; Neuling & Winfield, 1988; Rose, 1990; Smith et al., 1986). Spousal support and marital intimacy have been associated with better coping and patient self-esteem and depression scores (Douglass, 1997; Feigin et al., 2000). In addition, partners in good marriages often experience improvements in their relationship, specifically in areas of emotional closeness and communication (O'Mahoney & Carroll, 1997).

Indeed, relationship quality appears to be an important factor in how both caregivers and care recipients cope with impairment, over and above being in a marital relationship. As Lichtman, Taylor and Wood (1987) show, women with breast cancer who are in loving, supportive marriages prior to the onset of illness are more likely to adjust to, and cope better with, sickness. Specifically, among married women in their sample ($n = 55, 70\%$), the majority (75%) perceived "a great deal" of support from their spouse. Women who shared their concerns with their husbands or reported open and honest communication with their husbands were better adjusted.[1] Walker's (1997) results also speak to the impact of good marital

---

[1] Lichtman et al. (1987) employed 10 individual measures of adjustment, including patient self-report, total Profile of Mood States score, ratings on the Global Adjustment to Illness Scale, Index of Well-Being score, and Locke-Wallace Marital Adjustment Test.

relations (i.e., open communication) on coping with illness. Investigating how the spousal relationship affects fear of recurrence and emotional distress among women with breast cancer and their husbands, the author found that the amount of communication about the illness accounted for most of the variance in adjustment for both spouses.

More recently, Allen, Goldscheider, and Ciambrone (1999) investigated the role of emotional closeness in the unequal representation of husbands and wives as spousal caregivers to cancer outpatients ($n = 353$). Consistent with previous research, they found that men are more likely to name their spouse, both as confidant and as primary caregiver, while women also named daughters and friends, despite husbands' availability. The importance of marital intimacy was evident in that both husbands and wives who named their spouse as confidant were three times more likely to name them as primary caregiver than respondents who named someone other than their spouses as confidant, or who did not name anyone at all.

Being in a good marriage also helps husbands positively deal with traumatic cancer-related events, such as surgery. For example, the men in one study of spouses' reactions to breast cancer who reported having a satisfactory pre-mastectomy sexual relationship reported little change after the operation. However, men who reported having a less than satisfactory pre-mastectomy sexual relationship reported decreased sexual functioning post-mastectomy (Wellisch, Fawzy, Landsverk, Pasnau, & Wolcott, 1983). And Hoskins and colleagues (1996) found that marital support significantly predicted husbands' emotional and physical adjustment.

Further, marital satisfaction appears to be a good indicator of patient distress over time (Weihs, Enright, Howe, & Simmens, 1999). In their study of emotional adjustment after breast cancer, Weihs et al. found that marital satisfaction predicted change in patient distress from 15 to 34 months following diagnosis. Women who perceived that their marriages were unsatisfactory were at greater risk for future elevated distress than those who were satisfied with their marriage, regardless of their reports of distress at time of diagnosis.

Like the illness experience itself, however, the effect of cancer on interpersonal relationships is not uniform. The diagnosis may exacerbate marital problems and strain relationships or it may strengthen bonds (Cupp, 1998). In all likeliness, many couples may experience periods of strain and greater intimacy at different points throughout the course of the wife's illness. Although a diagnosis of breast cancer generally does not result in marital dissolution (Dorval, Maunsell, Taylor-Brown, & Kilpatrick, 1999), husbands report cancer-related stressors, such as poorer sexual relations and increased communication problems (Burman & Weinert, 1997; Northouse, 1994; Wellisch, Jamison, & Pasnau, 1978; Zahlis & Shands, 1991).

Contextual variables or challenges may make it difficult for spouses to meet their partners' caregiving expectations. An extremely difficult aspect of being a husband to a woman with cancer is having to help her cope with the psychosocial impact of illness, because many men may feel ill prepared to deal with their wives' emotional response to illness (Northouse, 1994). Similar to the housekeeper role, some male care providers are forced to take on unfamiliar expressive caregiving roles. The tension between men's traditional gender expectations and the "feminine" nature of caregiving often affects their performance in caring roles. As one woman remarked, "I do not get what you might call strong emotional support from my husband, I get more emotional support from my two daughters" (Allen, Petrisek, & Ciambrone, 2000). In fact, although women with breast cancer generally describe their husbands as supportive, some report that they are uncertain about their partners' ability to cope with their illness *over time* (Cameron & Horsburgh, 1998).

Husbands' attempts at emotionally supporting their wives may fall short of wives' expectations, despite genuine efforts. For example, in their study of husbands' reactions to their wives' mastectomies, Sabo, Brown, and Smith (1986) found that although men were emotionally invested in their wives' cancer experiences, they masked their true feelings and assumed a protective role. What these men intended as supportive behavior was perceived as insensitivity and distancing by their partners. A lack of discussion about cancer, for instance, may be perceived by husbands as a loving attempt to divert their wives' attention from her illness, but their wives may interpret this action as a thoughtless act, which invalidates their concerns. Despite their efforts to be supportive, husbands in Lewis and Deal's (1995) qualitative study of women with recurrent cancer often did not want to discuss issues their wives deemed important, particularly death, illustrating the difficulty husbands have discussing such sensitive topics. In Gotay's (1984) study of partners of women with early stage gynecologic cancer or advanced stage breast cancer, men reported much more concern with women's premature death than the patients themselves. Thus, it is likely that husbands are deeply concerned with such issues but avoid them in an attempt to minimize their wives' as well as their own distress.

Indeed, dissimilar notions of what constitutes positive support may lead to negative caring experiences for both the caregiver *and* the care recipient. Although marriage generally acts as a buffer for adverse events, if one partner cannot cope well with the disease, the benefits of an intimate relationship may be threatened. It is understandable that loving husbands, like other informal caregivers, may want to avoid topics like death and dying to minimize women's emotional pain as well as their own distress. It is also not surprising that some wives may want to discuss their mortality as they prepare for the end of their illness trajectory, and interpret their husbands' avoidant behaviors as insensitivity.

The difficulty some husbands experience providing emotional support to their wives may be due, in part, to adherence to socially prescribed gender roles and dissimilar expectations. In addition, as discussed below, men's own emotional state impacts the ways in which they perceive and respond to their wives' illness.

Men's Experience as Caregivers

The above discussion reviewed the importance of spousal caregiving to women with cancer as well as the potential barriers to positive spousal support. As such, it draws on literature largely from the patient's perspective. Important practical and theoretical questions stemming from this literature include: How do husbands perceive their role as primary care providers to their wives? How do husbands cope with their wives' illness? How are they affected by caregiver strain? It is difficult to paint a detailed picture of husbands' cancer caregiving experiences because the literature regarding men's involvement, and caregiver burden in particular, is relatively scarce and focuses largely on aged husbands (e.g., Chan & Chang, 1999; Gilbar, 1999; Stetz, 1987). It is clear, however, that a diagnosis of cancer is a family issue (Cassileth & Hamilton, 1979; Gotay, 1984; Lewis, 1990) and that spouses' unique position puts them at high risk for caregiver burden. For example, spousal caregivers typically provide more extensive and comprehensive care over longer periods of time than other informal caregivers (Siegel, Raveis, Mor, & Houts, 1991). In addition, intense care provision often demands that they make drastic lifestyle changes, such as reducing work hours (Siegel et al.). Moreover, changes in men's work environment and quality of their job performance has been associated with their emotional adjustment to their wives' cancer (Hoskins et al., 1996).

Research shows how the cancer experience profoundly affected husbands caring for their wives with cancer, even though they are disease-free. For example, Baider and De-Nour (1988) and Northouse, Dorris, and Charron-Moore (1995) found that among women with breast cancer, partners' adjustment scores were significantly correlated, suggesting that couples influence one another's adjustment. And Baider, Walach, Perry, and Kaplan-De-Nour (1998) found that couples in which both spouses have cancer were *no* more distressed than couples where only one partner is ill. Studies examining husbands' reactions and adjustment to their wives' cancer consistently show that husbands are faced with crises and adjustment difficulties, albeit of somewhat different nature than their wives'. For example, Northouse, Templin, Mood, and Oberst (1998) found that women and their partners perceived similar levels of role problems, underscoring that the diagnosis of breast cancer affects both partners.

The major concerns of women with cancer, such as uncertainty and fear of recurrence, are also concerns of their husbands (Samms, 1999; Zahlis & Shands, 1991). Chekryn's (1984) small descriptive study among patients with recurrent gynecologic or breast cancer and their spouses (n = 12 couples), for example, showed that recurrence and related uncertainty often signified a crisis for husbands. In fact, upon recurrence, half of the men experienced a grief response (e.g., crying, agitation, and withdrawal).

In addition to these ever-present concerns, specific cancer-related events, such as surgeries, are major stressors for husbands. Following their wives' breast surgery, for instance, husbands have reported psychosomatic sequelae, such as sleep disturbances and eating disorders (Wellisch et al., 1978). In addition, because wives are generally husbands' primary source of support, many men grieve the impending loss of their partner and confidant (Lutzky & Knight, 1994; Ptacek, Pierce, Dodge, & Ptacek, 1997). Similar to studies of female informal caregivers, research suggests that relative to non-caregiving husbands, caregiving husbands exhibit poorer psychological well-being such as greater levels of depression and less happiness (Kramer & Lambert, 1999).

Further, research strongly suggests that the elevated levels of distress experienced by spouses of cancer patients do not necessarily wane during the later stages of the disease (Lewis, 1990). There is evidence that caregivers continue to experience distress even when their ill partner's psychological state improves (Given & Given, 1992). For example, following cancer patients and their husbands over a 3-year period, Baider and De-Nour (1984) found that husbands' scores worsened whereas women's distress levels and adjustment scores improved over time. Northouse and Swain (1987) investigated the experience of newly diagnosed breast cancer patients and their husbands. They found that a month after their wives' mastectomies, husbands' were experiencing as much psychological distress as their partners. Husbands in another study exhibited heightened anxiety and depression over the course of a year following their wives' surgery (Maguire, 1981).

Husbands' distress may be difficult for informal others to gauge as female and male caregivers tend to report distress differently, and men are often hesitant to acknowledge stress at all (Lutzky & Knight, 1994). Caregiver burden among male care providers, therefore, may be underestimated due to underreporting. Husbands who are constrained by socially prescribed gender roles may be reluctant to report that they are experiencing stress in an attempt to uphold a masculine identity ascribing weakness to men who acknowledge and disclose feelings of helplessness (Blood, Blood, Bennett, Simpson, & Susman, 1994). For instance, focus group participants noted how traditional gender roles hindered their husbands' ability to reach out to them emotionally (Allen, Petrisek, & Ciambrone, 2000). As one woman stated:

He was terribly upset, but he could not talk to me about it. He's not an outward person . . . so I could do a lot of talking to him and he would talk a little bit but [he] could never express how he felt. I found out through two of our best friends [that] he was upset about this or was upset about that, or, you know, he is really behind you 100% no matter what you need to do, but he couldn't actually tell me how he was feeling. I mean he was there for everything, he came to as many appointments as he could come to.

Husbands may be especially vulnerable to caregiver burden because the intimate nature of the marital relationship may be strained by illness (Northouse, 1994; Wellisch et al., 1978). In fact, they may be more vulnerable than other informal helpers because they reside in the household and have daily contact with their wives, thus giving them greater, repeated exposure to patient stress (Baider et al., 1998). Discussing women with breast cancer, Pederson and Valanis note that "family members are strongly attuned to her feelings and tend to suffer with her" (1988, p. 98). Thus, in addition to proximity, it is likely that husbands who have a stronger emotional connection with their wives also are more prone to psychological distress.

Because they are emotionally invested in the marital relationship and hence affected by their wives' illness, they may inadvertently contribute to their wives' distress. Not surprisingly, husbands often feel powerless and are forced to "sit back" and watch their wives' health deteriorate as the disease progresses (Baider & DeNour, 1988; Siegel et al., 1991). Those who feel powerless over their wives' disease may consciously or unconsciously avoid their condition (Allen et al., 2000). Emotion-focused coping strategies, however, such as avoidance, denial, and self-blame tend to be counter-productive and increase caregiver strain relative to problem-focused coping styles (Kramer, 1997b). If husbands have difficulty facing their wives' cancer, they may be less able to provide assistance as doing so may bring their wives' disease to the fore. In discussing avoidance issues, two women commented:

My husband would probably say that I was the one doing the isolating. He would say that I was centered down on myself and he felt helpless. He probably had a tougher time emotionally.

My husband was in automatic denial that anything could possibly be wrong with me . . . He's a wonderful guy, don't get me wrong, he's a wonderful guy.

Another respondent noted that the difficulty her husband is experiencing in discussing her cancer is strongly related to his fear of losing her. As she said: "My cancer's still a threat of abandonment."

In addition to denial, it is not uncommon for patients and their loved ones to react to the cancer diagnosis with fear and anger (Aldredge-Clanton, 1998; Glasdam, Jensen, Madsen, & Rose, 1996; Pederson & Valanis, 1988). This may be especially true for those who have less experience and hence feel less comfortable with expressing emotions (Allen et al., 2000). As one woman remarked:

> My husband was mad all the time . . . until like basically we went to counseling. Then my daughter, had to deal with her, you know, she had nightmares and all this, and finally that brought us to counseling. And he finally woke up and realized that we have to face this.

Given that support from one's spouse is critical in helping wives cope with illness and that husbands may have difficulty assuming the caregiving role and experience distress, how do they manage to provide instrumental and emotional support? The men in Gotay's (1984) study responded by *taking action*; for example, obtaining information about the disease. Similarly, in order to better negotiate the illness experience, the men in Zahlis & Shands' (1991) sample became educated about cancer and participated in treatment decisions, by accompanying their partners to treatment sessions, for instance. They also made lifestyle changes (e.g., altering their work schedules to accommodate new responsibilities such as child care, cooking, shopping, and laundry). Being a supportive mate was an important, albeit the most difficult, part of the cancer experience for many men. To this end, they tried to be more attentive and emotionally available. Interestingly, men were often critical of their own efforts, noting that they feel they "could be more understanding" (Zahlis & Shands, 1991, p. 89). Moreover, although husbands were cognizant of their partners' distress, husbands were not sure of how to help and worried that they were ineffective.

Support from others may help alleviate men's anxiety. For example, the majority of men in Hirsch's (1996) sample of caregivers to aged relatives reported that they received support for their caring roles from family and friends and that this support appeared to help them thrive in the caregiving role. Men who do not receive support may be less able to deal with their wives' illness and hence be less competent caregivers. As one woman explained, husbands may be unfairly excluded from an experience that affects the entire family (Allen et al., 2000):

> It really didn't hit me until afterward how little support my husband got. My husband's from a family that's very businesslike and kind of cold . . . It wasn't until afterward that I realized that nobody from my husband's family really helped him through it. I was too busy worrying about me, and he was too busy worrying about me. But never his brother nor his parents really

came and said to him, "How are you?" and "How are you dealing with this?" and "Can we help?" Or, "What can we do for you?" . . . I don't know about anybody else's husbands, but I think they kind of get lost.

Male caregivers, like their female counterparts, are also vulnerable to unmet caregiver need. For example, caregivers to women with cancer reported feeling that they did not have enough information about the disease and often felt alone in dealing with their wives' illness (Burman & Weinert, 1997). Similarly, care-related needs and communication issues were key for husbands of women newly diagnosed with breast cancer (Kilpatrick, Kristjanson, Tataryn, & Fraser, 1998). The authors also found that husbands whose wives had undergone their first mastectomy reported approximately three times more unmet needs than those whose wives had undergone previous surgery, suggesting that the initial crises are likely to heighten needs that abate as men adjust to the experience.

Samms' (1999) small qualitative study ($n = 9$) investigating the needs of husbands of women with breast cancer revealed that just as women's needs change over time, husbands concerns changed over the course of their wives' illness. For example, when their wives were initially diagnosed, husbands felt helpless. During the treatment phase, husbands recognized the need to be instrumentally and emotionally supportive. Interestingly, in describing husbands' experiences during this stage, Samms writes, "husbands reported that their anxiety started to build during the treatment phase as they tried to read their wives' signals and danced around their wives' changing moods and needs" (1999, p. 1356). Feeling unsure of their wives' needs, they had a difficult time responding in a way their wives deemed supportive and, therefore, felt as if their efforts at providing emotional support were inadequate. The tension between wanting to be emotionally supportive and protect their wives yet feeling inadequate caused distress for the husbands in this study.

Although caregiving may lead to higher levels of strain and burden, there are also positive outcomes associated with caring labor. And just as women have described the advantages of providing care to their loved ones, including an increased sense of efficacy and the strengthening of interpersonal bonds (Thompson & Pitts, 1992), men also report benefit from caregiving. Qualitative accounts among husbands caring for their wives with dementia, for example, suggest that men derive many gains from the caregiving experience, including personal esteem rewards and the development of closer relationships to their wives (Kramer, 1997b). Among the respondents in Kramer's (1997b) study of predictors of negative and positive appraisals among older spousal caregivers, gain or positive appraisals were predicted by educational level and problem-focused coping. This finding highlights the importance of helping caregivers feel comfortable with and competent in the caregiver role.

CONCLUSION

Given the role of spousal support in adjusting to, coping with, and managing chronic illness, it is important to gain a better understanding of spousal caregiving to women with cancer as well as other illnesses. Our review suggests mixed findings regarding the nature and perceived effectiveness of spousal care to women with cancer. For example, some studies show that women with spouses turn to their husbands for practical assistance and that husbands assume nonconventional roles, such as helping with household chores (Allen et al., 2000; Kramer & Lambert, 1999). Other investigations suggest that married women with impairment are at elevated risk for not receiving practical support in line with their expectations (Allen, 1994; Morgan et al., 1984). Similarly, literature concentrating on emotional aid illustrates that the support offered by spouses is very important to how women react to, and cope with, their disease. Some men, however, appear to have a difficult time providing emotional support because they are not accustomed to doing so. These men conceive of the concept in a different way than their wives (Northouse, 1994), or they are unable to be emotionally available because they, too, are experiencing psychological distress (Baider et al., 1998; Northouse et al., 1995).

Thus, it appears that although women with cancer generally benefit from spousal support, some husbands may need assistance in mastering caregiving skills, particularly those most at odds with masculine gender role ideologies. It is not merely a matter of men renouncing the caregiver role, but rather discordance between men and women's socially constructed expectations. This is especially evident in the case of emotional succor, such as reassurance and validation support. Several of the studies discussed above (e.g., Chekryn, 1984; Lewis & Deal, 1995; Sabo et al., 1986) note that women's partners acted in a way that they believed was supportive, yet women did not interpret their behavior as such and at times perceived them as unhelpful. For example, downplaying the affects of cancer and minimizing discussion about cancer-related issues in order to ease women's worries are not effective coping strategies and may actually heighten anxiety as couples deal with disease *and* interpersonal relations. Indeed, even supportive husbands can have difficulty dealing with the sensitive issues illuminated by cancer.

Men's emotional responses to their wives' cancer affects the ways in which they approach and cope with the situation. Studies have shown that men and women have different ways of coping (e.g., Lutzky & Knight, 1994), however, they are not necessarily ineffective coping strategies. For example, in their investigation of caregivers of older adults, DeVries et al. (1997) found that although men and women used different types of coping, there were no gender differences in the perceived helpfulness of strategies (i.e., cognitive, behavioral, and avoidance). Contrary to the belief that women are apt to use less effective coping strategies, these authors found no gender difference in the use of avoidance coping. Further, although female caregivers were more likely to employ a wider range of strategies than male caregivers, they did not differ on their ratings of strategy usefulness (DeVries et al.).

Men's experiences with caregiving may also be influenced by changes associated with life course stages, specifically the relaxation of stereotyped gender roles in later life. Older husbands may be more comfortable assuming nontraditional gender roles, younger husbands may not. Further, as pointed out by Kramer (1997a), the benefits of caregiving reported by older men, including emotional gratification, suggest that caregiving may provide men with a vehicle to maintain meaningful familial roles, such as preserving family cohesion.

Because ill women typically desire high levels of emotional support from their husbands, couples' pre-illness relationship is of great importance. As discussed above, marital quality is a far more important indicator of spousal caregiving than spousal availability (Allen et al., 1991; Lichtman et al., 1987; Weihs et al., 1999). Just as we have come to challenge one dimensional (i.e., positive) views of informal care receipt and caregiver burden, and now investigate negative support and caregiver gain, so too must we question conceptions of caregivers based solely on the relationship to the care recipient. In terms of spousal caregiving, generally speaking, good marital relations provide an important base for positive social support and caregiving.

However, husbands are also faced with the challenges associated with cancer and are often simultaneously unexpectedly thrust into unfamiliar roles. As discussed above, cancer is a family affair, and spouses of women with cancer also experience a number of psychological responses that are shaped and altered over the course of their partner's illness trajectory. Thus, they may also need support to be "successful" in the caregiving role. It is reasonable to presume that many men are in the same position as the male caregivers in Zahlis and Shands' (1991) sample who wanted to help their wives but were not sure how. Support and encouragement from others in their social networks may help them incorporate the caring role into their lives. In addition to informal assistance, husbands also may benefit from formal support. An educational training program designed to introduce caregivers to pertinent instrumental and emotional support issues may provide husbands with greater information as well as role modeling. Such an endeavor comprises an overview of women's experiences of living and coping with cancer, including the psychosocial sequelae of the disease, the etiology and medical management of cancer, and peer or professional support to help men feel comfortable in their "new" role. Studies of psycho-educational support groups for other caregiver populations, for example, have reported decreased caregiving strain, enhanced competence, greater use of positive coping strategies (Cummings, Long, Peterson-Hazan, & Harrison, 1998), and enhanced problem-solving ability (Bucher, Houts, Nezu, & Nezu, 1999).

A lack of literature regarding working-age male caregivers relative to female and aged male care providers, however, makes it difficult to suggest recommendations that may facilitate men's involvement and competency in caregiving roles. To understand the male caregiving experience and the consequences of men's caring labor for themselves and those they help, a research agenda is needed that focuses specifically on men's caregiving activities. For example, studies that examine specific sources of support, rather than lumping husband's contributions into "familial" or "informal support," would provide a more comprehensive profile of male caregivers and the nature of the assistance they provide. Qualitative studies of the lived experiences of husband care providers would provide rich narrative data regarding a myriad of caregiving issues. The qualitative studies cited in this paper offer interesting descriptive and conceptual data with which we can begin to construct a more complete portrait of male caregivers. Most have relied, however, on small sample sizes (e.g., < 30) that methodologically may not allow for conceptual saturation (Gerhardt, 1990). A greater number of cases would add to our confidence that the results are closer to those found in the population of interest.

Substantively, studies are needed that explore how men come to occupy primary caregiving roles, how they evaluate their masculinity vis-à-vis traditionally female caring roles, the advantages of assuming the caregiving role, and their perceptions of role conflict and strain. Although there is evidence that male caregivers of older adults do benefit from providing care to their wives (Kramer, 1997b), we need more research on working-age husbands to see if they obtain the same benefits when occupying multiple, often competing, social roles.

In addition, longitudinal research is needed in order to address husbands' participation over time, identifying changes in caregiving activities, predictors of adjustment to the caregiving role, indicators of burden as well as subjective and objective care recipient outcomes (e.g., satisfaction with care and functional status, respectively). These are fertile areas of research that would enrich the cancer, caregiving, and gender-focused literatures. Inquiries into such areas would help us to better understand the contributions of husband caregivers. It would also allow us to assess the challenges male caregivers face and prescribe changes that may ease their distress, strengthen their caregiving skills, and better enable them to meet wives' needs as they go through one of life's most traumatic experiences.

REFERENCES

Aldredge-Clanton, J. (1998). *Counseling and pastoral theology.* Louisville, KY: Westminster John Knox Press.

Allen, S. M. (1994). Gender differences in spousal caregiving and unmet need for care. *Journal of Gerontology, 49,* S187–S195.

Allen, S. M., Goldscheider, F., & Ciambrone, D. (1999). Gender roles, marital intimacy, and nomination of spouse as primary caregiver. *The Gerontologist, 39,* 150–158.

Allen, S. M., & Mor, V. (1997). The prevalence and consequences of unmet need: Contrasts between older and younger adults with disability. *Medical Care, 35,* 1132–1148.

Allen, S. M., Petrisek, A. C., & Ciambrone, D. (2000). Unpublished data, Brown University.

American Cancer Society. (2000). *Cancer facts and figures, 2000.* Atlanta, GA: ACS.

Baider, L., & De-Nour, A. K. (1984). Couples' reactions and adjustment to mastectomies. *International Journal of Psychiatry in Medicine, 14,* 265–276.

Baider, L., & De-Nour, A. K. (1988). Adjustment to cancer: Who is the patient—the husband or the wife? *Israel Journal of Medical Sciences, 24,* 631–636.

Baider, L., Walach, N., Perry, S., & Kaplan-De-Nour, A. (1998). Cancer in married couples: Higher or lower distress? *Journal of Psychosomatic Research, 45,* 239–248.

Bailar, J. C., & Gornik, H. L. (1997). Trends in cancer mortality: Perspectives from Italy and the United States. *La Medicina del lavoro, 88,* 274–286.

Blood, G. W., Blood, I. M., Bennett, S., Simpson, K. C., & Susman, E. J. (1994). Spouses of individuals with laryngeal cancer: Caregiver strain and burden. *Journal of Communication Disorders, 27,* 19–35.

Bucher, J. A., Houts, P. S., Nezu, C. M., & Nezu, A. M. (1999). Improving problem-solving skills of family caregivers through group education. *Journal of Psychosocial Oncology, 16,* 73–84.

Burman, M. E., & Weinert, C. (1997). Concerns of rural men and women experiencing cancer. *Oncology Nursing Forum, 24,* 1593–1600.

Cameron, S., & Horsburgh, M. E. (1998). Comparing issues faced by younger and older women with breast cancer. *Canadian Oncology Nursing Journal, 8,* 40–44.

Cassileth, B. R., & Hamilton, J. N. (1979). The family with cancer. In B. R. Cassileth (Ed.), *The cancer patient: Social and medical aspects of care* (pp. 233–247). Philadelphia: Lea & Febiger.

Chan, C. W., & Chang, A. M. (1999). Stress associated with tasks for family caregivers of patients with cancer in Hong Kong. *Cancer Nursing, 22,* 260–265.

Chang, C. F., & White-Means, S. I. (1991). The men who care: An analysis of male primary caregivers who care for frail elders at home. *Journal of Applied Gerontology, 10,* 343–348.

Chekryn, J. (1984). Cancer recurrence: Personal meaning, communication, and marital adjustment. *Cancer Nursing, 7,* 491–498.

Cummings, S. M., Long, J. K., Peterson-Hazan, S., & Harrison, J. (1998). The efficacy of a group treatment model in helping spouses meet the emotional and practical challenges of early stage caregiving. *Clinical Gerontologist, 20,* 29–45.

Cupp, P. (1998). Intimacy in the face of catastrophic illness. *Journal of Couples Therapy, 7,* 63–67.

Dempsey, K. (1997). Women's perceptions of fairness and the persistence of an unequal division of housework. *Family Matters, 48,* 15–19.

DeVries, H. M., Hamilton, D. W., Lovett, S., & Gallagher-Thompson, D. (1997). Patterns of coping preference for male and female caregivers of frail older adults. *Psychology and Aging, 12,* 263–267.

Dorval, M., Maunsell, E., Taylor-Brown, J., & Kilpatrick, M. (1999). Marital stability after breast cancer. *Journal of the National Cancer Institute, 91,* 54–59.

Douglass, L. G. (1997). Reciprocal support in the context of cancer: Perspectives of the patient and spouse. *Oncology Nursing Forum, 24,* 1529–1536.

Feigin, R., Greenberg, A., Ras, H., Hardan, Y., Rizel, S., Ben Efraim, T., & Stemmer, S. M. (2000). The psychosocial experience of women treated for breast cancer by high-dose chemotherapy supported by autologous stem cell transplant: A qualitative analysis of support groups. *Psycho-Oncology, 9,* 57–68.

Gerhardt, U. (1990). Qualitative research on chronic illness: The issue and the story. *Social Science & Medicine, 30,* 1149–1159.

Gilbar, O. (1999). Gender as a predictor of burden and psychological distress of elderly husbands and wives of cancer patients. *Psycho-Oncology, 8,* 287–294.

Given, B., & Given, C. W. (1992). Patient and family caregiver reaction to new and recurrent breast cancer. *JAMWA, 47,* 201–212.

Glasdam, S., Jensen, A., Madsen, E. L., & Rose, C. (1996). Anxiety and depression in cancer patients' spouses. *Psycho-Oncology, 5,* 23–29.

Goodman, M. (1989). Managing the side effects of chemotherapy. *Seminars in Oncology Nursing, 5,* 29–52.

Gotay, C. C. (1984). The experience of cancer during early and advanced stages: The views of patients and their families. *Social Science & Medicine, 18,* 605–613.

Hirsch, C. (1996). Understanding the influence of gender role identity on the assumptions of family caregiving roles by men. *International Journal of Aging and Human Development, 42*, 103–121.

Hoskins, C. N., Baker, S., Budin, W., Ekstrom, D., Maislin, G., Sherman, D., Steelman-Bohlander, J., Bookbinder, M., & Knauer, C. (1996). Adjustment among husbands of women with breast cancer. *Journal of Psychosocial Oncology, 14*, 41–69.

Irvine, D., Crooks, D., & Browne, G. (1991). Psychosocial adjustment in women with breast cancer. *Cancer, 67*, 1097–1117.

Kaye, L. W., & Applegate, J. S. (1990). *Men as caregivers to the elderly: Understanding and aiding unrecognized family support.* Lexington, MA: D.C. Heath.

Kilpatrick, M. G., Kristjanson, L. J., Tataryn, D. J., & Fraser, V. H. (1998). Information needs of husbands of women with breast cancer. *Oncology Nursing Forum, 25*, 1595–1601.

Knobf, M. T. (1990). Symptoms and rehabilitation needs of patients with early stage breast cancer during primary therapy. *Cancer, 66*, 1392–1401.

Kramer, B. J. (1997a). Differential predictors of strain and gain among husbands caring for wives with dementia. *The Gerontologist, 37*, 239–249.

Kramer, B. J. (1997b). Gain in the caregiving experience: Where are we? What next? *The Gerontologist, 37*, 218–232.

Kramer, B. J., & Lambert, D. (1999). Caregiving as a life course transition among older husbands: A prospective study. *The Gerontologist, 39*, 658–667.

Lamanna, M. A., & Riedmann, A. C. (1997). *Marriages and families: Making choices in a diverse society.* Belmont, CA: Wadsworth.

Lee, C. O. (1997). Quality of life and breast cancer survivors: Psychosocial and treatment issues. *Cancer Practice, 5*, 309–316.

Lewis, F. M. (1990). Strengthening family supports. *Cancer and the Family, Cancer Supplement, 65*, 752–759.

Lewis, F. M., & Deal, L. W. (1995). Balancing our lives: A study of the married couple's experience with breast cancer recurrence. *Oncology Nursing Forum, 22*, 943–953.

Lichtman, R. R., Taylor, S. E., & Wood, J. V. (1987). Social support and marital adjustment after breast cancer. *Journal of Psychosocial Oncology, 5*, 47–74.

Love, R. R., Leventhal, H., Easterling, D. V., & Nerenz, D. R. (1989). Side effects and emotional distress during cancer chemotherapy. *Cancer, 63*, 604–612.

Lutzky, S. M., & Knight, B. G. (1994). Explaining gender differences in caregiver distress: The roles of emotional attentiveness and coping styles. *Psychology and Aging, 9*, 513–519.

Maguire, P. (1981). The repercussions of mastectomy on the family. *International Journal of Family Psychiatry, 1*, 485–503.

Messeri, P., Silverstein, M., & Litwak, E. (1993). Choosing optimal support groups: A review and reformulation. *Journal of Health and Social Behavior, 34*, 122–137.

Morgan, M., Patrick, D. L., & Charlton, J. R. (1984). Social networks and psychosocial support among disabled people. *Social Science & Medicine, 19*, 489–497.

Moyer, A., & Salovey, P. (1999). Predictors of social support and psychological distress in women with breast cancer. *Journal of Health Psychology, 4*, 177–191.

National Cancer Institute. (2000). *Breast Cancer Physician Data Query (PDQ)*. CancerNet.

Neuling, A., & Winfield, H. R. (1988). Social support and recovery after surgery for breast cancer: Frequency and correlates of supportive behaviors by family, friend and surgeons. *Social Science & Medicine, 27*, 385–392.

Northouse, L. L. (1994). Breast cancer in younger women: Effects on interpersonal and family relations. *Journal of the National Cancer Institute Monograph, 16*, 183–190.

Northouse, L. L., Dorris, G., & Charron-Moore, C. (1995). Factors affecting couples' adjustment to recurrent breast cancer. *Social Science & Medicine, 41*, 69–76.

Northouse, L. L., & Swain, C. (1987). Adjustment of patients and husbands to the initial impact of breast cancer. *Nursing Research, 36*, 221–225.

Northouse, L. L., Templin, T., Mood, D., & Oberst, M. (1998). Couples' adjustment to breast cancer and benign breast disease: A longitudinal analysis. *Psycho-Oncology, 7*, 37–48.

O'Mahoney, J. M., & Carroll, R. A. (1997). The impact of breast cancer and its treatment on marital functioning. *Journal of Clinical Psychology in Medical Settings, 4*, 397–415.

Paci, E., Cariddi, A., Barchielli, A., Bianchi, S., Cardona, G., Distante, V., Giorgi, D., Pacini, P., Zappa, M., & Del-Turco, M. R. (1996). Long-term sequelae of breast cancer surgery. *Tumori, 82*, 321–324.

Pederson, L. M., & Valanis, B. G. (1988). The effects of breast cancer on the family: A review of the literature. *Journal of Psychosocial Oncology, 6*, 95–118.

Ptacek, J. T., Pierce, G. R., Dodge, K. L., & Ptacek, J. J. (1997). Social support in spouses of cancer patients: What do they get and to what end? *Personal Relationship, 4*, 431–449.

Rose, J. H. (1990). Spousal support and cancer: Adult patients' desire for support from family, friends, and health professionals. *American Journal of Community Psychology, 18*, 439–464.

Rose-Rego, S., Strauss, M. E., & Smyth, K. A. (1998). Differences in the perceived well-being of wives and husbands caring for persons with Alzheimer's disease. *The Gerontologist, 38,* 224–230.

Sabo, D., Brown, J., & Smith, C. (1986). The male role and mastectomy: Support groups and men's adjustment. *Journal of Psychosocial Oncology, 4,* 19–31.

Samms, M. C. (1999). The husband's untold account of his wife's breast cancer: A chronologic analysis. *Oncology Nursing Forum, 26,* 1351–1358.

Shelton, B. A., & John, D. (1993). Ethnicity, race and difference: A comparison of white, black and Hispanic men's household labor time. In J. C. Hood (Ed.), *Men, Work and Family* (pp. 131–150). Newbury Park, CA: Sage.

Siegel, K., Raveis, V. H., Mor, V., & Houts, P. (1991). The relationship of spousal caregiver burden to patient disease and treatment-related conditions. *Annals of Oncology, 2,* 511–516.

Smith, E. M., Redman, R., Burns, T. L., & Sagert, K. M. (1986). Perceptions of social support among patients with recently diagnosed breast, endometrial, and ovarian cancer: An exploratory study. *Journal of Psychosocial Oncology, 3,* 65–81.

Stetz, K. M. (1987). Caregiving demands during advanced cancer: The spouse's needs. *Cancer Nursing, 10,* 260–268.

Thoits, P. A. (1995). Stress, coping and social support processes: Where are we? What next? *Journal of Health and Social Behavior* (extra issue), 53–79.

Thompson, S. C., & Pitts, J. S. (1992). In sickness and health: Chronic illness, marriage and spousal caregiving. In S. Spacapan & O. Oskamp (Eds.), *Helping and being helped* (pp. 115–151). Newbury Park, CA: Sage.

Vinokur, A. D., & Vinokur-Kaplan, D. (1990). "In sickness and in health": Patterns of social support and undermining in older married couples. *Journal of Aging and Health, 2,* 215–241.

Walker, B. L. (1997). Adjustment of husbands and wives to breast cancer. *Cancer Practice, 5,* 92–98.

Weihs, K., Enright, T., Howe, G., & Simmens, S. J. (1999). Marital satisfaction and emotional adjustment after breast cancer. *Journal of Psychosocial Oncology, 17,* 33–49.

Wellisch, D. K., Fawzy, F. I., Landsverk, J., Pasnau, R. O., & Wolcott, D. L. (1983). Evaluation of psychosocial problems of the home-bound cancer patient: The relationship of disease and the sociodemographic variables of patients to family problems. *Journal of Psychosocial Oncology, 1,* 1–15.

Wellisch, D. K., Jamison, K. R., & Pasnau, R. D. (1978). Psychological aspects of mastectomy: The man's perspective. *American Journal of Psychiatry, 135,* 543–546.

Zahlis, E. H., & Shands, M. E. (1991). Breast cancer: Demands of the illness on the patient's partner. *Journal of Psychosocial Oncology, 9,* 75–93.

Services and Interventions

IV

Professional Sensitivity to Religion-Spirituality Among Male Caregivers

14

Jacqueline M. Stolley
Joan Chohan

INTRODUCTION

When men take on the responsibilities of caring for a cognitively or physically impaired spouse, do they draw upon their spirituality and religious beliefs? Are religion and spirituality an important underpinning to men's ability to provide care? Listen to a few men.

> The thing (about religion) that helps me the most is you enter the sanctuary and sit quietly for a while and I think sitting quietly before the service probably is the most religious moment of the morning. It helped me in my thoughts. Just some silent prayers. Religion is such a private thing.

> My spirituality certainly has helped (with the caregiving experience). I have more patience than you normally would have. My personal religiousness, prayer, faith in God, that's what keeps me going. . . . I guess moral support and spiritual support is what the church gives me.

> I just turned (the caregiving experience) over to the good Lord. You're never given any more than you can handle. And I had a group of men, young ones, old ones, the same thing they would say is "We're praying for you." My faith has gotten deeper. Now that I'm older, I can see why the good Lord prepared me for all of these things ahead of time.

> I would pray in the morning and wonder what now, am I doing the right thing? I almost got the feeling somebody was trying to tell me something.

These comments were made by older male caregivers in response to a question about what *most* helped them cope with the experience of caring for a person with Alzheimer's disease (Stolley, 1997). Their remarks certainly provide insight into the active coping of some male caregivers; more important, their comments signal the salience of religion and spirituality in helping the men persevere in the caregiving experience. Mentioned were organized religious activities, as well as the role the congregation plays in support of men's caregiving efforts. Private spiritual and religious activities such as sitting quietly in a sacred place or praying while caregiving were revealed. So was the men's reliance on a higher power for strength and guidance. In addition, those men who specifically identified prayer as a coping activity believed that prayer was effective in helping them (Stolley). The observation that religion may help strengthen men's caregiving is not unique to the chronic stress of caregiving. Prayer, affiliation with a religious community, and spirituality are important in mediating men's stress (Ellison & Levin, 1998; Maltby, Lewis, & Day, 1999; Pargament et al., 1990a, 1992; Ross, 1990). In view of the importance of religion and spirituality to a person's mental and physical health, this chapter examines the place of spiritual and religious coping among male caregivers.

MALE CAREGIVER SPIRITUALITY

When considering men's religiosity-spirituality, it is necessary to first have an understanding of the two terms "religiosity" and "spirituality." Important distinctions have been made between the two concepts. Religiosity entails the beliefs and practices associated with a person's affiliation with an organized religious group, such as a belief in an afterlife or routinely attending religious services. Measures of religiosity describe the motivational, cognitive, and behavioral aspects of "being religious" (cf., Batson & Ventis, 1982; Futterman & Koenig, 1995). Spirituality, by comparison, refers to an awareness of a higher power; it is a personal experience and may or may not include membership in a faith community. Spirituality has to do with the search for meaning, an ongoing process through which an individual becomes increasingly aware of meaning and life's ultimate significance (Ellison, 1983; Tillich, 1957). As much as religious involvement has traditionally been a means for the expression of spirituality, spirituality is ". . . more basic than, prior to, and different from traditional expressions of religiosity" (Elkins, Hedstrom, Hughes, Leaf, & Saunders, 1988, p. 6).

Paloutzian and Ellison (1982) and others have theorized spirituality as having two dimensions. A horizontal dimension is more existential and encompasses the individual's growing awareness of the ultimate meaning inherent in relationships and all activities of life; the vertical dimension moves the individual into a deeper and closer relationship with a higher being. Researchers are beginning to recognize that individuals may only develop the horizontal and not the vertical process, or vise versa (Black & Rubenstein, 1999; Payne, 1994). Some persons may define their spirituality in terms of relationships, the arts, nature, or another meaningful activity and never acquire a relationship with a deity. Sometimes, when an individual has a spiritual experience, that person will then begin to express spirituality through a religious tradition. Other individuals are drawn into a relationship with a higher being and may not develop ordinary methods of spiritual expression. Put simply, individuals subjectively define their own spirituality and religiousness, based on their concepts of being religious but not spiritual, being spiritual but not religious, or being both religious and spiritual (Zinnbauer et al., 1997).

Religion and spirituality are most likely bound in the caregiver's religious and ethnic culture. Although the majority of persons living in the United States are of the Judeo-Christian tradition, the variability of beliefs and practices is wide. For example, research on the religiosity and spirituality of African Americans shows that in most cases, religion is central to their lives (Levin & Taylor, 1993; Levin, Taylor & Chatters, 1994), although this finding seems to be more pronounced for women than men. Also, they found that differences exist between Southern and Northern Blacks in that Southern Blacks tend to be more devoted than those in the North. Also, the United States has experienced periodic influxes of immigrants who practice religious and spiritual traditions much different from the more common Judeo-Christian perspective. These include traditions such as Buddhism, Islam, and Hinduism. Not every tradition has the same concept of God and the purpose of life, and it is important for health care and social service providers to be sensitive to both ethnic and religious culture when considering the spirituality of male caregivers.

To date, there is a dearth of research on men's spirituality or religiosity in general, or male caregiver spirituality in particular. Research examining adults' religiousness provides sufficient evidence to conclude that men do value religion more in later life than in earlier life stages (e.g., Gallup & Lindsay, 2000), even though, on average, they are less religious than their wives and sisters (Bergan & McConatha, 2000). Research shows the gender gap in religiosity narrowing in older age (deVaus & McAllister, 1987). It remains unclear why there is more religious activity and greater spirituality among men who reach older ages. It could be the premature death of nonreligious men, the freedom of older men to engage in spiritual questing, the emergence of a particular need to find meaning in late life, or some combination of the three. Research also has shown religiosity is reliably associated with men's gender orientation (Francis & Wilcox, 1996; Remmes & Thompson, 2000). Greater religious belief and practice are reported by men with a developed feminine outlook, as operationally defined by their self-assessment on the Bem Sex-Role Inventory. By comparison, men with an undeveloped feminine and a strong masculine orientation have been described as religious risk-takers, because they are less likely to invest their identities and daily lives in the religious world (Miller & Hoffmann, 1995; Stark, 2000). Such men do not seriously consider religion or spirituality as part of the human condition (Black, 1995; Culbertson, 1994). Much of this depends on the ethnic and spiritual-religious culture of the male, however, and individualized assessment is imperative.

Men who become caregivers, therefore, are not always going to turn to religious and spiritual resources for coping when faced with the physical and emotional demands of caring. This was what Chang, Noonan, and Tennstedt's (1998) findings suggest. Men caregivers in their study were less engaged in religious-spiritual coping than women caregivers. But there are serious reservations that ought to be raised about this finding and ones like it. Researchers have routinely found women more religiously involved than men (deVaus & McAllister, 1987). Religion, it is sometimes argued, is a woman's calling. Therefore, using a single item measure of religious-spiritual coping ("My religion or spiritual beliefs have helped me handle this whole experience"), and comparing men to women, we will not learn much about the men caregivers who do use religious-spiritual coping. The gender-comparative methodology pushes to the background those men who use religious-spiritual coping compared with the women and the nonreligious men in a study. Men who have faith or who seek religious-spiritual relief become, statistically, the comparative-other with more religious women and the nonreligious men.

However, when separate estimates for men are calculated, as Ferraro and Kelley-Moore did in their analysis of the first two waves of American Changing Lives longitudinal survey, researchers can uncover the unique reasons men seek religious or spiritual meaning, comfort, and inspiration. As Ferraro and Kelley-Moore reported, co-morbidity, or the combination of diseases, especially serious or life-threatening ones, was key to religious consolation among men, whereas functional limitation dampened seeking spiritual or religious comfort. Depression and unemployment resulted in men turning to spiritual and religious sources. In effect, "men faced with physical and mental health problems turn to spiritual or religious sources for meaning and comfort" (p. 231).

RELIGION-SPIRITUALITY AND THE COPING PROCESS

Coping is a complex process that is initiated in response to an event or situation that is appraised by the individual as being either irrelevant, benign-positive, or stressful (Lazarus & Folkman, 1984). Depending on this appraisal, the individual mobilizes coping activities that mediate the effect of the event or situation, resulting in outcomes of social functioning, morale, and somatic health. This process can be applied to the caregiving situation, and spirituality and religion must be viewed as major variables affecting the coping process. A foundation of spirituality or religiousness can be viewed as a coping resource. Religious-spiritual beliefs or activities are mechanisms to help the individual caregiver cope. Spirituality and religiosity can fit into the process of coping in three ways: as an element of the coping process, as a contributor to the process, and as a product of the process. Therefore, an individual's spirituality or religiousness can influence the appraisal of the stressor and provide a context in which to mobilize coping activities. The health care and social service provider must understand that wide variations exist between beliefs and practices within a denomination that encompasses both liberal and conservative perspectives (e.g. Catholicism and Judaism), or Christians who are "fundamentalists" versus moderate or more liberal denominations. Buddhists, Hindus, and Moslems may have perspectives that are very foreign to the traditional Judeo-Christian majority but must be incorporated to adequately evaluate coping resources, interventions, and outcomes.

Coping resource.   Depending on the beliefs of the caregiver, religiousness or spirituality can be a resource or a constraint to coping (Pargament, 1990). For example, Mickley, Pargament, Brant, and Hipp (1998) found that hospice caregivers who appraised their experience as part of God's plan or as a way of becoming stronger and closer to God, reported positive mental and spiritual health outcomes. But caregivers who viewed their situation as an unjust and unfair punishment from God, or felt God had deserted them, had poorer mental and spiritual health.

Numerous studies have investigated the general importance of spirituality-religiosity in coping. Cox and Hammonds (1988) found that those persons who remain religiously active tend to have greater life satisfaction. Ferraro and Kelley-Moore (2000) reported that, for the most part, those men who are most likely to turn to religious or spiritual sources are those who are already religious. It was more the effects of men's religious participation than the salience of religious or spiritual beliefs that proved to be a stronger predictor of seeking religious consolation (p. 230). Other studies equally show that existing religious attitudes and beliefs appear to affect mental and physical health outcomes (Conway, 1985; Koenig, George, & Siegler, 1988; Manfredi & Pickett, 1987).

A sense of spirituality or religiousness can thus be a resource for caregivers when they face a situation appraised as stressful. Beliefs about God and personal control influence the individuals' appraisal and evaluation of the caregiving situation as something they can manage. More positive appraisal results in optimistic assessment of caregiving, and in turn results in better health outcomes, such as lower levels of depression and powerlessness (Cohen & Eisdorfer, 1988). Religious or spiritual beliefs contribute to the experience of caregivers finding meaning in the caregiving situation. Farran, Miller, Kaufman, and Davis (1994) reported that finding meaning, which is an expression of spirituality, had a direct effect in predicting caregiver depression and role strain, with persons who reported higher levels of provisional meaning reporting lower levels of detrimental outcomes.

Coping mediator.   Researchers have studied quite extensively the value of being religious or spiritual, both in the general population and among caregivers. They list religious-spiritual activities as forms of coping for older adults (e.g., Krause, 1992; Rosen, 1992; Stolley, Buckwalter, & Koenig, 1999; Whitlach, Meddaugh, & Langhout, 1992) and in numerous studies of ill populations (cf., Koenig & Futterman, 1995). Within the past two decades, there has been a general acceptance of research that examines the place of spirituality and religious involvement in health outcomes, particularly physical and mental health status, health care use, and adjustment to functional decline or aging (e.g., Koenig, 1995; Levin, 1994). Ironically, most of this work has treated spirituality and religiosity as the same phenomenon. That is, spiritual-religious coping typically comprises one of three forms: person's organized religious activity such as participating in religious services; the frequency of nonorganized religious activity such as prayer and reading religious material; or, the salience of religious belief, whether called "faith" or "intrinsic" beliefs. The working assumption is either faith or participation offers consolation.

Male caregivers may apply many different skills and techniques for their spiritual-religious coping. Dossey (1996) discusses the different methods in which persons use prayer in their daily lives. Many follow the formalities of a particular religious group and may pray for specific events to occur. They may pray to a personal god or goddess, a higher being. Some may pray to an impersonal Universe or Absolute. Others may not pray in any conventional sense but experience a deeply interiorized sense of the sacred, being attuned or aligned with "something higher." Similarly, Strawbridge, Shema, Cohen, Roberts, and Kaplan (1998) observed that religiosity-spirituality can buffer some stressors, but it may well exacerbate others. The health care or social service professional must understand these attitudes and the cultural context from which they emerge.

Spirituality must not be thought of as uncommon among men (cf., Katz, 1999). Men who are caregivers at times draw directly upon religious and spiritual resources when faced with the demands of caring (Black &

Rubenstein, 1999; Koenig, Pargament, & Nielsen, 1998). From interviews with men who were the primary caregivers to their wives, Black and Rubenstein found that older men search for meaning, and at times depend upon a high power. Using multi-item measures of caregiving men's religious-spiritual beliefs and their religious practices, Folkman and colleagues determined that religiosity-spirituality held importance for many of the gay men who were primary caregivers to their partners. Folkman, Chesney, Cooke, Boccellari, & Collette (1994) observed that HIV-positive men who cared for a partner with AIDS had higher levels of burden than HIV-negative men, and their religion-spirituality helped ease their caregiving burden. Richards and Folkman (1997) reported that experiences of the presence of the deceased partner, and a transcendent connection with people and events, were common during bereavement. These spiritual experiences and religious beliefs provided the emotional and cognitive resources to cope with the partner's death.

Studies have shown that the use of coping activities to mediate stress can be stable over time (Vitaliano, Maiuro, Ochs, & Russo, 1989) and vary by length of caregiving (Killeen, 1990). That is, spiritual-religious coping can vary with the type of stressor more than the duration of the stressor, or caregivers can change coping strategies as the care recipient deteriorates physically or mentally (cf., Williamson & Schulz, 1993). Although the men in their study used spiritual-religious coping less than the women, Chang et al. (1998) reported that men and women caregivers who used religious-spiritual beliefs to cope tended to have healthier relationships with the care recipient and displayed less evidence of their own depression.

In view of the likely importance of both religious involvement and spirituality as mediators in caregivers' stress-and-coping process, perhaps we need to pay greater attention to caregiver's spiritual needs. Long (1997) invites nurses to rethink what the promotion of spirituality would mean to the health of patients and caregivers. Stolley et al. (1999) recognized the importance of pastoral counselors and clergy in assisting men caregivers who are already religiously involved and not likely to directly report their distress with caregiving. Interventions to ensure these caregivers' spiritual well-being, which in turn assures the possibilities of effective coping, require appropriate assessment of both caregiver distress and spiritual health.

Outcomes: Religious-Spiritual Conservation and Transformation

Longitudinal studies have shown that religiousness or spiritual orientation is fairly stable throughout the life span, until late life when men are more likely to be open to spiritual growth. Cross-sectional studies have shown that people turn to religious and spiritual sources for coping when faced with the physical and emotional stresses of caregiving. What is not as clearly known is how stressful life events and caregiving combine and influence one's spirituality or religious involvement. Pargament (1997) theorizes that stressful life events often prompt spiritual-religious conservation (e.g., faith remains unchanged) or transformation (e.g., spiritual questing occurs, and the change is either positive or negative for the per son questing). When we consider the impact of the experience of caregiving—for example, the blow of the care-recipient's continued deterioration, or the drudgery of the daily responsibilities—on a man's spiritual-religious orientation, we might find changes in particular spiritual-religious activities or change altogether. Caregivers who are caring for an individual whose condition deteriorates progressively are likely to participate in fewer and fewer organized religious activities. Assuming that their faith is not rocked, they are as likely to increase their participation in nonorganized, personal religious activities. On the surface, their spiritual-religious involvement changes in forum, yet their spirituality or religiousness has conserved. Alternatively, male caregivers may become more spiritual and employ nonorganizational activities for coping, to provide them with the strength to deal with a progressively deteriorating care-recipient.

While these presumed pathways are logical and even evident among gay men who cared for a dying partner (Richards, Acree, & Folkman, 1999; Richards & Folkman, 1997), it is important for researchers to systematically examine the range of outcomes experienced by men engaged in caregiving. Recent research reported that older men who entered the caregiving role actually participated in more religious social events than a comparison group of non-caregivers (Kramer & Lambert). It remains unclear why there is more religious activity and greater spirituality among older men caregivers. Kramer and Lambert suggested that religious involvement may replenish social contact and emotional support that often diminishes in caregiving. Alternatively, it could be that the control group of non-caregivers comprises men who are religious risk-takers and thus not engaged in spirituality or a faith; it could be the emergence of a particular need among caregivers to find meaning; or, it may be some combination of the three.

Spiritual and religious conservation or transformation also may be a reflection of morale, and it may have an effect on morale. Changes in overall spirituality or religiousness are foreseeable outcomes in the stress and coping process (Pargament, 1990). For example, the male caregiver may feel closer to God and experience a deepening of faith as a result of the coping process, representing a religious response that many clergy might call "healthy." Several of the male caregivers cited at the beginning of this chapter illustrated this. On the other hand, the male caregiver may feel estranged from God, representing existential doubt and spiritual questing that many clergy may perceive as an "unhealthy" response. Thus, both the nature of the stressor and coping process and the caregiver's spiritual-religious resources can influence whether the individual experience changes that conserve current faith or transform belief (Pargament, 1997). Again, this conserve versus transform alternative points to the importance of health care and social service professionals' ability to assess a caregiver's spiritual well-being and, perhaps, spiritual need.

Because religious conservation or transformation can be considered outcomes, experienced in a different way by men than women caregivers, as well as considered resources in the ongoing stress-and-coping process, researchers and caregiving professionals need to become more attentive to men's unique needs. Specific religious and spiritual outcomes that evolve to become coping resources (or the loss of resources) need to be recognized as important to our research agenda. The influence of cultural factors must also be integrated. Outcome evaluation can provide more information about whether the caregiver is coping effectively, and whether spiritual-religious outcomes prove to be coping resources.

THE HEALTH AND SOCIAL SERVICE PROFESSIONAL ROLE

Professionals in nursing, medicine, social work, clinical psychology, and pastoral care have recognized the importance of attending to caregivers' spiritual or religious needs (cf., Hatch, Burg, Naberhaus, & Hellmich, 1998; Kaye & Robinson, 1994; Long, 1997; McSherry, 1987). Health and social service professionals can assess a male caregiver's spiritual and religious resources, determine his use of these resources for coping, and evaluate his spiritual-religious outcomes and their effectiveness. We will discuss these issues in the remainder of this chapter, along with relevant components of assessment, diagnosis, intervention, and outcomes. Not all professionals have the time or relationship with caregivers to perform a spiritual assessment or to develop a plan of care, but each discipline is becoming aware of either the necessity or value of planning religious and spiritual care for caregivers. The following has a decidedly Judeo-Christian bias, because very few studies have considered nontraditional spiritual-religious involvement.

Assessment and Religious History Taking

Spiritual-religious assessment essentially involves determining the caregiver's need to find meaning in existence. This type of assessment, or history taking (Rizzuto, 1996) includes both objective and interpretative data and incorporates both the horizontal and vertical processes described by Paloutzian and Ellison (1982) and Fitchett (1993). For example, a health professional may describe spiritual distress as a caregiver's inability to practice his spiritual-religious rituals. The objective assessment may include the male caregiver requesting spiritual materials or sacraments. In either case, the professional needs to interpret, determining if the caregiver is seeking a continuity of his spiritual-religious experience, is discouraged and exhibiting a feeling of emptiness, or is lacking an ability to forgive others and find meaning for himself. Often in this case, characteristic features are easily identifiable behavioral signs and symptoms, such as mood changes, psychomotor agitation, or disorientation.

Health care and social service professionals can evaluate both the horizontal and vertical processes of spirituality-religiosity to determine if the caregiver is where he wants to be. Evaluation of the horizontal process includes the male caregiver's values and relationships. The caregiver who has optimum outcomes in the horizontal process will express positive views of his future and a belief in himself. He may also express a sense of inner peace and self-control, as well as a zest for life. In addition, he may display a belief in others, whether it is his religious or spiritual group, a circle of friends, or his backup caregivers. He is able to forgive himself and others. This horizontal process may or may not include activity in a religious organization, but it definitely encompasses spiritual values that point to his own worth and the worth of others.

Evaluation of the vertical process may include many of the components of the horizontal process, but specifically the male caregiver's spirituality-religiosity. For healthy outcomes, he expresses hope and faith, the usefulness of prayer or meditation, and perhaps his participation in religious activities.

One most influential work on spiritual assessment is *The Minister as Diagnostician* (Pruyser, 1976). Pruyser wanted to encourage pastors to include spiritual assessment in their work. His model lists seven themes and key questions and has become the foundation of many other models of spiritual assessment. The method of information gathering in Pruyser's model addresses several significant aspects of spiritual life. The model uses open-ended questions and encourages insight into the reality of the caregiver's world. Once this information is gathered, the process of interpretation is left to the professional. Although this model is a dynamic approach to spiritual assessment, it is time-consuming and considerable training is required for effective use.

Another model, developed by a physician, is directed toward developing a clinical science in pastoral care and to assist chaplains in planning such care (McSherry, 1987). The information gathered can be also used by health disciplines. In addition to assessing health status, the model adds the Spiritual Profile Assessment, which caregivers can complete themselves, and the Semi-Structured Interview, which is a series of questions asked by the professional. McSherry's model seeks to be systematic and easy to administer. It does employ a Protestant Evangelical orientation and thus modifications are necessary to be helpful with caregivers of other Christian backgrounds or other faiths. Furthermore, in using this model, the healthcare professional must provide empathic understanding of the caregiver's unique experiences and needs.

Fitchett (1993) also developed what is called the 7 x 7 model of spiritual assessment for caregivers. This model envisions two dimensions of caregiver need: the holistic and the spiritual. The holistic dimension is subdivided into factors that range from intrapersonal to interpersonal, and the spiritual dimension incorporates a range of the intrinsic and behavior aspects of a caregiver's spirituality and religiosity. Assessment of both dimensions within the 7 x 7 model is perceived as vital to appreciate the individual caregiver's own perspective and to avoid imposing one's own values on the caregiver. The model encompasses such intrinsic characteristics as experiences, emotional tone, and feelings of obligation. The model is applicable in many settings; however, it also may be somewhat cumbersome for busy healthcare and social service professional to employ.

In addition to these three general models to assess spiritual-religious involvement and beliefs, several multi-item scales that index person's spirituality have become available over the past two decades. For example, the widely known Spiritual Well-Being Scale (SWBS; Ellison, 1983) measures spiritual and existential well-being, and the Spiritual Experience Index (SEI; Genia, 1991) measures spiritual development from an object relations perspective. Another strategy called the Nursing Outcomes Classification (NOC; Johnson, Maas, & Moorehead, 2000) provides indicators of "personal expressions of connectedness with self, others, and a higher power." This "spiritual well-being" assessment determines how compromised the caregiver's spirituality-religiosity is in Likert-type scales. One measure developed specifically to assess African American spirituality is the Spirituality Scale (Jagers & Smith, 1996). Another often used instrument assessing spiritual-religious motivation, the Religious Life Inventory (Batson, 1976), incorporates assessments of a person's intrinsic and extrinsic motivations and a third, called questing.

Whatever model or technique the professional chooses to use to assess the religiosity-spirituality of the male caregiver, it is vital that the professional be mindful of the demands and sensitivity needed to engage in spiritual assessment and religious history taking. A simple determination of religious belief and practice does not provide an adequate account of the caregiver's spirituality or the role of religion in the caregiver's life.

Diagnosis

In 1978, the North American Nursing Diagnosis Association (NANDA) approved "spiritual distress" as a nursing diagnosis and has since added "potential for enhanced spiritual well-being" (1994) and "risk for spiritual distress" (1998). Spiritual Distress (or Distress of the Human Spirit) is "disruption in the life principle that pervades a person's entire being and that integrates and transcends one's biological and psychosocial nature" (NANDA, 1999, p. 69). A nursing diagnosis is made based on evidence gleaned from assessment data (symptoms or defining characteristics) and related factors. For example, the diagnosis of Spiritual Distress may be related to challenged belief and value system (e.g., illness of the care recipient), as evidenced by behaviors such as anger, crying, withdrawal, or hostility. Among other evidence for this diagnosis is his expressions of concern with the meaning of life and death, his belief system, or his questions about the meaning of suffering.

The male caregiver may not have an actual response to caregiving that contributes to a problem such as spiritual distress, but the professional identifies risks for spiritual distress or the potential for him to grow spiritually through the caregiving experience. A diagnosis of Risk for Spiritual Distress, in which he is "at risk for an altered sense of harmonious connectedness with all of life and the universe in which dimensions that transcend and empower the self may be disrupted" (NANDA, 1999, p. 68). Some factors gleaned from the assessment data that may indicate he is at risk for spiritual distress are low self-esteem, energy-consuming anxiety, substance abuse, and loss of a loved one. Opportunities for enhancing the male caregiver's strengths can be incorporated using the nursing diagnosis Potential for Enhanced Spiritual Well-Being, which is ". . . the process of an individual's developing-unfolding of mystery through harmonious interconnectedness that springs from inner strengths" (NANDA, p. 68). Evidence may be his inner strengths or his connectedness with himself, others, a higher power, and the environment.

The NANDA diagnoses of spiritual distress, well-being, and risk for spiritual distress are very practical. They enable health care and social service professionals to understand the likelihood of "spiritual pain" and "religious pathology," and diagnosis affords ways to address the caregiver's spiritual needs. Although initially designed to be used by nurses, NANDA diagnoses have been developed in such a way that other disciplines can use them for spiritual assessment and diagnosis. The specificity of the defining characteristics, or symptoms, is also a major strength of this particular approach.

The American Psychological Association (1994) included a diagnostic category in the 4th edition of the *DSM* (the *Diagnostic and Statistical Manual of Mental Disorders*) under "other conditions that may be a focus of clinical attention." The *DSM* diagnosis has been criticized because of the potential for the clinician's lack of sensitivity to culture within diagnoses, resulting in misdiagnosing a culturally bound condition as pathology. For example, Turner, Lukoff, Barnhouse, and Lu (1995) strongly encourage the clinician to consult with a religious professional or traditional healer when one encounters a person with a belief system that differs markedly from the clinician's. This sensitivity to nontraditional spirituality-religiousness or to caregiver's with traditional religious involvement but with spiritual problems, enables the mental health professional to recognize a component of mental health need that had previously been ignored or pathologized. Again, the importance of ethnic and religious culture cannot be minimized.

Intervention

Potts (1998, p. 509) would argue that during the course of caregiving, men "may have inadvertently become disengaged from involvement with a community of faith, or suspended spiritual practices which had been as source of strength and comfort in the past." When the caregiver's spirituality is at risk, is distressed, or can be enhanced, the nurse, health psychologist, or social service professional can intervene in ways that are comfortable for both the professional and the caregiver himself. Spiritual or religious interventions may well be uncomfortable for professionals in the United States, where spiritual and religious beliefs are personal and diverse, and rights are fiercely guarded. Religious and spiritual practices may reflect cultural traditions that are foreign to the "mainstream." However, spirituality and religiousness have become widely recognized as components of legitimate health care, and despite one's comfort level, it is the responsibility of each health care and social service professional to address rather than ignore caregivers' spiritual needs. Accrediting agencies such as the Joint Commission for Accreditation of Healthcare Organizations stress the need for spiritual and cultural assessment and intervention in health care facilities.

Nursing Interventions Classification (NIC) has compiled a number of standardized interventions that are nurse driven, along with possible nursing activities that support the intervention (McCloskey & Bulechek, 2000). NIC interventions are relevant for other health care professionals such as occupational therapists and rehabilitation therapists. Among the most relevant interventions for male caregivers is providing spiritual support to address "spiritual distress." Among examples of supportive interventions include "being open to patient's expressions of loneliness and powerlessness," and "Listen carefully to patient's communication, and develop a sense of timing for prayer or spiritual rituals" (p. 607).

These interventions can be adapted to traditional Judeo-Christian practices as well as to those religious and ethnic cultures less common in the United States.

Spiritual support refers to assisting the caregiver to feel balanced and connected to a higher power (McCloskey & Bulechek, 2000). By contrast, spiritual growth facilitation is another intervention wherein the health psychologist, nurse, social worker, or physician facilitates the caregiver's capacity to identify, connect with, and call upon his spirituality. Professionals can help the male caregiver by developing with him a plan to resume his spiritual-religious preferences, beliefs, and commitment. Religious reframing (Pargament, 1997) or constructing an account of the caregiver's experience as parallel to one found in religious texts may trigger a renewed sense of meaning, coherence, and hope.

A third intervention assists the caregiver as he explores his beliefs about a punishing, unforgiving God or about a benevolent, supportive God. It is important to explore the way the caregiver interprets forgiveness, and whether forgiveness is an important part of the caregiver's accounts. Black (2000), however, cautions that the subject of forgiveness is a problematic topic, perhaps because it presupposes the caregiver did something "wrong" or a "wrong" was committed against the caregiver. Forgiveness can be a powerful force that enhances personal well-being and alleviates inappropriate anger and bitterness (McCullough, Pargament, & Thoresen, 2000; Rye et al., 2000). All health care and social service professionals can be attentive to this issue and can refer the caregiver to a trained health psychologist, social worker, or religious leader.

Many religious congregations have on-site nurses or volunteers who can be a tremendous influence on the male caregiver's religious and spiritual well-being. These individuals are educated to assist persons from the faith community. Both health care and social service professionals can initiate the use of these resources and can facilitate their participation in supporting the religious and spiritual care of the male caregiver. Referring the caregiver to his pastor or spiritual leader, or eliciting the support of his religious congregation, can be powerful activities to facilitate spiritual growth, especially in view of findings that male caregivers tend to participate in social religious events (Kramer & Lambert, 1999). Depending on the extent and type of interaction with the caregiver, the health care or social service professional can implement the intervention according to a needs-specific spiritual assessment.

Outcomes

Outcomes associated with men caregivers' spirituality-religiosity can be envisioned in a variety of ways, such as the men's level of social functioning or expressions of meaning, hope, and communion with a higher power. An outcome identified by Nursing Outcomes Classification (NOC) (Johnson et al., 2000) is Spiritual Well-Being. Each outcome "label" is defined, with a series of indicators that are periodically scored on a Likert-type scale on a continuum from 1 (extremely compromised) to 5 (not compromised). The professional can assess progress toward an outcome using this scale. The NOC outcome label of Spiritual Well-Being is defined as "personal expressions of connectedness with self, others, higher power, all life, nature, and the universe that transcend and empower the self" (p. 407). Among the indicators are "expressions of faith," "interaction with spiritual leaders", and "connectedness with others to share thoughts, feelings, and beliefs." These indicators are germane to spirituality or religiosity of many ethnic and spiritual traditions.

NOC allows the health care professional to reassess and evaluate the caregiver's spiritual and religious needs and progress, and to identify specific areas that need attention. As with NIC, NOC can be used as an interdisciplinary tool for measuring outcomes and the effects of interventions.

As noted earlier, religion-spirituality can be powerful resources for caregiver coping, but they also can become a constraint (Pargament et al., 1990). For example, if the male caregiver believes that the situation is "punishment from God" because of some religious teaching or belief, he may develop attitudes that make him take his punishment (conservation), or he may find ways to replace this attitude so that his interpretation is less harsh, more healthy, and transformed. It is noteworthy that a male caregiver with no religious or spiritual inclination may emerge from his experience as someone who now bases life on the spiritual. Someone else who has a rich spiritual-religious life may experience a deepening of faith and spirituality. Understanding the caregiver's ethnic and spiritual culture is an important component of assessing outcomes in a holistic way.

SUMMARY AND CONCLUSIONS

This chapter provides a selection of operational theories and models that can assist health care and social service professionals in their understanding of the spiritual-religious needs of men involved in caregiving. The importance of religiosity and spirituality in the stress and coping process, particularly for male caregivers whose caregiving is as often ignored as are their spiritual needs, cannot continue to be ignored. Health care professionals must be sensitive to these areas, perform a spiritual assessment, and develop a plan of care for the caregiver derived from this assessment along with assessment of the culture of the caregiver. As the number of male caregivers increases, the health and social service professions will be eventually called upon to assess and intervene.

The role of spirituality and religiosity in mental and physical health is an emerging area of study. Much more research is needed to identify the conditions under which spirituality-religiosity is and is not a coping resource, a useful mediator balancing the stresses of caregiving, and a transformed outcome that recycles to become a positive or negative coping resource. In particular, research must be done on how male caregivers can best use these resources to meet both their caregiving and their spiritual needs. This chapter has demonstrated that a systematic body of research on men's spirituality-religiosity and caregiver well-being does exist and can assist professional assisting caregivers. By taking a functional perspective to understand that religious and spiritual activities and beliefs can successfully sustain meaning and promote caregivers' resilience and adjustments, health care and social service professionals can become more sensitive to the religious, spiritual, and cultural needs of the male caregiver and can facilitate the care recipient's continued care.

REFERENCES

American Psychological Association. (1994). *Diagnostic and statistical manual of mental disorders,* (4th ed.) Washington, DC: American Psychological Association Press.

Batson, C. D. (1976). Religion as prosocial: Agent or double agent? *Journal for the Scientific Study of Religion, 15,* 29–45.

Batson, C. D., & Ventis, W. L. (1982). *The religious experience: A social-psychological perspective.* New York: Oxford University Press.

Bergan, A., & McConatha, J. T. (2000). Religiosity and life satisfaction. *Activities, Adaptation, and Aging, 24*(3), 23–34.

Black, H. K. (1995). "Wasted lives" and the hero grown old: Personal perspectives of spirituality by aging men. *Journal of Religious Gerontology, 9*(3), 35–48.

Black, H. K. (2000). *To forgive is—amazing: Elders' narratives of forgiveness.* Paper presented at the annual meeting of the Gerontological Society of America, Washington, DC.

Black, H. K., & Rubenstein, R. (1999). *No one laughs his way through life: The spiritual value of suffering in aged men.* Paper presented at the annual meeting of the Gerontological Society of America, San Francisco.

Chang, B. H., Noonan, A. E., & Tennstedt, S. L. (1998). The role of religion/spirituality in coping with caregiving for disabled elders. *The Gerontologist, 38,* 463–470.

Cohen, D., & Eisdorfer, C. (1988). Depression in family members caring for a relative with Alzheimer's disease. *Journal of the American Geriatrics Society, 34,* 493–498.

Conway, K. (1985). Coping with the stress of medical problems among black and white elderly. *International Journal of Aging and Human Development, 21*, 39–48.

Cox, H., & Hammonds, A. (1988). Religiosity, aging, and life satisfaction. *Journal of Religion and Aging, 5*(1/2), 1–21.

Culbertson, P. (1994). *Counseling men.* Minneapolis, MN: Fortress Press.

deVaus, D., & McAllister, I. (1987). Gender differences in religion: A test of the structural location theory. *American Sociological Review, 51*, 472–481.

Dossey, L. (1996). *Prayer is good medicine: How to reap the healing benefits of prayer.* New York: HarperCollins.

Elkins, D. N., Hedstrom, L. J., Hughes, L., Leaf, J. A., et al. (1988). Toward a humanistic-phemenological spirituality: Definition, description, and measurement. *Journal of Humanistic Psychology, 28*(4), 5–18.

Ellison, C. W. (1983). Spiritual well-being: Conceptualization and measurement. *Journal of Psychology and Theology, 11*, 330–340.

Ellison, C. G., & Levin, J. S. (1998). The religion-health connection: Evidence, theory, and future directions. *Health Education & Behavior, 25*, 700–720.

Farran, C. J., Miller, B., Kaufman, J. E., & Davis, L. (1994). *Finding meaning as a moderator of caregiver distress: A comparison of African American and white caregivers of persons with dementia.* Unpublished manuscript.

Ferraro, K. F., & Kelley-Moore, J. A. (2000). Religious consolation among men and women: Do health problems spur seeking?. *Journal for the Scientific Study of Religion, 39*, 220–234.

Fitchett, G. F. (1993). *Assessing spiritual needs: A guide for caregivers.* Minneapolis, MN: Augsburg Fortress.

Folkman, S., Chesney, M. A., Cooke, M., Boccellari, A., & Collette, L. (1994). Caregiver burden in HIV positive and HIV negative partners of mens with AIDS. *Journal of Consulting and Clinical Psychology, 62*, 764–756.

Francis, L. J., & Wilcox, C. (1996). Religion and gender orientation. *Personality and Individual Differences, 20*, 119–121.

Futterman, A. M., & Koenig, H. G. (1995). Measuring religiosity in later life: What can gerontology learn from the sociology and psychology of religion? In *Methodological approaches to the study of religion, aging and health.* Washington, DC: National Institute of Aging.

Gallup, G., & Lindsay, D. M. (2000). *Surveying the religious landscape: Trends in U.S. beliefs.* New York: Morehouse.

Genia, V. (1991). The Spiritual Experience Index: A measure of spiritual maturity. *Journal of Religion and Health, 30*, 337–347.

Hatch, R. L., Burg, M. A., Naberhaus, D. S., & Hellmich, L. K. (1998). The Spiritual Involvement and Beliefs Scale: Development and testing a new instrument. *Journal of Family Practice, 46*, 476–486.

Jagers, R. J., & Smith, P. (1996). Further examination of the spirituality scale. *Journal of Black Psychology, 22*, 429–442.

Johnson, M., Maas, M., & Moorehead, S. (2000). *Nursing outcomes classification (NOC)*, (2nd ed.) St. Louis, MO: Mosby.

Katz, J. (1999). *Running to the mountain: A journal of faith and change.* New York: Broadway Books.

Kaye, J., & Robinson, K. M. (1994). Spirituality among caregivers. *IMAGE: Journal of Nursing Scholarship, 26,* 218–221.

Killeen, M. (1990). The influence of stress and coping on family caregivers' perceptions of health. *International Journal of Aging and Human Development, 30,* 197–211.

Koenig, H. G. (1995). *Research on religion and aging.* Westport, CT: Greenwood.

Koenig, H. G., & Futterman, A. M. (1995). Religion and health outcomes: A review and synthesis of the literature. In *Methodological approaches to the study of religion, aging and health.* Washington, DC: National Institute of Aging.

Koenig, H. G., George, L. K., & Siegler, I. C. (1988). The use of religion and other emotion-regulating coping strategies among older adults. *The Gerontologist, 28,* 303–310.

Koenig, H. G., Pargament, K. I., & Nielsen, J. (1998). Religious coping and health status in medically ill hospitalized older adults. *Journal of Nervous & Mental Disease, 186,* 513–521.

Kramer, B. J., & Lambert, J. D. (1999). Caregiving as a life course transition among older husbands: A prospective study. *The Gerontologist, 39,* 658–667.

Krause, N. (1992). Stress, religiosity, and psychological well-being among older blacks. *Journal of Aging and Health, 4,* 412–439.

Lazarus, R. S., & Folkman, S. (1984). *Stress, appraisal, and coping.* New York: Springer.

Levin, J. S. (1994). *Religion in aging and health.* Thousand Oaks, CA: Sage.

Levin, J. S., & Taylor, R. J. (1993). Gender and age differences in religiosity among Black Americans. *The Gerontologist, 33,* 16–23.

Levin, J. S., Taylor, R. J., & Chatters, L. M. (1994). Race and gender differences in religiosity among old adults: Findings from four national surveys. *Journal of Gerontology: Social Sciences, 49,* S137–S145.

Long, A. (1997). Nursing: A spiritual perspective. *Nursing Ethics, 4,* 496–510.

Maltby, J., Lewis, C. A., & Day, L. (1999). Religious orientation and psychological well-being: The role of the frequency of personal prayer. *British Journal of Health Psychology, 4,* 363–378.

Manfredi, C., & Pickett, M. (1987). Perceived stressful situations and coping strategies utilized by the elderly. *Journal of Community Health Nursing, 4,* 99–110.

McCloskey, J. C., & Bulechek, G. M. (2000). *Nursing interventions classifications (NIC).* St Louis, MO: Mosby.

McCullough, M. E., Pargament, K. I., & Thoresen, C. E. (2000). The psychology of forgiveness: History, conceptual issues, and overview. In M. E. McCullough & K. I. Pargament (Eds.), *Forgiveness: Theory, research, and practice* (pp. 1–14). New York: Guilford.

McSherry, E. (1987). The modernization of chaplaincy. *Care Giver, 4*(1), 1.

Mickley, J. R, Pargament, K. I., Brant, C. R., & Hipp, K. M. (1998). God and the search for meaning among hospice caregivers. *Hospice Journal, 13*(4), 1–17.

Miller, A. S., & Hoffmann, J. P. (1995). Risk and religion: An explanation of gender differences in religiosity. *Journal for the Scientific Study of Religion, 34*, 63–75.

North American Nursing Diagnosis Association (NANDA). (1999). *Nursing diagnoses: Definitions and classifications.* Philadelphia: North American Nursing Diagnosis Association.

Paloutzian, R., & Ellison, C. W. (1982). Loneliness, spiritual well-being, and the quality of life. In A. Peplau & D. Perlman (Eds.), *Loneliness: A source book of current theory, research, and therapy* (pp. 224–237). New York: Wiley.

Pargament, K. I. (1990). God help me: Toward a theoretical framework of coping for the psychology of religion. *Research in the Social Scientific Study of Religion, 2*, 195–224.

Pargament, K. I. (1997). *The psychology of religion and coping.* New York: Guildford.

Pargament, K. I., Ensing, D. S., Falgout, K., Olsen, H., Reilly, B., van Haitsma, K., & Warren, R. (1990). God help me (I): Religious coping efforts as predictors of the outcomes to significant negative life events. *American Journal of Community Psychology, 18*, 793–824.

Pargament, K. I., Ensing, D. S., Falgout, K., Olsen, H., Reilly, B., van Haitsma, K., & Warren, R. (1992). God help me (II): The relationship of religious orientation to religious coping with negative life events. *Journal for the Scientific Study of Religion, 31*, 504–513.

Payne, B. P. (1994). Faith development in older men. In E. Thompson (Ed.), *Older men's lives* (pp. 85–103). Thousand Oaks, CA: Sage.

Potts, R. G. (1998). Spirituality, religion, and the experience of illness. In P. Camic & S. Knight (Eds.), *Clinical handbook of health psychology: A practical guide to effective interventions* (pp. 495–522). Kirkland, WA: Hogrefe & Huber.

Pruyser, P. (1976). *The minister as diagnostician.* Philadelphia: Westminster.

Remmes, K. R., & Thompson, E. H. (2000). *The differential effects of gender orientation and masculinity ideology on older men's religious involvement.* Paper presented at the annual meeting of the Gerontological Society of America, Washington, DC.

Richards, T. A., Acree, M., & Folkman, S. (1999). Spiritual aspects of loss among partners of men with AIDS: Postbereavement follow-up. *Death Studies, 23,* 105–127.

Richards, T. A., & Folkman, S. (1997). Spiritual aspects of loss at the time of a partner's death from AIDS. *Death Studies, 21,* 527–552.

Rizzuto, A. (1996). Psychoanalytic treatment and the religious person. In E. P. Shafrankse (Ed.), *Religion and the clinical practice of psychology* (pp. 409–431). Washington, DC: American Psychological Association.

Rosen, C. C. (1982). Ethnic differences among impoverished rural elderly in use of religion as a coping mechanism. *Journal of Rural Community Psychology, 3,* 27–34.

Ross, C. E. (1990). Religion and psychological distress. *Journal for the Scientific Study of Religion, 29,* 236–245.

Rye, M. S., Pargament, K. I., Ali, M. A., Beck, G. L., Dorff, E. N., Hallisey, C., Narayanan, V., & Williams, J. G. (2000). Religious perspectives on forgiveness. In M. E. McCullough & K. I. Pargament (Eds.), *Forgiveness: Theory, research, and practice* (pp. 17–40). New York: Guilford.

Stark, R. (2000). *Sociology* (8th ed.). Belmont, CA: Wadsworth.

Stolley, J. M. (1997). *Religiosity and coping for caregivers of persons with Alzheimer's disease and related disorders.* Unpublished doctoral dissertation. Iowa City: University of Iowa.

Stolley, J. M., Buckwalter, K. C., & Koenig, H. G. (1999). Prayer and religious coping for caregivers of persons with Alzheimer's disease and related disorders. *American Journal of Alzheimer's Disease, 14,* 181–191.

Strawbridge, W. J., Shema, S. J., Cohen, R. D., Roberts, R. E., & Kaplan, G. A. (1998). Religiosity buffers effects of some stressors on depression but exacerbates others. *Journal of Gerontology: Social Sciences, 53,* S118–S126.

Tillich, P. (1957). *Dynamics of faith.* New York: Harper.

Turner, R. P., Lukoff, D., Barnhouse, R. T., & Lu, F. G. (1995). Religious or spiritual problem: A culturally sensitive diagnostic category in the DSM–IV. *Journal of Nervous and Mental Disease, 183,* 435–444.

Vitaliano, P. P., Maiuro, R. D., Ochs, R. D., & Russo, J. (1989). A model of burden in caregivers of DAT patients. In E. Light & B. Lebowitz (Eds.), *Alzheimer's disease treatment and family stress: Future directions for research* (pp. 267–291). Washington, DC: U.S. Government Printing Office.

Whitlatch, A. M., Meddaugh, D. I., & Langhout, K. J. (1992). Religiosity among Alzheimer's disease caregivers. *American Journal of Alzheimer's Disease and Related Disorders and Research, 7*(6), 11–20.

Williamson, G., & Schulz, R. (1993). Coping with specific stressors in Alzheimer's disease caregiving. *The Gerontologist, 33,* 747–755.

Zinnbauer, B. J., Pargament, K. I., Cole, B., Rye, M. S., Butter, E. M., Belavich, T. G., Hipp, K. M., Scott, A. B., & Kadar, J. L. (1997). Religion and spirituality: Unfuzzing the fuzzy. *Journal for the Scientific Study of Religion, 36,* 549–564.

Principles and Interventions for Working Therapeutically With Caregiving Men: Responding to Challenges

15

Sam Femiano
Aimee Coonerty-Femiano

The needs of men who are caregivers are determined by a variety of factors, including the impact of prior gender socialization, the emotional and psychological development of the caregiver, the family constellation within which the man is living, and the particular stressors and challenges that he must face. In this chapter, the caregiver will be understood as any man who is charged primarily or secondarily with the informal care of another. Although male caregivers provide care in any number of settings, the focus of this chapter will be on clinical and informational needs of men giving care to family members, and gay men caring for their partners or friends. This chapter will review common challenges facing male caregivers, will articulate principles and interventions for responding to these challenges, and is intended to serve as a resource for individual therapists and counselors, social service providers, and facilitators of informal and formal support groups.

As noted earlier in this volume (e.g., see chaps. 4 and 5) and by other scholars (Jackson, Chatters, & Taylor, 1993), little empirical attention has been given to the experiences of culturally diverse subpopulations of male caregivers. One comparative study suggested that African American men may be more comfortable shifting into the caregiving role than Caucasian men (Miller & Kaufman, 1996). Although several studies have included samples that cross class lines (Arber & Gilbert, 1989; Harris, 1995; Szinovacz, 1989), we have gained little insight regarding specific needs of men that vary by socioeconomic status. Gaps in knowledge seriously limit understanding of culturally appropriate and relevant interventions for diverse groups of men. As suggested interventions reviewed in this chapter are primarily based on prior research, they are likely to be biased to Caucasian, middle-class samples. There is clearly a need to attend to these gaps in knowledge in future research if culturally sensitive interventions are to be developed.

MALE GENDER SOCIALIZATION

The social construction of "gender" is a pervasive reality that affects not only men's own psychological and emotional well-being, but also the ways in which society is structured, and the demands and expectations placed on men. As such, it is essential that clinicians understand the construct of gender socialization and the implications for working with the male caregiver. Without this basic understanding, men's roles and contributions to care risk being misconstrued and undervalued. In the literature on caregivers, gender issues and male caregivers are receiving more attention. Often, however, this attention sees gender as simply another trait, without recognizing the complexity in how males view themselves and how they are engaged in their roles and in the world. In this chapter we consider the intrapsychic and interpersonal effects of gender socialization as necessary considerations in clinical assessment and intervention processes.

The sociological picture of the past two decades that portrayed caregiving solely as a "woman's issue" is changing as we become more cognizant of men's divergent and growing contributions to caregiving, and as definitions of caregiving are expanded to include a broader scope of tasks, responsibilities, and approaches (Dwyer & Coward, 1992; Harris, 1995; Morano, 1998; Neal, Ingersoll-Dayton, & Starrels, 1997). As dimensions of men's caregiving roles evolve, public perception needs also to evolve and to accept and expect that men will and do take on caregiving functions (Kramer, 1997; Marks, 1996; Thompson, 1994; Walker, 1992). One role of clinicians will be to help men by elucidating the parameters of their caregiving function as their evolving public role is defined (Arber & Gilbert, 1989; Kramer & Lambert, 1999).

As this evolution takes places, one must beware of merely interchanging the roles of men and women and seeing that as a reversal of the traditional gender paradigm. A true understanding of gender requires that both men's and women's roles be seen not as interchangeable polarities, but rather as the manifestations of the needs and capacities of the individuals themselves, with whatever patterns of behavior and personality configurations fit their own sense of self and the social situation in which they function (Harris, 1995; Levant & Pollack, 1995).

The range of male caregiving is broad, and men will approach caregiving tasks differently according to their understanding of their roles, their sense of maleness, expectations of others, and their relationships (Harris, 1995). For some men, re-education and reconceptualizing their self-concept may be part of that task and clinicians will need to work with men in a context that is consonant with their own self-concept and understanding of the male role while helping them accept new demands and changes in their lives. For other men, their understanding of themselves and the meaning of maleness may be more contemporary and they will approach their tasks with a more complex perspective, thus allowing clinicians a wider range of intervention. In either case, however, male socialization will play a role and its repercussions will need to be taken into account.

Anyone wishing to intervene in men's lives must act not out of prede-termined notions about men, but rather seeing individual men in their uniqueness and individuality. For example, an older man caring for an ailing spouse may show his care and loving attention differently from a younger man caring for a long-term partner with AIDS, or from an adult son caring for a father with Parkinson's disease. The underlying desire to respond to the needs of a loved one, however, may be the same and vali-dating that desire and the experiences and challenges of caregiving is essen-tial. As in all therapeutic interventions, knowing that you are not deviant or unusual is the first step to accepting yourself and your experience.

It is equally important to understand how men perceive themselves in their caregiving roles. For example, contrary to stereotypical representations of men, Kaye and Applegate (1990) reported that older male caregivers described their attitudes and behaviors as more affective than instrumental. This finding may give clinicians pause when they assess men in compari-son to the masculinity stereotype. Male caregivers may seek support from clinicians or support groups to affirm their nontraditional self-image. As Kaye and Applegate warn, "the degree of androgeny reflected in our find-ing suggests that those planning policies, programs and services for male elder caregivers should not restrict themselves to traditional conceptions of the male gender role. Rather, planners should be guided by a flexible view of mid- and late-life that takes men's nurturant, expressive strivings into consideration. Such a view makes it possible to help men benefit from elder caregiving as a potentially gratifying developmental opportu-nity" (p. 224).

Any discussion of the clinical and informational needs of men then, must not only take into consideration the impact of gender stereotypes and gender socialization, but also the societal structures that dictate how we view men in the caregiving system (Arber & Gilbert, 1989; Meth & Pasick, 1990). Thompson makes the point that male caregivers are consid-ered deviant because, if they approach their caregiving differently from that of women, they are seen as deviant from women, but if they function as caregivers in the same mold as women, they are seen as deviant from men (Thompson, 2000). This prejudice about men's abilities and men's roles has led many people to overlook men's contributions or to dismiss them as not relevant. The lens through which one looks at a phenomenon determines how one sees the phenomenon, and looking at caregiving through the lens of gender socialization enriches our understanding of the caregiving population and the ways in which they care.

COMMON CHALLENGES

Challenges facing male caregivers have direct bearing on the concomitant needs to be met and subsequent interventions for responding to those needs. Each of these challenges and ways of responding to these challenges will need to be individually assessed and tailored. We will briefly highlight common challenges experienced and reported by male caregivers, followed by an articulation of principles and interventions that professionals may utilize in responding to these challenges.

Stressors

The stressors of informal caregiving are well documented through decades of research. In their review of the literature on stressors studied specifically among male caregivers, Carpenter and Miller in chapter 5 of this text note that illness variables (e.g., cognitive impairment, memory and behavior problems among elders with dementia), and physical and psychosocial deterioration of the care receiver have significant detrimental impacts on the well-being of male caregivers. Men who enter the caregiving role are often challenged to respond to and manage a variety of illness symptoms brought on by progressively debilitating physical, emotional, or cognitive impairments.

New Tasks and Skills

A related challenge is that many illness symptoms require male caregivers to learn and engage in new tasks and skills. For example, although health care providers typically spend years in training to learn about illnesses and how to manage and treat them, most adults receive little or no preparation for these functions. In addition, as men enter the caregiving role they may need to learn how to engage in household tasks that were previously performed by the care-receiver. For example, several large- and small-scale studies have reported the presence of traditional gender differentiation in the division of household responsibilities in later-life families (Ade-Ridder & Brubaker, 1988; Szinovacz, 1989). Spouses become more involved in household tasks that are not traditional for their gender if their partner has serious health problems (Kaye & Applegate, 1994; Wright, 1993). Husbands who entered the caregiving role reported approximately 7 more hours per week on average performing the tasks of meal preparation, dishes, cleaning, shopping, and laundry compared with husbands with well spouses (Kramer & Lambert, 1999). For some men, the challenge of learning several new skills while at the same time coping with multiple losses associated with caregiving may provoke a tremendous sense of anxiety (Kramer, 2000).

Detriments to Well-Being

The strains of caring for another person often bring about fatigue, feelings of insecurity, and general declines in psychological well-being (Schulz & Williamson, 1991; Zarit, Todd, & Zarit, 1986). The most common effects of caregiver stress are depression, anxiety, guilt, self-blame, psychosomatic disorders, and the exacerbation of long-standing interpersonal problems (Gottlieb, 1997; LeBlanc, Aneshensel, & Wight, 1995; Marquis, 1993; Toseland & Rossiter, 1989). When compared with noncaregiving males, male caregivers to persons with dementia and AIDS reported higher levels of depression (Folkman, Chesney, & Christopher-Richards, 1994; Fuller-Jonap & Haley, 1995); more difficulty sleeping and taking regular exercise; more respiratory problems; using more over-the-counter medications; and higher levels of psychoticism (Fuller-Jonap & Haley). Older men who transitioned into the caregiving role reported less happiness and more depression than husbands with well spouses (Kramer & Lambert, 1999).

Grief

Critical to any understanding of men's needs as caregivers is the pervasiveness of grief as an underlying dynamic to be dealt with (Rudd, Viney, & Preston, 1999; Walker & Pomeroy, 1996). Several studies have documented a grief response among caregiving men (e.g., Folkman, Chesney, & Christopher-Richards, 1994; Harris, 1993, 1995; Kaye & Applegate, 1990; Siriopoulos, Brown, & Wright, 1999). Grief is the emotional reaction to loss (Kramer, 2000; Weiss & Richards, 1997), and caregiving is fraught with a multitude of losses. Men whose wives experience debilitating illness for example, may suffer the simultaneous loss of a partner, a confidant, and a companion as well as finding themselves thrust into dramatic changes in lifestyle imposed by new sets of demands. Exacerbating their grief may be other losses of friends and family. Gay men who lose their partners are more susceptible to complicated grief because they have usually lost many close friends over the course of the years resulting in the accumulation of losses. Unanticipated loss or loss in relationships that were already troubled can be even more difficult to assimilate. An additional factor making grief a challenge is society's lack of acknowledgment of the grief process in those who are caregiving because their partner is still present (Rudd et al. 1999, Walker & Pomeroy, 1996). Grief in men, particularly older men whose socialization fostered emotional restraint, is not always immediately evident, and their need to grieve may even be met with resistance. It is incumbent upon professionals working with grieving men that they themselves be comfortable with grief and have the ability to be fully present to the grief response of men.

Changes in Social Life

Several qualitative studies have noted the challenges regarding changes in the male caregiver's social life such as increased sense of social isolation (Harris, 1993, 1995), and declines in social and recreational activities (Revenson & Majerovitz, 1991), and emotional support (Kramer & Lambert, 1999). Older husbands who transitioned into the caregiving role reported greater declines in marital happiness and perceptions that their marriages were in trouble than non-caregiving men with well spouses (Kramer & Lambert). As a result of illness or of placement of care-receivers in institutional settings, male caregivers may experience changes in their sexual relationships that exacerbate feelings of isolation.

Lack of Attention to Self-Care

The tendency to ignore one's physical, emotional, and psychological needs is an often unacknowledged challenge facing many male caregivers (Sabo & Gordon, 1995). Men are socialized to be self-reliant, confident, uncomplaining, rational, courageous, focused on solving problems, good providers, able to endure stress and pain, and dependable (Staudacher, 1991). These are all qualities that serve men, their families, and society well, but they also may make take a serious toll, preventing the kinds of self-care that might make their lives easier and, ultimately, longer. As a group, men tend to ignore physical complaints until they have become serious and impair their functioning (McFarland & Sanders, 1999), and often guard their feelings, remain silent, or become immersed in activity when confronted with challenging emotions (Staudacher, 1991). As noted by Adler, Patterson, and Grant (chap. 6), several studies have noted a greater level of physiological disturbance among caregiving men than among caregiving women. These studies, however, have not addressed the extent to which emotional restraint may contribute to these higher levels of disturbance among male caregivers.

Going Against the Mainstream

For adult sons who assume full-time responsibility for a parent, there is the issue of being outside of the career mainstream of their friends and relatives (Harris, 1993). This lack of consonance with their peers can bring with it a lowering of their self-esteem and questions about their manliness. It is not easy going against the mainstream of gender stereotypes, and it requires emotional strength as well as an intellectual understanding of the role.

Gay caregivers, more so than other caregivers, feel the stresses that arise from gender role expectations. There are few role models to help them in their task of caring for a loved one who is terminally ill (DeCarlo & Folkman, 1996; Frediksen, 1999). In general, they are still working, which makes full-time care more stressful, and their sense of the orderliness of the world, which has been destroyed by the presence of the disease, disorients them in their vision of life and brings on feelings of depression and despair (Clipp, Adinolfer, Forrest, & Bennett, 1995; Folkman, Chesney, Cooke, Boccellari, & Collette, 1994). Further, fears about their own physical well-being and their susceptibility to being HIV+ affect their mental and emotional states and, as a corollary, their caregiving capacity. As a result, these fearful and grieving caregivers find themselves with even more stress and they need particular attention paid to their situation (O'Connor, 1997; Park & Folkman, 1997). LeBlanc et al. (1995) reported that increased levels of depression among gay caregivers were caused by secondary stressors such as work-related strain and financial hardship more so than the effects of providing primary care.

In sum, there are a multitude of challenges facing men caregivers that are related to the tasks, demands, responses, changes, and effects of caregiving, and that are influenced by gender socialization processes and expectations of others. The needs of caregivers that accompany these challenges include the need for validation, emotional and social support, information and education, assistance with practical concerns, and skills training. The following principles and interventions are designed with these needs in mind.

PRINCIPLES FOR WORKING WITH MEN

There are several general principles that practitioners should consider when responding to the challenges of male caregivers. Although the focus of this chapter is on "clinical" and direct service approaches, service providers are obliged to see their clients not only in the context of their individual lives, but to advocate for systems and social policy changes that will benefit informal caregivers more broadly (e.g., paternal and elder care leave).

Validate the Individual's Approach and Experience

As noted previously, men may approach their caregiving tasks with a style different from women. For example, they may be more active and show their affection by doing rather than by talking (Kaye & Applegate, 1990). Such an approach is not wrong, but simply different, and men need to be validated by clinicians and other service providers. Clinicians should honor unique approaches and give caregivers permission to pave their own path. Professionals should be aware of their own biases about males, should validate the contributions these men seek to make, and should acknowledge the beneficial experiences of caregiving as well as the challenges.

Build on Strengths and Foster Sense of Control

Although caregivers often must to learn new skills and face new challenges in caregiving tasks, it is essential that we acknowledge not only their capability of making changes but also their unique strengths (e.g., qualities, traits, values, and coping skills) to do so. Clinicians should strive to identify and help caregivers to recognize the unique strengths and skills that they bring to their role. Even amidst many challenges, many men creatively adjust, learn, and do quite well. They may take on new challenges in much the same way that they have approached prior jobs (e.g., determining a task approach), but this does not negate the affective foundation of their caregiving nor lessen their commitment and competence (Harris, 1993). Indeed, their approach may allow them to succeed in their caregiving role. Men, generally, are task-oriented and enjoy problem solving. Interventions with men need to build on the skills that men already have and, through these skills, help them to move ahead into new areas of functioning (Davies, Priddy, & Tinklenberg, 1986). In enlisting the strengths and skills that men have already developed, clinicians will put men at ease and give them a sense of competence and success. In so doing, they may ease insecurities and allow for the expression of more challenging emotions. Beginning with men's socialized expectation of themselves is the most effective way to expand men's horizons and allow them to grow.

It is essential that men feel respected and that their feelings and experiences are not pathologized (Gwyther, 1992; Kramer, 2000). It may be necessary for clinicians to approach their interactions with caregivers more as partners in problem solving, rather than as "expert." Clinicians who are accustomed to treating mental and emotional disturbances must be cautious to avoid the hierarchical stance often common in traditional therapeutic situations. The relationship of the clinician to the caregiver needs to be more facilitative with the clinician listening attentively to the caregiver, placing emphasis on his capabilities and strengths, and enlisting his aid in problem solving or working through feelings and other challenges (Folkman, Chesney, Christopher, & Richards, 1994). This approach especially suits men who are accustomed to task- oriented work relationships, and is more likely to engender a sense of control.

Conduct Comprehensive Psychosocial Assessments

Psychosocial assessments should minimally include attention to stressors, appraisals of stressors, resources available to the caregiver (e.g., social and financial support, coping strategies), and attention to the potential impacts of caregiving (i.e., depression, burden, well-being). Exploring the caregiver's assessment of the ways in which their life has changed as a result of caregiving, and the challenges and needs they currently face, is central to individualizing the approach for responding to those needs. Professionals should distinguish between grief and depression and, in the area of depression, between clinical depression and "transient dysphoric mood" (Walker & Pomeroy, 1996). They also need to share this diagnostic information with caregivers in order to explore treatment options and plans. Among caregivers of persons with AIDS clinicians need to assess for signs of AIDS-Related Burnout such as constant fatigue, frequent illness, depression, isolation, carelessness, addictive behaviors, and emotional flatness (Clipp, Adinolfe, Forrest, & Bennett, 1995). Severe burnout can be doubly harmful because it often leads to physical and emotional harm to the caregiver, and interferes with effective caregiving (Kairos, 1999).

In planning for clinical and informational interventions, it is useful to know which coping strategies caregivers themselves already use (McFarland & Sanders, 1999). Several coping instruments are available for use (e.g., see Kramer & Vitaliano for a review); however, even simple inquiries such as "What is most stressful to you about caring for your partner?" and "How have you been coping with this stress?" may be most revealing. Are they coping by drinking alcohol? Taking medications? Exercising? Expressing anger? It is also useful to determine how effective they perceive their coping strategies have been and to explore other strategies they have used in the past to cope with challenging situations. A study by DeVries and Hamilton (1997) on older male and female caregivers, which differentiated active cognitive and active behavioral coping approaches, reported a combination of approaches. Practical and concrete strategies such as "took things one day at a time" and "knew what had to be done and tried harder" were the most frequently endorsed responses. Interestingly, "talked with a professional person" was at the bottom of the list of strategies chosen by these caregivers.

Recognize the Depth and Breadth of Unexpressed Feeling

Another important principle for working with male caregivers is the recognition that men have a depth and breadth of caring and feeling that is not always immediately evident to the outside observer (Lynch & Kilmartin, 1999). Davies et al. (1986) reported that in their male caregiver groups, "Most men . . . were more interested in the interpersonal aspects of the group than in the development of more problem-solving methodologies." Men who are caregivers for older adults reported affection and concern for the caregiver as the most common motive for caregiving (Caregiver of the Year; Kramer, 1997; Schulz & Williamson, 1991). For gay men, this issue is also salient because the affectional base of their caring is often at the core of their caring efforts (Clipp et al., 1995).

As noted previously, men may find it challenging to express but may nevertheless be experiencing profound loss, grief, sadness, frustration, anxiety, and a sense of insecurity. Grief often underlies other feelings and is best treated through psychoeducational means and therapeutic support (Gilbar, 1997; Walker & Pomeroy, 1997). It is important to aid expression of thoughts and feelings to the extent that the caregiver is willing, be alert to their need to talk (Kramer, 2000), and identify and give names to feelings because men have generally not been socialized to identify these types of feelings even when they are experiencing them (Levant & Pollack, 1995; Lynch & Kilmartin, 1999). Normalizing and validating these feelings, explaining why they come about, and seeing them as manageable are the first steps a clinician should undertake when working with male caregivers.

Consider Developmental Needs

Various cohorts of men present with different sets of values and developmental needs. Older men who were raised in a generation when stereotypical male roles were more the norm may find it much harder to recognize their needs and to talk about them, and may have less experience engaging in household tasks traditionally performed by older wives (Davies et al., 1986). By comparison, younger caregivers who have lived through the various revolutions of the 1960s and '70s may be more accustomed to role changes and expression of feelings. As noted previously they also may be experiencing other strains such as launching careers and concomitant work role strains. Older men may be more accustomed to taking life as it comes without questioning and not complaining, and their caregiving may become knotted with issues of transition into retirement and the practical reality that their own deaths are now closer. Different age groups will vary in their receptivity to psychotherapeutic interventions and perceptions of social welfare services. Interventions will need to take into consideration the particular life tasks, values, attitudes, experiences, and approaches of men at different phases of the life cycle.

Foster Emotional and Social Support

As noted previously, male caregivers often feel isolated and alone in the caregiving role and that as social support declines, caregiver depression increases (Schulz & Wiliamson, 1991). Howard Shapiro (Caregiver of the Year) reported that the most difficult part of caregiving is "Going alone, doing it all yourself. The loneliness of being a care person. You're a one man band, you play all the instruments." Clinicians and other service providers need to assist men with practical concerns and emotional support (Folkman, Chesney, & Christopher-Richards, 1994; Wrubel & Folkman, 1997). Clinicians "should work to foster supportive relationships among this population and to educate other family members about the importance of social contact" (Kramer, 2000, p. 22). Practitioners should help men understand the essential role of social support to their well-being and work with them to determine the best strategies to enhance this resource. Later in this chapter we will provide several suggestions for fostering support through individual psychotherapy and group-based interventions. Other strategies for fostering a sense of support are to provide linkages for men to connect with other caregivers through buddy systems, male support groups, and phone support. In addition, many male caregivers are finding the Internet a valuable way to connect with a virtual support group (Caregiver of the Year).

Provide Information and Education

Information and education are essential needs of all caregivers. In the literature on caregiving, a distinction often is made between the degree to which men and women seek information, with men considered more instrumental and less engaged (Dwyer & Coward, 1992) and their need for data and facts a way of managing care from a distance. From the perspective of gender socialization, however, this trait is better understood not as distancing, but as functional. Information for men is a way of entering into a situation more deeply, understanding the context, and then being able to provide for the needs of the care-recipient more fully. Their liking for information is not a way of avoiding personal involvement, but rather providing a foundation for more fully connecting with their care-recipients (Harris, 1993). Men feel more secure if they know the context, the lay of the land, as it were, which can then allow them to take personal risks and be more vulnerable. It provides men with a way of structuring their world and providing a context within which they can deal with the other needs they have (Harris, 1993; McFarland, & Sanders, 1999; Morano, 1998).

Depending on the situation, informational needs can range from learning about the course and presentation of the illness and medical procedures that will be used, such as administering injections, to knowing the types, range, and availability of support services (Folkman, Chesney, & Christopher-Richards, 1994). This need for medical data and training is particularly important for caregivers of persons with complex medical needs (e.g., late-stage Alzheimer's disease and AIDS), or persons with challenging cognitive or behavioral symptoms (e.g., dementia). Often, knowing how to react in a particular situation or knowing what is happening medically with the care-recipient is sufficient to lessen the worry and concern that accompany caregiving. For men, particularly, this is an important need because they are accustomed to obtaining facts and data before acting and will be more inclined to seek out support services, for example, if they are well informed of the usefulness and scope of such services (Stommel, Collins, Given, & Given, 1999)

Assist with Practical Concerns and Future Planning

Responding to the caregiver's day-to-day practical concerns is not only necessary but serves as a vehicle to foster the therapeutic alliance. Providing information about financial resources or community supports may help caregivers to navigate confusing service systems. Planting seeds of information about practical resources should be done prior to the time that formal services are required to allow time to process and explore options. Educating caregivers about illness trajectories and the ways in which they might prepare legally and financially for the future may facilitate a sense of control. One husband caregiver explained that the hardest part of caregiving was "Knowing what to expect next. With any form of dementia, you never know . . . what's around the corner. If I knew what was coming, then I could anticipate and get the necessary medical supplies. I could structure my life more quickly to adapt. And, if I knew about how much time was left, I could do some financial planning to make sure we could make it. I would feel more in control. Now, I'm always reacting" (Caregiver of the Year). Men often worry about their financial resources and how often they will last. They should be encouraged to have Advanced Directives, wills, and other documents in place in the event that they or their partners die or need invasive medical treatments.

Provide Skills Training and Encourage Self-Care Strategies

As noted previously, many illness symptoms require male caregivers to learn and engage in new tasks and skills. These men may benefit from active engagement in training sessions or classes to teach these skills. Caregivers of persons with dementia will often need to learn how to manage challenging behaviors and symptoms of the illness and how to communicate best with this population. Men who are just learning how to cook, clean, do laundry, and shop for groceries may appreciate the opportunity to formally learn these skills and share strategies with other caregivers. Given the stressful nature of informal caregiving in all contexts, stress management techniques such as progressive relaxation, visualization, and biofeedback may be helpful.

INTERVENTIONS

In addition to understanding the challenges facing male caregivers, and the principles that will allow clinicians to respond to their common needs, there are additional considerations for determining how to best intervene with men caregivers. First, depending on the stage of caregiving and the particular characteristics of the caregiver, interventions for male caregivers will range widely (Siriopoulos et al., 1999). As noted by Pearlin and Aneshensel (1994) caregiving may be conceptualized as a "career" that involves several stages and transitions. In the initial stage, the caregiver must cope with the impact of the diagnosis. Practical information about the disease, community resources, and treatment options are very important, as is information of the course of the illness and its prognosis (Cummings, 1996). The following stages of care, during which decisions about continuing to be a caregiver and the place in which care will be given, require both informational interventions and support for dealing with emotions (Dello Buono et al., 1999). The final stages of dealing with the death of the loved one and moving on with life again require a new set of coping mechanisms and interventions (Pfeiffer, 1999).

Second, the choice of intervention will be determined by the particular characteristics, values, motivations, and needs of the caregiver. For example, in a qualitative study of older husbands caring for wives with dementia, Harris (1993) reported that these men fell into four categories with each benefiting from alternative interventions and approaches. For those men who approach caregiving as an extension of their work life, men who are task oriented and rational, pragmatic interventions are most useful. For those caregivers who see their caregiving as a "labor of love" and expend all their time and energy on the care-recipient, social isolation is a serious risk and they need encouragement in seeking out social supports. For men who care out of a "sense of duty," the third category, volunteerism, has been found to be a helpful support because it extends their basic stance into the world where they can receive validation and support. "Men at the crossroads," the fourth group, are those trying to make a decision about possible placement of their care recipient. These men are in crisis and need immediate assistance in the form of information and problem solving (Rosenthal, Sulman, & Marshall, 1993).

Third, the caregivers sense of spirituality or religiosity may serve as a resource for intervention approaches. A study done by Kramer and Lambert (1999) found that men who entered the caregiving role reported an increase in time spent in religious social events as compared with non-caregiving men. Data drawn from a longitudinal study of caregiving and bereavement among partners of men with AIDS revealed that "spiritual beliefs and experiences provided emotional and cognitive resources for coping with high levels of distress" (Richards, Acree, & Folkman, 1999). Religious institutions that play a role in the lives of male caregivers may be utilized more often as places where interventions can take place. Richards and her colleagues found that gay caregivers who had a strong spirituality were more able to enter into and work through the grieving process. Their spirituality, which remained with them and informed their lives after bereavement, made their healing process shorter and more peaceful. Given the importance of religion, religious institutions, and spirituality in the lives of older caregivers, it seems that clinicians and other professionals might begin to make more use of these supports as they plan interventions.

Two specific forms of intervention include psychotherapy and group work. The research on the use and usefulness of psychotherapy for caregiving populations is limited and ambivalent. DeVries and Hamilton (1997) reported that psychotherapy is very low on the list of coping strategies used by older husbands and adult sons. Gay caregivers, on the other hand, use psychotherapy extensively to deal with depression (LeBlanc et al., 1995). These results are sparse and difficult to interpret because there is little information on the types of therapy in question or on the attitudes of the therapists toward the caregivers. Nonetheless, the decision to provide individual therapy may be an appropriate one for particular caregivers. Even though there is some commonality among male caregivers, there is also considerable individual difference because of their diverse backgrounds and psychological development (Harris, 1995; Scher, Stevens, Good, & Eichenfield, 1987). At times these differences may require the privacy of individual therapy, where the client can speak without fear of being misconstrued or where personal issues that would have no relevance in a group can be discussed and dealt with (see LeBlanc et al.). If psychotherapy is to be effective with male caregivers, it must be practical and focused on the particular characteristics of the male socialization process. The usefulness of individual psychotherapy should not be underestimated but its form will depend on the needs of the individual caregiver in question (Folkman et al., 1994).

The entry point to working with men and their feelings in therapy may be difficult because men are frequently unwilling to disclose what they perceive as negative affect, which might then be construed as making them appear weak or vulnerable (Davies et al., 1986). In addition, because of their socialization, many caregivers may not have learned the skills they would need to talk about the feelings causing them distress. This reticence to reveal self-doubt and lack of skill to disclose their distress and feelings can be a challenge to planning services because the clinician is called upon to see through the mask of control to the vulnerability beneath it. Depending on the type of intervention in question, a variety of techniques can be used. It is often helpful for clinicians to describe the underlying feelings directly and ask the caregiver if the description has any relevance to their current emotional state. Encouraging men to talk about their caregiving experiences provides a non-threatening way for clinicians to explore feelings (Folkman, 1997). Teaching men relaxation techniques as a way of becoming more centered and introspective also may be helpful (Femiano, 1992). For clinical interventions to be therapeutic, the clinician must be flexible and creative, able to keep the caregiver's context in mind and willing to shift gears as crises arise.

Group interventions are an important service for any caregiving population (Cummings, 1996; Gilbar, 1997; Toseland & Rossiter, 1989). They are seen as mutual support systems in which members share their concerns, find acceptance of their feelings, learn problem-solving and coping skills, learn about resources, and gain practical skills (McFarland & Sanders, 1999). Caregiver groups can be organized with or without professional facilitators. To be optimally helpful, the goals of the group must be clear from the beginning. Support groups with their emphasis on information, teaching coping skills and sharing experience, should be distinguished from therapeutic groups with their focus on interpersonal dynamics and feelings. Again, the distinction between grief and depression is useful for determining the focus of a group. Caregivers who are grieving would do best with information about the disease and about community resources as well as an understanding of their feelings, whereas caregivers whose main difficulty is depression would do better with a cognitive group focussed on alleviation of symptoms (Gendron, Poitras, Dastoor, & Perodeau, 1996; Walker & Pomcroy, 1996). An evaluative study of 29 groups (Toseland & Rossiter, 1989) reported the most common themes in educational and support groups included:

- medical information about the care-receiver's situation
- the emotional impact of caregiving and its adverse effects
- self-care
- dealing with problematic interpersonal relationships between caregiver and care-receiver
- home care skills
- the development and use of outside support systems

Psychotherapy groups will have a different set of expectations and characteristics. The focus will be more personal, delving into the motivations and psychological issues of the men in the group and helping them to function more effectively as caregivers through giving them a better understanding of their own inner dynamics. Such groups require a higher level of psychological insight on the part of the participants and a consistent commitment of time. They also require a willingness to be vulnerable and open about one's own inner life. For older men, in general, such groups may be less appealing because their socialization did not include such expectations. Nonetheless, such groups may be helpful because they provide access to deeper healing work, and participants may gain a sense of inner calm that will help them weather the storm of their caregiving work.

Participant characteristics will always be an initial consideration in forming a group. It is frequently useful to do an initial assessment in the early group sessions, asking the participants to articulate their goals and expectations. This list can then serve as an informal agenda, to be revised as new members enter and the caregivers' concerns evolve. For the populations being considered in this chapter, groups made up only of men may well be the most appropriate intervention (Harris, 1995; Kaye & Applegate, 1990). Older men will often do best in an all-men's group because they will feel less constrained to maintain their façade of self-sufficiency and will not be intimidated by the verbal proficiency of women (Davies et al., 1986; Kaye & Applegate, 1990). Men's groups also have the advantage of fostering mutuality and minimizing competitiveness as men discover they are not alone in their concerns and fears.

In providing clinical and informational groups for men, clinicians must remember that, although the needs of men are much the same as those of women, men use a different language to express their needs. The language they use to communicate their care and concern may be more instrumental than that of women, and it will be important to look through the surface to the meaning underneath. It will also be important to look at men's actions and evaluate them as the expression of their thinking and feeling even when they cannot articulate those same feelings and thoughts. An often neglected aspect of working with men is their ability to use humor and laughter as a way of talking about difficult topics (Caregiver of the

Year). The traditional psychotherapeutic view of laughter would see it as an avoidance technique, but, in support groups, it can bring men together and help them speak about their issues. For this reason, it should be fostered. Group cohesiveness is important for the success of any group and, to this end, members should be encouraged to be supportive and open, sharing their own experiences and knowledge. Group members should also feel free to contact each other outside of the group.

In planning groups, several logistical considerations need to be kept in mind. Because many caregiving situations are long term, long-term groups are often preferable (Gendron et al., 1996; Harris, 1993). Groups should also be organized to allow men flexibility in attendance. Men who are caring for ill partners, whether aged or not, will have times of crisis when group participation is not possible because of other demands on their time. Also, men who are caring for someone long term may occasionally not come to group because they need a break from therapeutically oriented activities. For these reasons, a group that is open will serve them best.

Depending on the population, the time at which groups meet may also be a consideration. For example, employed caregivers may find it difficult to meet during the day. Group cost may also be a factor in determining the extent of their participation, so subsidized groups may be the only way to attract certain men in need. Finally, since men are often more hesitant to join groups, the advertising and the promotion of the group needs to be done in a way that will attract them. Several useful marketing strategies are noted by Kaye (chap. 16) late in this volume. Davies, Priddy, and Tinklenberg promoted their all-male groups by telling the prospective participants that they were seeking volunteers to pilot a new intervention for male caregivers and were asking the men to provide them with feedback concerning the relevance of the concepts and interventions tested in the new groups (Davies et al., 1986).

CONCLUSION

The changing understanding of the meanings of masculinity and the appreciation of the impact of gender socialization is redefining the roles our society has assigned to men and women in the past and has given a new freedom for both men and women to express their own potential. As this evolution takes place, the numbers of informal male caregivers in our health care system is increasing, their roles are becoming more important, and their unique contributions more apparent. These changes challenge service providers to broaden their own understanding of the significant difficulties facing male caregivers. In this chapter, we have articulated several principles for therapeutically responding to the common needs of male caregivers to facilitate these efforts. As noted earlier, much work remains to be done to identify the unique experiences and needs of diverse subpopulations of men caregivers so that culturally and economically relevant interventions may be developed and evaluated.

REFERENCES

Ade-Ridder, L., & Brubaker, T. (1988). Expected and reported division of responsibility of household tasks among older wives in two residential settings. *Journal of Consumer Studies and Home Economics, 12*, 59–70.

Arber, S. & Gilbert, N.. (1989). Men: The forgotten caregivers. *Sociology 23*(1), 111–118.

Clipp, E. C., Adinolfe, A. J., Forrest, L., & Bennett, C. L. (1995). Informal caregivers of persons with AIDS. *Journal of Palliative care, 11*(2), 10–18.

Cummings, S. M. (1996). Spousal caregivers of early stage Alzheimer's patients: A psychoeducational support group model. *Journal of Gerontological Social Work, 26*(3/4), 83–98.

Davies, H., Priddy, J. M., & Tinklenberg, J. R. (1986). Support groups for male caregivers of Alzheimer's patients. *Clinical gerontologist, 5*(3/4), 385–395.

DeCarlo, P., & Folkman, S. (1996). *Are informal caregivers important in AIDS care?* [on-line]. Available: www.hivpositive.com/index.html.

Dello Buono, M., Busato, R., Mazzetto, M., Paccagnella, B., Aleotti, F., Zanetti, O., Bianchetti, A., Trabucchi, M., & De Leo, D. (1999). Community care for patients with Alzheimer's disease and non-demented elderly people: Use and satisfaction with services and unmet needs in family caregivers. *International Journal of Geriatric Psychiatry, 14*, 915–924.

DeVries, H. M., & Hamilton, D. W. (1997). Patterns of coping preferences for male and female caregivers of frail older adults. *Psychology and Aging, 12*(2), 263–267.

Dwyer, J. W., & Coward, R. T. (Eds.). (1992). *Gender, families and elder care.* Newbury Park, CA: Sage.

Femiano, S. D. (1992). The role of affect in therapy with men. *The Journal of men's studies, 1*(2), 117–124.

Folkman, S. (1997). Introduction to the special section: Use of bereavement narratives to predict well-being in gay men whose partners died of AIDS—four theoretical perspectives. *Journal of Personality and Social Psychology, 72*(4), 851–854.

Folkman, S., Chesney, M. A., & Christopher-Richards, A. (1994). Stress and coping in caregiving partners of men with AIDS. *Psychiatric Clinics of North America, 17*(1), 35–53.

Folkman, S., Chesney, M. A., Cooke, M., Boccellari, A., & Collette, L. (1994). Caregiver burden in HIV-positive and HIV-negative partners of men with AIDS. *Journal of Consulting and Clinical Psychology, 62*(4), 746–756.

Frediksen, K. I. (1999). Family caregiving responsibilities among lesbians and gay men. *Social work, 44*(2), 142–155.

Fuller-Jonap, F., & Haley, W. E. (1995). Mental and physical health of male caregivers of a spouse with Alzheimer's Disease. *Journal of Aging and Health, 7,* 99–118.

Gendron, C., Poitras, L., Dastoor, D. P. & Perodeau, G. (1996). Cognitive-behavioral group intervention for spousal caregivers: Findings and clinical considerations. *Clinical Gerontologist, 17*(1), 3–19.

Gilbar, O. (1997). Cancer caregiver support group: A model for intervention. *Clinical Gerontologist, 18*(1), 37.

Gottlieb, B. (Ed.). (1997). *Coping with chronic stress.* New York: Plenum.

Gwyther, L. (1992). Research on gender and family caregiving: Implications for clinical practice. In J. W. Dwyer & R. T. Coward (Eds.), *Gender, Families, and Elder Care.* Newbury Park, CA: Sage.

Harris, P. B. (1993). The misunderstood caregiver? A qualitative study of the male caregiver of Alzheimer's disease victims. *The Gerontologist 33*(4), 551–556.

Harris, P. B. (1995). Differences among husbands caring for their wives with Alzheimer's disease: Qualitative findings and counseling implications. *Journal of Clinical Geropsychology, 1*(2), 97–106.

Jackson, J. S., Chatters, L. M., & Taylor, R. J. (Eds.). (1993). *Aging in Black America.* Newbury Park, Sage.

Kairos support for Caregivers. (1999). *Are you ARB+* [on-line]. Available: www.The-Park.com/Kairos.

Kaye, L. W., & Applegate, J. S. (1990). *Men as caregivers to the elderly: Understanding and aiding unrecognized family support.* Lexington, MA: D. C. Heath and Company.

Kaye, L. W., & Applegate, J. S. (1994). Older men and the family caregiving orientation. In E. H. Thompson, Jr. (Ed.), *Older men's lives* (pp. 218–236). Thousand Oaks, CA: Sage.

Kramer, B. J. (1997). Differential predictors of strain and gain among husbands caring for wives with dementia. *The Gerontologist, 37*(2), 239–249.

Kramer, B. J. (2000). Grief and bereavement in older men. *Geriatric Care Management Journal, 10*(1), 17–23.

Kramer, B. J., & Lambert, J. D. (1999). Caregiving as a life course transition among older husbands: A prospective study. *The Gerontologist 39*(6), 658–667.

Kramer, B. J., & Vitaliano, P. P. (1994). Coping: A review of the theoretical frameworks and the measures used among caregivers of individuals with dementia. *Journal of Gerontological Social Work, 23*, 151–174.

LeBlanc, A. J., Aneshensel, C. S., & Wight, R. G. (1995). Psychotherapy use and depression among AIDS caregivers. *Journal of Community Psychology, 23*, (April 1995), 127–142.

Levant, R. F., & Pollack, W. S. (1995). *A new psychology of men.* New York: BasicBooks.

Lynch, J., & Kilmartin, C. (1999). The pain behind the mask: Overcoming masculine depression. New York: The Haworth Press.

Marks, N. F. (1996). Caregiving across the lifespan: National prevalence and predictors. *Family Relations, 45*, 27–36.

Marquis, S. (1993). Death of the nursed: Burnout of the provider. In Richard Kalish (Ed.), *The Final Transition* (pp.17–33). Amityville, NY: Baywood.

McFarland, P. L., & Sanders, S. (1999). Male caregivers: Preparing men for nurturing roles. *American Journal of Alzheimer's Disease 14*(5), 278–282.

Meth, R. L., & Pasick, R. S. (1990). *Men in therapy: The challenge of change.* New York: Guilford.

Miller, B., & Kaufman, J. E. (1996). Beyond gender stereotypes: Spouse caregivers of persons with dementia. *Journal of Aging Studies, 10*(3), 189–204.

Morano, C. (1998). Special focus: Identifying the special needs of male caregivers. *Continuum, July-August*, 8–13.

Neal, M. B., Ingersoll-Dayton, B., & Starrels, M. E. (1997). Gender and relationship differences in caregiving patterns and consequences among employed caregivers. *The Gerontologist, 37*(6), 804–816.

O'Connor, M. F. (1997). Treating gay men with HIV. In M. O'Connor (Ed.), *Treating the psychological consequences of HIV.* San Francisco: Jossey-Bass.

Park, C. L., & Folkman, S. (1997). Stability and change in psychosocial resources during caregiving and bereavement in partners of men with AIDS. *Journal of Personality, 65*(2), 421–447.

Pearlin, L. I., & Aneshensel, C. S. (1994). Caregiving: The unexpected career. *Social Justice Research, 7*, 373–390.

Pfeiffer, E. (1999). Stages of Caregiving. *American Journal of Alzheimer's Disease, 14*(2), 125–127.

Revenson, T. A., & Majerovitz, S. D. (1991). The effects of chronic illness on the spouse: Social resources as stress buffers. *Arthritic Care and Research, 4*(2), 63–72.

Richards, A., Acree, M., & Folkman, S. (1999). Spiritual aspects of loss among partners of men with AIDS: Postbereavement follow-up. *Death Studies, 23*(2), 105–127.

Rosenthal, C. J., Sulman, J., & Marshall, V. W. (1993). Depressive symptoms in family caregivers of long-stay patients. *The Gerontologist, 33*(2), 249–257.

Rudd, M. G., Viney, L. L., & Preston, C. A. (1999). The grief experienced by spousal caregivers of dementia patients: The role of place of care of patient and gender of caregiver. *International Journal of Aging and Development, 48*(3), 217–240.

Sabo, D., & Gordon, D. F. (1995). *Men's health and illness: Gender, power and the body.* Thousand Oaks, CA: Sage.

Scher, M., Stevens, M., Good, G., & Eichenfield, G. A. (1987). *Handbook of counseling and psychotherapy with men.* Newbury Park, CA: Sage.

Schulz, R., & Williamson, G. M. (1991). A 2-year longitudinal study of depression among Alzheimer's caregivers. *Psychology and Aging, 6*(4), 569–578.

Shapiro, H. [on-line]. Available: http://www.caregiving.com, accessed 5/3/2000. *Caregiver of the Year.*

Siriopoulos, G., Brown, Y., & Wright, K. (1999). Caregivers of wives diagnosed with Alzheimer's disease: Husbands' perspectives. *American Journal of Alzheimer's Disease, 14*(2), 79–87.

Staudacher, C. (1991). *Men and grief: A guide for men surviving the death of a loved one: A resources for caregivers and mental health professionals.* Oakland, CA: New Harbinger.

Stommel, M., Collins, C. E., Given, B. A., & Given, C. W. (1999). Correlates of community service attitudes among family caregivers. *The Journal of Applied Gerontology, 18*(2), 145–161.

Szinovacz, M. (1989). Retirement, couples, and household work. In S. J. Bahr & E. T. Peterson (Eds.), Aging and the family (pp. 33–58). New York: Lexington Books.

Thompson, E. H., Jr. (Ed.). (1994). *Older men's lives.* Thousands Oaks, CA: Sage.

Thompson, E. H. (2000). The gendered caregiving of husbands and sons and the social construction of men caregivers as deviants. In E. Markson & L. Hollins (Eds.), *Intersections of aging: Readings in social gerontology.* Los Angeles: Roxbury.

Toseland, R. W., & Rossiter, C. M. (1989). Group interventions to support family caregivers: A review and analysis. *The Gerontologist, 29*(4), 438–448.

Walker, A. J. (1992). Conceptual perspectives on gender and family caregiving. In J. W. Dwyer & R. T. Coward (Eds.), *Gender, families and elder care.* Newbury Park, CA: Sage.

Walker, R. J., & Pomeroy, E. (1996). Depression or grief? *Health and Social Work, 21*(4), 247–254.

Walker, R. J., & Pomeroy, E. (1997). The impact of anticipatory grief on caregivers of persons with Alzheimer's disease. *Home Health Care Services Quarterly, 16*(1/2), 55–76.

Weiss, R. S., & Richards, T. A. (1997). A scale for predicting quality of recovery following the death of a partner. *Journal of Personality and Social Psychology, 72*(4), 885–891.

Wright, L. K. (1993). *Alzheimer's disease and marriage: An intimate account.* Newbury Park, CA: Sage.

Wrubel, J., & Folkman, S. (1997). What informal caregivers actually do: The caregiving skills of partners of men with AIDS. *AIDS care, 9*(6), 691–706.

Zarit, S. H., Todd, P. A., & Zarit, J. M. (1986). Subjective burden of husbands and wives as caregivers: A longitudinal study. *The Gerontologist, 26*(3), 260–266.

INTERNET RESOURCES

Elder Care

www.caregivers.on.ca
www.caregivers.com

Gay Men and Gay Concerns

www.caps.ucsf.edu/index.html
www.hivpositive.com/
http://the-park.com/kairos

Service Utilization and Support Provision of Caregiving Men

16

Lenard W. Kaye

INTRODUCTION

Significant interest has been shown in better understanding the experiences of informal caregivers during the past 10 to 15 years by both the professional and lay communities. Of more recent origin has been attention given by researchers and other human service professionals to the community service utilization patterns of caregivers (cf., Pedlar & Smyth, 1999). The available research not withstanding, our knowledge of service use by family caregivers remains incomplete. Given the continuing bias in caregiver research toward interpreting the experience of women, information that speaks to male caregivers' service consumption patterns and needs is even scarcer.

This chapter will explore our current, albeit incomplete, understanding of male caregivers as community service consumers. It will consider the classic features of the male caregiving perspective and the associated implications for men accessing and consuming formal (organizationally sponsored) forms of assistance. Potential barriers to service utilization will be highlighted and programmatic strategies for overcoming such barriers will be explored. The preferred services of male caregivers and the special case of support groups for informal caregivers will be considered in delineating concrete strategies for making interventions increasingly male gender-sensitive. I will close by revisiting a series of society-wide trends, many of which were discussed in chapter 1, that are predicted to influence the scope and breath of male caregiving in the future. I will consider especially the implications of such trends for service utilization and support.

MALE CAREGIVERS AND THEIR SERVICE CONSUMPTION PATTERNS

Anderson's (1968) behavioral model of health services posits that predisposing, enabling, and need factors determine service use. A person has to be predisposed (influenced by age, gender, race, ethnicity, etc.), to use services, able to do so (have the necessary health insurance, income, transportation, etc.), and need the service (perceive there to be a disability or illness requiring intervention). The extent to which gender is a predisposing factor that interacts with other predisposing, enabling, and need factors to influence service utilization among male caregivers has not been well defined.

Provision of formal caregiver service aims to reduce the burden of care carried by all informal providers. The philosophy is one in which formal assistance aims to supplement rather than substitute for the care provided by informal supports. Biegel, Sales, and Schulz (1991) classify caregiver interventions into three types. Support group interventions emphasize emotional support, informational support, and enhancement of coping skills. Educational interventions emphasize the provision of cognitive, self-enhancement, and behavioral management information and skills usually in group format. Clinical interventions are direct services and can include counseling-therapy, respite, hospice, day hospital, behavioral-cognitive stimulation, and psychosocial interventions.

Reducing the burden or stress of informal caregiving by the formal service community has tended to focus on the provision of respite-type interventions for providers. Indeed, services related to respite have traditionally been highest on the priority lists of care providers and the offerings made available through community agencies. But not all informal providers consume services with the same intensity. Caregivers of dementia patients, for example, have been found not only to consume fewer services than caregivers of nondemented individuals (Straw, 1991) but to delay their use of those services for longer periods of time (Lawton, Brody, & Saperstein, 1989). Toseland et al. (1999) in their analysis of primary caregivers of community-residing people with dementia in New York State found that outpatient and inpatient health care, home health aides, and visiting nurse services were the most frequently used health services by caregivers. Human services used most frequently were homemaker, legal, information and referral, and sectarian caregiver support services. Their analysis did not, however, differentiate between the service consumption patterns of men and women, and the vast majority of their subjects were women.

Harris (1993), on the other hand, found that the use of respite care represented a major coping strategy of men who had been caring for their wives for extended periods of time. Harris's subjects also believed that they needed to talk to men in similar situations. Specialized services for men were needed because they were uncomfortable discussing such issues as sex, platonic female companionship, the personal hygiene of their wives, and their lack of housekeeping skills in traditional support groups. Kosloski, Montgomery, and Karner (1999) also found that predisposing factors were more important with respect to day care use. White male caregivers compared with females and older and working African American caregivers were more likely to use in-home respite services. Among White and African American caregivers, working full-time increased the likelihood of day care use. Their research underscores how ethnicity can moderate male (and female) caregivers' perceptions of need, which are then most likely to affect the use of services that involve high levels of individual discretion such as in-home respite care, meal services, and adult day care.

BARRIERS TO SERVICE AND SUPPORT CONSUMPTION

Although millions of older adults (approximately one in five persons 65 years and older) use one or more community-based services in any given year, studies of service utilization continue to document that many individuals eligible for such assistance don't make use of it (Cox, 1999). Why don't informal caregivers use services, especially respite and support services? Biegel, Farkas, and Wadsworth (1994) noted the lack of financial resources made available by agencies because these organizations are likely to see such services as adjunctive or secondary in importance to interventions directly needed by care-recipients themselves.

Negative and discriminatory service experiences, traditional values and norms, and lower income are some of the predisposing and enabling factors that deter utilization of formal services by caregivers. Lack of service knowledge and perceptions that a particular service is not relevant to a caregiver's need can inhibit usage as well (Cox, 1999). Strain and Blandford (1999) found male caregivers significantly more likely than female caregivers to be unaware of the availability of community-based services. In the Toseland et al. (1999) analysis, service ignorance or not knowing where to obtain services stood out as the primary factor impeding service use by family caregivers of people with dementia. Of significantly less importance were such factors as cost and willingness to use a particular service. Access (i.e., lack of transportation and other physical impediments, inconvenient location or hours of operation, strict eligibility rules) proved also not to be a significant barrier except in the case of using support groups and educational programs. Wykle et al. (1999)

found that for both Black and White caregivers, the knowledge of services and frailty of the elderly person predict an increased use of formal services. Although not studying caregivers, the findings of Epure, Murdaugh, Joseph, and Masaki (1999) affirm that increased use of health care services is precipitated by elderly with worse functional status and cognitive impairment.

Alzheimer's caregivers report that resistance on the part of care-recipients to accept outside help combined with reluctance on the part of caregivers, because of concerns over quality and finances, can be major deterrents to accepting aid (Winslow, 1999). Male (and female) caregivers of persons with dementia and other mental health problems may, in particular, use services less because the increased demand of such care typically promotes social isolation and reduced contact with outside sources of information. In addition to the difficulty in caring for individuals with dementia, the fact that there remains a scarcity of providers trained in dementia management and a tendency for informal providers to socially withdraw due to shame and efforts to conceal the illness, also tend to reduce formal service usage (Aneshensel, Pearlin, Mullan, Zarit, & Whitlatch, 1995; Birkel & Jones, 1989; Cotrell & Engel, 1998).

Service delivery barriers have been found to be especially significant for older persons of color and their caregivers. In an analysis of hospice access and use by African Americans, Reese, Ahern, Nair, O'Faire, and Warren (1999) highlighted a number of cultural and institutional barriers to service, including differences in values regarding medical care and differences in spiritual beliefs between African Americans and European Americans. Institutional barriers included lack of knowledge of services, economic factors, lack of trust by African Americans in the health care system, and lack of diversity among health care staff. Not surprisingly, Hinrichsen and Ramirez (1992) reported that Black caregivers of dementia patients express more unmet need than White caregivers and that Medicaid patients and patients from higher social class position reported more formal care network utilization. Kosberg and Morano (2000) and others (Valle, 1998; Yeo & Gallagher-Thompson, 1996) underscored the powerful and differential impact that cultural origin (including considerations of race, ethnicity, social class, and religion) can have on men's help-seeking behavior and various aspects of the service network response, including problem identification, worker-client relationships, assessments and care planning, formal service provider characteristics, and group treatment dynamics.

Attitudes toward service use of male caregivers can differ in significant ways from their female counterparts. Stommel, Collins, Given, and Given (1999) found male caregivers more concerned about the opinion of others, more inclined to favor family independence in providing care, more likely to reject government provision of community services, and less confident in those same services. Miller and Mukherjee (1999) also reported that male caregivers have a lesser likelihood of accepting government and community services. A national survey of facilitators of caregiver support groups found that the most frequently mentioned deterrent to men joining was the traditional attitude that men should be able to manage caregiving without assistance (Kaye & Applegate, 1993). For many men, attending a support group was believed to constitute an admission of weakness, loss of control, and ultimately failure. Also voiced was the belief that men have either a resistance or inability to engage in personal sharing that was ascribed to internalized societal attitudes that men should not "go public" with their problems. Of lesser significance were such potential deterrents as health problems, lack of awareness of available groups, and misunderstandings about the group's purpose and function. It is noteworthy, however, that once men had joined a support group, they tended to remain members as long as women.

Kaye and Applegate (1994) found that caregiving men were not necessarily driven to seek outside resources to substitute for their own. Indeed, the men in their research (primarily spouses, and to a lesser degree sons) seemed to approach caregiving with a rather stoic, stiff-upper-lip orientation. Although recognizing that their care-recipients could benefit from additional measures of assistance, these men (and their care-recipients) tended to benefit minimally from family and community resources. In fact, it was rare for these men to be receiving secondary aid from more than one other relative. Furthermore, family aid declined significantly over time. Archer and MacLean (1993) documented similar observations and reported that the caregiving husbands and sons in their research even spoke of abandonment and neglect by family and friends.

The following list shows potential reasons for reluctance of male caregivers to use community services and other forms of professional assistance:

1. Men's inability to leave the care-recipient alone;
2. Men's lack of familiarity with certain services and programs;
3. Men's fear of appearing as if or admitting they can't handle the situation;
4. Men's reluctance to share personal feelings;
5. The lack of other men using or participating in a particular service or program;
6. Inconvenient hours, meeting times, or locations of certain programs;
7. Men's lack of identification with other caregivers;
8. The lack of clear-cut, concrete benefits to be derived from particular services; and
9. Ongoing pressures to be strong and independent (Kaye & Applegate, 1990).

These barriers to program participation and service utilization have implications for structuring and marketing community services to men. Strategies for addressing these barriers are discussed below. For this discussion the case of caregiver support group programs will be highlighted to illustrate relevant access and design issues as they apply to serving male caregivers.

STRUCTURAL STRATEGIES

Service planners and designers should give careful consideration to the manner in which programs are structured before they move to implementation. Key questions to ask during planning and implementation include: What groups and subgroups of caregivers and care-recipients are we trying to serve, and what characteristics will the various categories of caregivers–care-recipients display? In the case of caregiver support groups, the answers to these questions will influence group structure, frequency of meetings, meeting location, and group sponsorship.

Group facilitation. While most support groups have one facilitator, there are several benefits to be derived from co-facilitation. The use of co-facilitators allows one facilitator to focus on the presentation of information while the other deals with matters of group dynamics. If the facilitation team includes one male and one female, the likelihood increases that each group member will be able to relate to at least one of the leaders.

Group facilitators also should be trained in the influences that gender can have on group dynamics (Forsyth, 1999), differences between counseling men and women, gender-specific differences in the aging process, and the extent to which particular community services, entitlements, and benefits may be especially sensitive (or insensitive) to the needs of middle-age and older men. Facilitators should also be sensitized to variations in the customs and cultural traditions of men representative of different racial and ethnic groups residing within the community served by a particular program (cf., Aleman, Fitzpatrick, Tran, & Gonzalez, 1999; Kosberg & Morano, 2000; Valle, 1998).

Group sponsorship. The auspices under which programs operate, including caregiver support groups, may affect both the number and type of caregivers that participate. It is important for group organizers to evaluate whether sponsorship will positively or negatively bear on the male caregiver's decision to attend the support group. The following questions should be considered in assessing the impact of a potential sponsor: (a) Is the organization highly regarded within the community? (b) Will a group of male caregivers feel comfortable associating with the organization? and (c) Is the sponsoring body sufficiently neutral? Every effort should be made to ensure that male caregivers are not deterred from group participation because of its affiliation with a particular sponsor.

Group size.   The optimal size of a caregiver support group depends on a particular group's purpose. Most traditional support groups have a membership of 8 to 20 people. This is small enough to encourage caregivers to open up, yet large enough for people to share the responsibility of maintaining discussion. Groups whose primary purpose is to provide concrete information (these may be particularly appealing to male caregivers) can maintain a much larger membership. Lecture-style meetings will meet the needs of many male caregivers. They will not, however, meet the needs of those male caregivers that are looking for emotional support or individualized attention.

Group membership.   In recent years there has been some movement toward creating support groups and other caregiver services that serve particular subpopulations of caregivers such as those who are employed or caring for Alzheimer patients. The impetus behind this programmatic trend is the belief that group members may relate better to people like themselves (Toseland & Rivas, 2001). However, homogeneity among program participants may be less important once individuals have accessed programs. Group members often benefit from hearing about the experiences of people different from themselves in terms of learning about new coping strategies and being exposed to different skills and information about diverse resources. Gender homogeneity in particular may be less important once men have begun participating in a caregiver support group and similar such community services. In fact, facilitators have reported that ongoing mixed support group functioning is not significantly affected by gender (Kaye & Applegate, 1993). Neither sex dominated the group or expressed greater satisfaction or dissatisfaction with group process. Men reported that they felt comfortable sharing their thoughts and feelings with the group. They did not participate any more or less than the women in such groups. The major hurdle to overcome for the men in the Kaye and Applegate research was the initial effort required to reach out and commence participation in mixed groups. Yet, it is important to remember that although some men will find mixed groups satisfying, still others can be expected to express a clear preference for all male groups. In such cases, it is important that the personal wishes of potential group participants be respected.

The men in the Kaye and Applegate (1993) study identified the following preferred features of the caregiver support programs they were affiliated with:

- Being with people who have experiences and feelings similar to their own
- Receiving support from others
- Resolving problems
- Receiving information regarding community programs and resources
- Learning the skills of caregiving
- Learning how to deal with guilt, depression, and anger
- Helping others
- Being relieved of caregiving responsibilities for a brief period of time
- Learning what to expect in the future

Ensuring that programs emphasize the above experiences can be expected to promote men's engagement in such programming. On the other hand, these same men emphasized the following negative features of support programs:

- They are depressing and demoralizing
- Certain participants can dominate discussions
- It is a reminder that impairments are irreversible
- You learn what to expect in the future
- Some of the information provided is irrelevant

Such features, if allowed to dominate the process, may reduce the likelihood of men's continued engagement in support group programming.

Meeting time: The time of group meetings must be carefully selected to appeal to the type of caregiver targeted for participation. Older male caregivers often prefer daytime meetings because they are more comfortable driving or walking during the day and because formal respite services are more accessible during daytime hours. Evening meetings are most appropriate for employed men and for those male caregivers that depend on working family members for transportation or respite.

The number of times the group meets is also dependent upon the group's composition and functioning. Most support groups have monthly meetings. However, weekly meetings may be appropriate for male caregivers that are not burdened with the responsibility of obtaining respite care. Lecture-style groups may find a bimonthly meeting schedule preferable.

Meeting location.   Group meetings should be held at a central site that is easily accessible by both public and private transportation. Either gender-neutral locations for mixed groups or male-oriented locations for men's groups are recommended. Common locations include public buildings, facilities for the aged, churches, synagogues, community service buildings, and group members' homes.

Meeting format. The format of most support group meetings consists of several different activities. Given the observed interests of male caregivers in support group programs, it is recommended that components be offered in the following prioritized sequence:

Primary components	Information sharing and dissemination
	Problem solving
	Skills building
	Expert-Guest speakers
Secondary components	Personal sharing and ventilation
	Mutual support
	Socializing

MARKETING STRATEGIES

Different strategies may be employed by support group facilitators and leaders to combat the feelings of failure that some men associate with the need for caregiver services. It is important to market the group in a professional manner and stress expert advice and the provision of concrete information in your marketing campaign. Try using language that is "acceptable" to men to describe the group's process. Be pragmatic, emphasizing the provision of competency-enhancing information and tangible benefits such as lists of community programs and resources, legal and financial information, and expert speakers. The following techniques are suggested for increasing the group's appeal to men:

1. *Include men in your program outreach.* Many men believe that support groups and similar caregiver services are for women. They also fear they will be the only male participants in a support group. Include testimonials of male participants and the benefits that can accrue to men in press releases and other publicity.
2. *Have male participants contact other men.* Male "recruiters" and orientation "buddies" can reduce prospective participants' apprehensions and help them adjust to the group.
3. *Focus on the provision of concrete information and competency acquisition.* Initially, men will frequently be more responsive to a program that offers practical information than one that focuses on emotional support. Use informational seminars to attract men. Try skills-building sessions that emphasize enhancing competencies in such hands-on tasks as bathing,

grooming, and toileting as well as workshops on cooking, household maintenance, and comparative shopping. Men will likely be more accepting of other therapeutic benefits of support group programming after they have been exposed to a program's structure and membership.

4. *Utilize a credible male spokesperson.* A respected male figure will add credibility to caregiver programming. It will provide potential male participants with someone strong to identify with.

5. *Publicize the program in places where men affiliate.* Notices of services for men may best be placed in unconventional venues including: union and industry newsletters, accompanying monthly utility service billings; postings at sporting events, golf courses, bowling alleys, pool halls, stadiums, community taverns and pubs; presentations made at social, fraternal and civic organizations; information in church and synagogue bulletins; public service announcements on radio and television; ads in men's and sports magazines; and material distributed through veterans' clubs and organizations.

Barusch (2000) has summarized the characteristics of "male-friendly" interventions. Many of her principles parallel the elements inherent in the above model. To increase service utilization Barusch recommends that: (a) men present as leaders and participants; (b) services be offered at a comfortable location for men; (c) men have opportunities to contribute, to help others, and to serve as "experts"; (d) men have opportunities to take control and participate in decision making; (e) there be limits on spontaneous expressions of emotion and rather, the emphasis be placed on opportunities for ritualized expressions of emotion; (f) interventions be designed to provide information, not "therapy"; (g) opportunities be available for goal attainment; and (h) relationship-building skills be woven into, but not dominate, the intervention.

EMERGENT TRENDS AND THEIR IMPLICATIONS FOR SERVICES UTILIZATION AND SUPPORT

As discussed in chapter 1, a series of trends can be expected to influence the roles, functions, and stresses of caregiving males in the future. I would like to consider the implications of these and other demographic, social, familial, and technological trends for men's use of formal caregiver services and supports in the immediate years ahead (Kaye, 2000).

1. Consider first the increasing geographic dispersal of American families. Today's elderly are less likely to live with relatives and more likely to live alone than any previous cohort of older Americans (Friedland &

Summer, 1999; Muller & Honig, 2000). It is increasingly uncommon to find adult sons and daughters (and their families) living in the immediate vicinity of their parents. Consequently those men who live in close proximity to their care-recipients and are engaged in the caregiving enterprise will commonly have fewer and fewer relatives immediately available to help them with tasks requiring face-to-face contact. Accordingly, formal community services will likely become relatively more important sources of aid for these men. Those men who live at significant distances from the recipients of their care may benefit in particular from long-distance geriatric care management services and elder care resource and referral services offered on an increasingly frequent basis at the employed caregiver's work site (Kaye & Davitt, 1999).

2. We continue to witness the disintegration of traditional communities and neighborhoods in many regions of the nation. Some observers of the family caregiving phenomenon worry that this will inevitably lead to the weakening of alternative informal support networks for older adults (namely the help provided by neighbors and friends) at the very time when their assistance may be especially needed given the inclinations of blood relatives to live at increasingly greater distances from one anther. The changing face of communities may well result in male caregivers having fewer immediate informal supports to turn to for assistance. Pressure may mount for these men to consider accessing formal systems of community assistance with greater frequency.

3. A now well-established trend is the increasing number of women in the workforce (Friedland & Summer, 1999; Poulos & Nightingale, 1997; Quinn, in press). As each year passes, larger proportions of workforce women are assuming professional roles demanding even more of their time and energy. Some of these women may have been counted among the traditional corps of family caregivers and may no longer be as readily available to help because of competing responsibilities arising out of the workplace. More men can be expected to be called upon. The call for men to aid in family care may well not discriminate between those men who are well equipped and those who are less well equipped to assume the responsibilities of caregiving. Less well-equipped men may be expected to benefit in particular from supplemental forms of community program support, especially those forms of aid that emphasize caregiver education and training.

4. An even more recent trend is the changing shape and form that work is taking (that is, how and where work is done). In many fields, modern technology has permitted us to construct virtual offices and be productive outside of the traditional 9 to 5 framework. People are living through their computers not only in terms of performing their work but also in terms of the construction of their social worlds. This represents

both good news and bad news for the male caregiver. Although it offers a husband, son, son-in-law, or grandson some flexibility to provide caregiving for an incapacitated relative or friend in the middle of the workday, it also may result in the simultaneous extension of the workday and workweek. These employed caregivers run the risk of going nonstop virtually every waking hour, no longer able to construct separate spaces for work and caregiving. There also may be no such thing as a weekend or a day off according to this particular scenario. Such men may be in particularly urgent need of respite-type support services so as to avoid the risk of premature caregiver burnout.

5. A fifth trend, at least until recently, has been the decision by many women to have children later in their lives (Poulos & Nightingale, 1997). This increases the likelihood that these same women will become members of the now well-documented and exceedingly popularized sandwich generation, consumed by the responsibility of caring for two dependent generations residing at both ends of the life span continuum. At the same time, families tend to be smaller in size with fewer children available to serve as primary and supplementary providers of elder care. These developments translate into declining numbers of internal caregiving resources in the average family and have likely resulted in men being expected more and more frequently to assume the caregiving function. As already noted, men who engage in such activities may or may not be prepared to carry such responsibilities. The supplementary aid that can be offered by community service resources may be particularly helpful for those men who have been thrust into the role of caregiver with inadequate preparation.

6. Realize also that older adults are an increasingly sophisticated, educated, healthy, politically astute, mobile, and vocal cohort with higher expectations and more disposable income than any prior generation of older adults (Kaye, in press; Morrow-Howell, Hinterlong, & Sherraden, 2001). While we continue to see increasing disparity in the incomes of the rich and poor in this country, poverty rates among older adults are on the decline as people's sources of income and assets continue to expand (Muller & Honig, 2000), life expectancy continues to increase and disability rates among elders stabilize and in fact appear now to be decreasing (Federal Interagency Forum on Aging Related Statistics, 2000; Muller & Honig, 2000; Research Highlights, 1999). The *new aged*, if you will, are emerging as a significant force in today's world and will have much to say in terms of wanting a wide range of choices and options available to them in the way of community services and programs. Future cohorts of older adults will be even better off. They will continue to redefine concepts such as retirement and old age. Elders of the future will also be more ethnically and culturally diverse than in the past. Future caregiving husbands counted among the cohort of the new aged may be more forthcoming in

their willingness to access caregiver support services. To meet these men's needs, the formal community service system will have to be more responsive to the wide range of expectations, attitudes, and values exhibited by such a heterogeneous cohort of caregivers.

7. Health care reform and models of managed care represent a seventh trend bound to influence the nature of informal caregiving and the demand for men's engagement as caregivers in the home. Strict limitations that medical care reimbursement policies place on the length of available care in hospitals and similar facilities, combined with continued anti-institutional sentiment, are influencing our thinking about community-based and home-based care and the responsibilities placed on families to help older people remain out of institutional care settings. Increased responsibilities placed on families will translate, at least to some extent, on increased pressures for men to participate in caregiving whether or not they are prepared for such responsibilities. Men's transition into caregiving could be eased by the right blend of available community support services.

8. A final trend of relevance when thinking about men's need for community services pertains to the simple reality that women may be reaching their absorptive capacity in terms of their willingness and ability to assume the lion's share of informal caregiving responsibilities. Combine this with the continuing vertical expansion of families (as a result of expanding life span), the concurrent shrinkage of those same families horizontally (as a result of declining birthrates and high divorce rates) and one is compelled to speak to a predicted scarcity of family caregivers in the future and the increasing likelihood that caregivers themselves will be aging. A network of gender-sensitive community services could mean the difference between men surviving and thriving as care providers or failing in performing the necessary functions of family care.

SERVICE SECTOR RESPONSES

Several new categories of innovative programs and services have emerged in the past several years that have responded to some of the trends noted here. These services speak to the expectation of increased choice and the growing economic well-being of older adults and their families as consumers. These services can help relieve some of the burden felt by male caregivers (and other informal supports). Unfortunately, others services have not yet emerged but remain badly needed.

In response to the needs of long-distance male caregivers, geriatric care management services have flourished (Kaye, 1998). These professionals may operate out of public agencies or private firms and can help a husband, son, grandson, and other men with practical matters, deal with emotional issues, help secure needed services, and assess the older person's health and functional status. These professionals represent a neutral third party dealing with difficult and emotional decisions and mediating between spouses or adult male children and their older parents.

For employed male caregivers, more and more companies offer elder care resource and referral services that will help an employee locate needed services for an older relative regardless of whether that person lives down the street, or across the country (Fredricksen-Goldsen & Scharlach, 2001). Such services may be particularly useful in combination with a private geriatric care manager for sons and other male caregivers residing out of state. Elder care locator services and telephone hotlines offer similar services and may be available through certain local Area Agencies on Aging.

High-technology home health care services are increasingly available in the community offering sophisticated medical treatment in the home using technology that would only have been found in hospitals and nursing homes just a few years ago (Emerman, 2001; Kaye & Davitt, 1999; Wylde, 2001). The availability of miniaturized and portable nutrition and hydration equipment, mechanical ventilation, intravenous therapies, computerized health-monitoring equipment, and more is now widespread. Add to this list personal emergency response and related communications systems, telemedicine and telehealth computer technology, home robotics, and numerous other smart house applications and you can see that the boundaries between home and hospital and between hospital room and living room are becoming increasingly blurred.

Sophisticated, community creating service networks are also emerging whereby formal service providers are beginning to think rather creatively about novel shapes and forms of help being made available to older consumers and their families. Such innovative interventions include assisted living, continuing care retirement communities, Eden alternative nursing homes, home hospice and other end-of-life programs, and comprehensive one stop service centers.

MECHANISMS FOR ASSURING MEN'S ACCESS TO AND UTILIZATION OF SERVICES

The service delivery responses noted above hold considerable promise for easing some of the burdens placed on caregiving men and the recipients of their care. However, formulating creative programs that meet the needs of caregiving men is not enough. Programmatic strategies that encourage men to take the first step of reaching out to the services network are also necessary. Barusch (2000) put it simply and directly by pointing out that geriatric care settings are essentially feminine entities that focus on a feminine world view of an "ethic of caring." As a result, it may be no coincidence that men are underrepresented in the service delivery system and their unique needs largely unrecognized. Consequently, such settings are composed of primarily female providers serving primarily female recipients.

Several alternative models for helping isolated older adults access services in the community may be instructive in this regard. Consider first the development of neighborhood advocacy centers especially geared to serving caregivers. Crose and Minear (1998) describe Project CARE (Community Action to Reach the Elderly), which was developed as part of the National Eldercare Campaign of the Administration on Aging. The principles of Project CARE may be applicable in the context of caregiving. Those principles include: (a) raising the community level of awareness of the needs of frail and vulnerable elderly; (b) developing community-based steering committees and eventually neighborhood coalitions; and (c) finally, establishing neighborhood advocacy centers that emphasize the use of volunteers and referrals through informal support networks. These centers are exceedingly user friendly, informal in their structure, and welcoming to individuals who may ordinarily not reach out to the formal services sector for help such as minority elders and men.

Although the literature presents mixed findings on the matter, Cotrell and Engel (1998) found that informal supports can be important mediating forces in overcoming the barriers to caregiver use of formal services, especially respite, through the provision of information, encouragement, and instrumental activities. Their findings suggest that in the absence of relatives, friends, and neighbors performing such a mediating function, service use by caregivers can be expected to decline. This may especially be true for spousal caregivers, a category of caregiver more commonly occupied by men. Programmers may therefore want to consider ways in which networks of informal supports, significant others, and confidants of male providers can be bolstered in their efforts to serve as secondary caregivers and mediating forces between male caregivers and the formal services network. Given the emphasis of current caregiver support programming to focus on meeting the needs of primary caregivers, expanding that function to support others in the male's informal caregiver network would appear well advised. The gatekeeper program in Spokane, Washington, reflects such a philosophy (Raschko & Coleman, no date). This creative community organization effort was designed to systematically locate and identify high-risk elders, particularly those who are isolated, living alone, and in need of support. Through the use of nontraditional referral sources (employees of businesses and other organizations that have contact with isolated elders including bank tellers, police, property appraisers, pharmacists, telephone company personnel, utility company meter readers, postal carriers, and apartment house managers) serving as key intermediaries, lifelines are created between isolated elders in the community and the formal service system. The Spokane gatekeeper program has already recognized that older male caregivers may be particularly resistant to accepting outside help, especially husbands caring for spouses with Alzheimer's disease.

THE EVOLVING ROLE OF THE SERVICES NETWORK

Given the aforementioned trends that are predicted to impact elder caregiving, one is compelled to reevaluate the roles of professionals serving older adults and their caregivers. The predicted changing face of caregiving presents both challenges and opportunities for service providers in the health and human services. Taken in total, the highlighted trends result not only in a more gender, racially and ethnically diverse, but increasingly stressed cohort of informal providers of care. Despite it being a cliché, if it takes a community to raise a child, it will also take a community to support the informal providers of elder care. Clearly, informal caregivers will require support and services from the professional community as they seek at least temporary relief from some of their elder care responsibilities. Designing and implementing future services, however, needs to take into greater account caregiver attitudes, beliefs, and perceptions generally (Smyth & Pedlar, 1999), and specifically among subgroups of caregivers, especially in terms of the role gender, race, ethnicity, employment status, and related sociodemographic variables play in preference formation and demand for services. Service providers and practitioners must be willing to abandon the stereotype that all caregiving men want to "go it alone."

Certainly, most men need encouragement in innovative ways to make greater use of a range of community support services capable of supplementing their efforts at family caring. While there are significant opportunities for private practitioners and firms to provide services to this population on a fee-for-service basis, it remains imperative that services and programs of equivalent quality be made available to family caregivers lacking the economic clout to purchase private sector offerings. Whether through the nurturing of informal supports that may serve as constructive mediating forces for men engaged in the caregiving enterprise, or through neighborhood advocacy centers and gatekeeper programs that reach out to caregiving men who are hesitant to seek aid or uninformed about available supports, creative programming is pivotal. Such programming that is gender sensitive will be especially critical for men experiencing social isolation as a result of their caregiving efforts. Because substantial numbers of caregiving men may resist asking for assistance in performing their tasks, it is important for family members, human service practitioners, and others to recognize the warning signs of those men who may be especially in need of help. These sources of potential support need also to be willing to help men "step up" to their calling and permit them to "do caregiving" in their own way.

SUMMARY

The demographic imperative of a burgeoning aged population, managed care, increasingly enlightened perspectives on gender-appropriate behavior, and redefined principles of workplace performance, are all to be counted among the major influences destined to shape the caregiving experience for men in the years ahead. The role played by husbands, sons, and other males in caring for incapacitated relatives and other vulnerable individuals will continue to evolve. We will want to continue to refine our understanding of the male caregiver persona. At the same time, however, we must not overlook the importance of gaining a more enlightened and nuanced perspective on caregiving men's ambivalent relationship with the service network. Male caregivers need and can benefit enormously from caregiver services. To the extent that community services providers come to reflect less feminine bias in their structure and configuration and greater sensitivity to the distinctive attributes of masculinity then such interventive resources will come to represent genuine supports for men engaged in the caregiving experience.

REFERENCES

Aleman, S., Fitzpatrick, T., Tran, T.V., & Gonzalez, E. W. (1999). *Therapeutic interventions with ethnic elders: Health and social issues.* New York: The Haworth Press.

Anderson, R. M. (1968). *A behavioral model of families' use of health services* (Research Series 25). Chicago: The University of Chicago Center for Health Administration Studies.

Aneshensel, C. S., Pearlin, L. I., Mullan, J. T., Zarit, S. H., & Whitlatch, C. J. (1995). *Profiles in caregiving: The unexpected career.* San Diego, CA: Academic Press.

Archer, C., & MacLean, M. (1993). Husbands and sons as caregivers of chronically ill elderly women. *Journal of Gerontological Social Work, 21*(1/2), 5–23.

Barusch, A. S. (2000). Serving older men: Dilemmas and opportunities for geriatric care managers. *Geriatric Care Management Journal, 10*(1), 31–36.

Biegel, D. E., Farkas, K. J., & Wadsworth, N. (1994). Social service programs for older adults and their families: Service use and barriers. In P. K. H. Kim (Ed.), *Services to the aging and aged: Public policies and programs* (pp. 141–178). New York: Garland.

Biegel, D. E., Sales, E., & Schulz, R. (1991). *Family caregiving and chronic illness: Alzheimer's disease, cancer, heart disease, mental illness, and stroke.* Newbury Park, CA: Sage.

Birkel, R., & Jones, C. (1989). A comparison of the caregiving networks dependent elderly individuals who are lucid and those who are demented. *The Gerontologist, 29,* 114–119.

Cotrell, V., & Engel, R. J. (1998). The role of secondary supports in mediating formal services to dementia caregivers. *Journal of Gerontological Social Work, 30*(3/4), 117–132.

Cox, C. (1999). Race and caregiving: Patterns of service use by African American and white caregivers of persons with Alzheimer's disease. *Journal of Gerontological Social Work, 32*(2), 5–19.

Crose, R., & Minear, M. (1998). Project CARE: A model for establishing neighborhood centers to increase access to services by low-income, minority elders. *Journal of Gerontological Social Work, 30*(3/4), 73–82.

Emerman, J. (2001 January/February). Futurecare: The web, virtual services and even 'carebots.' *Aging Today XXII*(1), 11–12.

Epure, J. P., Murdaugh, C., Joseph, C., & Masaki, K. (1999, November). *Relationship between elder caregiver characteristics and patient health care utilization.* Poster session presented at the annual scientific meeting of the Gerontological Society of America, San Francisco, CA.

Federal Interagency Forum on Aging Related Statistics. (2000). *Health, United States, 2000.* Washington, DC: author.

Forsyth, D. (1999). *Group dynamics* (3rd ed.). Belmont, CA: Wadsworth.

Fredricksen-Goldsen, & Scharlach, A. E. (2001). *Families and work: New directions in the twenty-first century.* New York: Oxford University Press.

Friedland, R. B., & Summer, L. (1999). *Demography is not destiny.* Washington, DC: National Academy on an Aging Society, The Gerontological Society of America.

Harris, P. (1993). The misunderstood caregiver? A qualitative study of the male caregiver of Alzheimer's disease victims. *The Gerontologist, 33,* 551–556.

Hinrichsen, G. A., & Ramirez, M. (1992). Black and white dementia caregivers: A comparison of their adaptation, adjustment, and service utilization. *The Gerontologist, 32*(3), 375–381.

Kaye, L. W. (1998). Practicing geriatric care management: Getting back to basics. *Geriatric Care Management Journal, 8*(1), 2–5.

Kaye, L. W. (November 13, 2000). *Family transformations and demand for eldercare in America.* Annual Visiting Libra Professor University Lecture. Orono, ME.

Kaye, L. W. (in press). *Perspectives on productive aging: Social work practice with the new aged.* Washington, DC: NASW Press.

Kaye, L. W. & Applegate, J. S. (1990). *Men as caregivers to the elderly: Understanding and aiding unrecognized family support.* Lexington, MA: Lexington Books.

Kaye, L. W., & Applegate, J. S. (1993). Family support groups for male caregivers: Benefits of participation. *Journal of Gerontological Social Work, 20*(3/4), 167–185.

Kaye, L. W., & Applegate, J. S. (1994). Older men and the family caregiving orientation. In E. H. Thompson, Jr. (Ed.), *Older men's lives* (pp. 218–236). Thousand Oaks, CA: Sage.

Kaye, L. W., & Davitt, J. K. (1999). *Current practices in high-tech home care.* New York: Springer.

Kosberg, J. I., & Morano, C. L. (2000). Cultural considerations in care management with older men. *Geriatric Care Management Journal, 10*(1), 24–30.

Kosloski, K., Montgomery, R. J., & Karner, T. X. (1999). Differences in the perceived need for assistive services by culturally diverse caregivers of persons with dementia. *The Journal of Applied Gerontology, 18*(2), 239–256.

Lawton, M., Brody, E., & Saperstein, A. (1989). A controlled study of respite service for caregivers of Alzheimer's patients. *The Gerontologist, 29*(1), 8–16.

Miller, B., & Mukherjee, S. (1999). Service use, caregiving mastery, and attitudes toward community services. *The Journal of Applied Gerontology, 18*(2), 162–176.

Morrow-Howell, N., Hinterlong, J., & Sherraden, M. (2001). *Productive aging: Concepts and challenges.* Baltimore, MD: The Johns Hopkins University Press.

Muller, C., & Honig, M. (2000, April). *International longevity report: Charting the productivity and independence of older persons.* New York: International Longevity Center.

Pedlar, D. J., & Smyth, K. A. (Eds.). (1999). Caregiver attitudes, beliefs, and perceptions about service use. Special issue. *Journal of Applied Gerontology, 18*(2), 141–261.

Poulos, S., & Nightingale, D. S. (1997, June). *The aging baby boom: Implications for employment and training programs.* Washington, DC: The Urban Institute.

Quinn, J. (in press). *Retirement patterns and bridge jobs in the 1990s.* Washington, DC: Employee Benefit Research Institute.

Raschko, R., & Coleman, F. (no date). *Gatekeeper training manual.* Spokane, WA: Elder Services, Spokane Mental Health.

Reese, D. J., Ahern, R. E., Nair, S., O'Faire, J. D., & Warren, C. (1999). Hospice access and use by African Americans: Addressing cultural and institutional barriers through participatory action research, *Social Work, 44*(6), 549–559.

Research Highlights in the Demography and Economics of Aging. (1999, March). The declining disability of older Americans. *Research Highlights, 5,* 1–4.

Smyth, K. A., & Pedlar, D. J. (1999). Caregiver attitudes, beliefs, and perceptions about service use: Charting a course for further research. *Journal of Applied Gerontology, 18*(2), 257–261.

Stommel, M., Collins, C. E., Given, B. A., & Given, C. W. (1999). Correlates of community service attitudes among family caregivers. *Journal of Applied Gerontology, 18*(2), 145–161.

Strain, L. A., & Blandford, A. A. (1999, November). *Exploring reasons for not using community-based services.* Poster session presented at the annual scientific meeting of the Gerontological Society of America, San Francisco.

Straw, L. (1991). Support system participation in spousal caregiving: Alzheimer's disease versus other illness. *Journal of Applied Gerontology, 10,* 359–371.

Toseland, R. W., McCallion, P., Gerber, T., Dawson, C., Gieryic, S., & Guilamo-Ramos, V. (1999). Use of health and human services by community-residing people with dementia. *Social Work, 44*(6), 535–548.

Toseland, R. W., & Rivas, R. F. (2001). *An introduction to group work practice* (4th ed.). Boston: Allyn and Bacon.

Valle, R. (1998). *Caregiving across cultures.* Washington, DC: Taylor & Francis.

Winslow, B. W. (1999, November). *Benefits and barriers in the use of community services for dementia caregivers.* Poster session presented at the annual scientific meeting of the Gerontological Society of America, San Francisco.

Wykle, M., Fink, S., Constantino, L., Haug, M., Namazi, K., Picot, S., & Taylor, A. (1999, November). *Use of formal services in black and white caregivers.* Poster session presented at the annual scientific meeting of the Gerontological Society of America, San Francisco.

Wylde, M. (2001, January/February). Caring technology. *Aging Today XXII*(1), 9, 11.

Yeo, G., & Gallagher-Thompson, D. (Eds.). (1996). *Ethnicity & the dementias.* Washington, DC: Taylor & Francis.

Epilogue:
Implications for Practice
and Future Research

Betty J. Kramer

We developed this text to acknowledge the contributions of caregiving men and to enhance knowledge regarding their needs and experiences. This volume first examined the nature and extent of men as caregivers, identified the fundamental social and demographic trends that have implications for the future, and introduced what is potentially unique about men caregivers. Next, theoretical and methodological issues relevant to the study of men involved in caregiving were highlighted, followed by several chapters that critiqued the literature and presented original research on men caregivers in a variety of contexts. Finally this volume profiled gender-sensitive interventions, skills, supports, and services that are relevant to direct practice and program development. What have we learned from this exploration that might be helpful to service providers, and what are the implications for future research?

IMPLICATIONS FOR SERVICE PROVIDERS

There are several themes and emerging areas of inquiry that have surfaced in this volume that have clear implications for practice and future research. Perhaps the most far-reaching theme emerging from this volume that has implications for service providers is the breadth, depth, variation, and divergent experiences that caregiving men are engaged in. The stressors, resources, and outcomes of caregiving and how caregiving is approached by the subgroups of caregivers vary tremendously. Thompson (chap. 2) reviewed documented evidence relevant to the divergence in activities, motivations, approaches, and styles among men caregivers. Bookwala, Newman, and Schulz (chap. 4) and Carpenter and Miller (chap. 5) noted that the vast majority of studies of men caregivers have focused on care-givers of persons with dementia. Most of these men are spouses who are themselves older. How they respond to caregiving demands and what types of tasks challenge them, may be very different from what younger caregiving men will experience when their wives have breast cancer or their partners live with AIDS. We know that despite some change toward somewhat more egalitarian patterns of household work among younger cohorts of married couples (Deutsch, 1999; Walzer, 1998), several small- and large-scale investigations have demonstrated the presence of traditional gender differentiation in the division of household responsibilities in later-life families, which persist after taking employment status and retire-ment into consideration (Ade-Ridder & Brubaker, 1988; Keith, 1980, 1985, 1994; Szinovacz, 1989). How men respond to caregiving responsibilities involving household tasks and how stressful they may be perceived, will likely depend upon their personal experience with those activities and will-ingness and ability to restructure their relationship with the care-recipient.

Several chapters reviewed in this volume revealed that different sub-groups of caregiving men are confronted with unique challenges and are engaged in caregiving with very different patterns. The type of care-recipient illness or condition that requires care may drastically influence the challenges confronting the caregiver. Sipes (chap. 7) and Wight (chap. 8) revealed the complexities of caregiving among men caring for partners with AIDS. As contrasted with older spousal caregivers, these men were likely to be young to middle-aged gay males, many of whom were work-ing and experiencing sources of stress that are unique to AIDS caregiving. Wight revealed that sources of stress unique to AIDS caregiving (i.e., AIDS alienation, gay acceptance, young age, the caregiver's own poor health due to HIV infection) were critical determinants of stress and health. Men caring for persons with AIDS revealed dramatic needs for guidance in understanding and anticipating the course of disease, learning where and how to seek help, understanding what would be involved in caregiving, juggling work-role conflicts, and coping with the pervasive and multiple fears associated with AIDS caregiving. Practitioners working with HIV+ caregivers to persons with AIDS clearly will need to access resources for alleviating financial strain and for providing practical assistance.

Although Harris (chap. 9) noted several common caregiving themes between husband and son caregivers, she noted several important differ-ences as well. For example, she found that sons were more likely to set boundaries and time limits on caregiving, were less distressed emotional-ly, and were more willing to question health care providers. Sons wanted short-term educational workshops and information on how to navigate the service delivery system, while husbands wanted to talk to other men in similar situations and to learn skills for providing hands-on personal care. Essex, Seltzer, and Krauss (chap. 11) and Greenberg (chap. 12) revealed the unique and differential experiences of men as caregivers to adult children with mental retardation and mental illness, respectively. Findings suggested that men served important roles in both of these caregiving contexts, but that there were different patterns of caregiving involvement, sources of stress, amount and type of care provided, and outcomes experienced among father caregivers as contrasted with mother caregivers. Ciambrone and Allen (chap. 13) noted the unique emotional challenges and needs of partners who are coping with breast cancer. Studies reviewed suggested that these men often felt alone and without adequate information about the disease. In addition, although these men were deeply concerned about treatment issues associated with breast cancer, evidence reviewed suggested that they may mask their feelings and avoid discussing them in attempts to minimize their partner's distress. Unique interventions for this subgroup of men caregivers might include the initiation of networking interventions in oncology clinics, and the use of interdisciplinary teams to address the profound psychosocial issues facing couples that would routinely encourage dialogue regarding expectations, worries, needs, and fears, and provide education and practical assistance with care planning.

These points of divergence in the experience of men caregivers have essential implications for assessment processes and for designing interventions for particular subgroups of caregiving men. Femiano and Coonerty-Femiano (chap. 15), present principles for working with men that honor and value the individual variation that is so important to the caregiving experience. Clearly, assessment processes need to be individually tailored for competent and responsive practice to be enacted, and sources of stress unique to the caregiving subgroups and context must be considered (e.g., sources of stress unique to caring for wives with dementia, or partners with AIDS). As illustrated by Stolley and Chohan (chap. 14), attention to the ways in which spirituality and religious beliefs may influence the caregiving experience is an important consideration that is neglected.

Additional implications for service providers are clearly articulated in Part IV of this volume. Although there were many points of divergence in the caregiving experience, Femiano and Coonerty-Femiano (chap. 15) identified some of the common challenges that are documented across studies of caregiving men and general principles for working with men caregivers that practitioners could individually tailor in responding to these challenges. Principles included validating the individual's approach and experience, building on strengths, fostering a sense of control, conducting comprehensive psychosocial assessments, recognizing the potential depth and breadth of unexpressed feeling, considering developmental needs, fostering emotional and social support, providing information and education, assisting with practical concerns and future planning, and providing skills training. Chapter 15 additionally articulated several considerations for determining which interventions are most appropriate including the state of caregiving; the particular values, motivations, and needs of the caregivers, and the sense of spirituality or religiosity that may serve as a resource for intervention approaches. Finally, Kaye (chap. 16) noted several implications for service providers that are relevant to reducing service delivery barriers. He also challenged practitioners and program developers to think creatively to design services that "reflect less feminine bias in their structure and configuration," to reach out to men who are hesitant to seek aid, and to design and implement services that meet the needs of the poor and culturally diverse subgroups of caregivers.

IMPLICATIONS FOR FUTURE RESEARCH

There are six primary themes in this volume that point to implications for future research. First, several chapters noted the tendency, dilemmas, and serious limitations that result from viewing men caregivers through the lens of women's experiences, and called for an unbiased and fresh perspective in future research that attempts to understand the lived experience of men caregivers. Thompson (chap. 2) noted that the gender-comparative approach in research involving men has fostered stereotypical views of men caregivers and minimized understanding of their unique contributions and experiences. Stoller (chap. 3) and Matthews (chap. 10) provided examples of alternative ways to interpret research through expansion of our theoretical assumptions and considering alternative explanations for findings. Carpenter and Miller (chap. 5) reviewed several investigations that reported findings which contrasted sharply with traditional stereotypes and assumptions about men caregivers as less involved and emotionally distant. Qualitative investigations that generate theory and ground data in the unique and varied experiences of men caregivers in different contexts would facilitate advances in theory development specific to men caregivers.

Second, several authors noted that although there is a recent swell in sheer numbers of investigations focusing specifically on men caregivers, many methodological issues and problems need to be addressed for advances in knowledge to move us forward. These issues are similar to those that have plagued caregiving research more generally (Barer & Johnson, 1990), but have been more adequately addressed in studies of women caregivers. Specifically, Bookwala et al. (chap. 4), recommended the use of larger samples, greater use of random, probability sampling techniques, more sophisticated data analyses, longitudinal panel designs, and rigorous qualitative methodologies. Most research to date has been cross-sectional. As such, we know little about how men caregivers adapt over time, and how needs vary across the caregiving trajectory. Sipes (chap. 7) recommended that we more fully define, understand, and explain the many phases of caregiving in order to better anticipate and more appropriately respond to caregiving needs. In addition, Bookwala et al. (chap. 4) and Carpenter and Miller (chap. 5) suggested that we should move beyond descriptive accounts of experiences, encourage research that is more theoretically grounded and that illuminates understanding of patterns identified.

Third, several authors noted additional methodological challenges to research related to gender stereotypes and socialization. For example, Ciambrone and Allen (chap. 13) suggested that impacts of caregiving may be underestimated due to underreporting associated with socialized pressures to minimize or mask emotional responses viewed as more "feminine," which subjective measures of outcomes frequently encapsulate. Work needs to be done to develop non-gender-biased measures of caregiving outcomes. Researchers face the difficult challenge of building non-gender-biased measures that skirt self-report biases. Adler, Patterson, and Grant (chap. 6), noted that more "objective" physiological measures revealed a greater level of physiological disturbance among caregiving men than of women and that ample evidence indicated that men may be more physiologically reactive to psychosocial stressors than women. They suggested that we need further investigation for assessing the interaction of gender and caregiving on physical health and physiological responses to more definitively determine differences in caregiving impact between men and women. Future studies should seek to use a multimethod approach to measurement of caregiving impact that includes both subjective and objective measures when ever possible.

Fourth, as noted previously, the chapters in this text revealed tremendous variation and divergent experiences among men who occupy different caregiving roles, and suggested the need for further research on subgroups of caregiving men. Thompson (chap. 2), Bookwala et al. (chap. 4), Carpenter and Miller (chap. 5), and Ciambrone and Allen (chap. 13) noted that many sources of heterogeneity among men caregivers remains insufficiently explored, including men caring for persons with varied illnesses and who possess divergent forms of relationship to care recipients. As such, future studies should seek better understanding of differences that exist between subgroups of caregivers. How do men vary when they are husbands, partners, sons, brothers, or friends? How does the experience of caring for an adult child with Cerebral Palsy differ from caring for a child with mental retardation, or mental illness? How does type of illness differentially impact the experience of men caring for persons with Parkinson's disease, stroke, arthritis, advanced Congestive Heart Failure, or other terminal diseases? How does age, ethnicity, relationship, or other contextual variables influence motivations for caregiving, resources available to caregivers, coping processes, or impacts of caregiving?

Fifth, it is eminently clear that there is a substantial gap in our understanding of ethnic variation among men caregivers. No studies were identified in this volume that specifically addressed the needs and experiences of caregivers of color. Bookwala et al. (chap. 4) and Carpenter and Miller (chap. 5) both noted this gap and the need to explore ethnic variation, which is currently not represented in the descriptive research conducted to date. Findings reported in chapter 5 revealed significant differences between African American and Caucasian men caregivers in terms of depression and role strain. Cross-cultural comparisons of men caregivers are desperately needed.

Finally, work remains to be done to develop, design, and test interventions specifically for men. As described in chapter 1, we know that men are severely underrepresented in interventions designed for assisting caregivers (DeVries, Hamilton, Lovett, & Gallagher-Thompson, 1997; Toseland & Rossiter, 1989) and that there are several potential service delivery barriers. Kaye (chap. 16) noted that we have an incomplete understanding of men caregivers as consumers of community services and that there may be barriers that are especially salient to older caregivers of color (i.e., lack of trust, lack of diversity among staff of many agencies, lack of knowledge and economic barriers). Although we must be thoughtful in designing interventions appropriate for men, we must refrain from developing a "universal" model for men. As noted previously, experiences vary tremendously. What interventions and services are best suited to the African American, Hispanic American or Latino, or Asian American caregiver who is a husband, adult son, or partner? How does that compare to the reported needs of Caucasian caregivers? Qualitative and evaluation-research investigations are needed to explore formal service needs, desires, barriers, and effectiveness. It might be helpful if future investigations would routinely inquire about the kinds of services and interventions that men would find most helpful, seek insights from men regarding design issues as well as suggestions for overcoming potential barriers to service utilization.

It is our hope that the contributions in this volume will stimulate efforts to replicate, and extend the current research, and address these fundamental gaps in our knowledge and theories relevant to men caregivers.

REFERENCES

Ade-Ridder, L., & Brubaker, T. (1988). Expected and reported division of responsibility of household tasks among older wives in two residential settings. *Journal of Consumer Studies and Home Economics, 12*, 59–70.

Barer, B. M., & Johnson, C. L. (1990). A critique of the caregiving literature. *The Gerontologist, 30*, 26–29.

Deutsch, F. M. (1999). *Halving it all: How equally shared parenting works.* Cambridge, MA: Harvard University Press.

DeVries, H. M., Hamilton, D. W., Lovett, S., & Gallagher-Thompson, D. (1997). Patterns of coping preferences for male and female caregivers of frail older adults. *Psychology and Aging, 12*, 263–267.

Keith, P. M. (1980). Sex differences in household involvement of the unmarried. *Journal of Gerontological Social Work, 2*, 331–334.

Keith, P. M. (1985). Work, retirement and well-being among unmarried men and women. *The Gerontologist, 25*, 410–416.

Keith, P. M. (1994). A typology of orientations toward household and marital roles of older men and women. In E. H. Thompson, Jr. (Ed.), *Older men's lives* (pp. 141–158). Thousand Oaks, CA: Sage.

Szinovacz, M. (1989). Retirement, couples, and household work. In S. J. Bahr & E. T. Peterson (Eds.), *Aging and the family* (pp. 33–58). New York: Lexington Books.

Toseland, R. W., & Rossiter, C. M. (1989). Group interventions to support family caregivers: A review and analysis. *The Gerontologist, 29*, 438–448.

Walzer, S. (1998). *Thinking about the baby: Gender and transitions into parenthood.* Philadelphia: Temple University Press.

Index